HEARING

HEARING

An Introduction to Psychological and Physiological Acoustics

SECOND EDITION, REVISED AND EXPANDED

Stanley A. Gelfand

Department of Communication
Arts and Sciences
Queens College of the
City University of New York
Flushing, New York

MARCEL DEKKER, INC.   New York and Basel

ISBN: 0-8247-8368-9

This book is printed on acid-free paper.

MARCEL DEKKER, INC.
270 Madison Avenue, New York, New York 10016

Current printing (last digit):
10 9 8 7 6 5 4 3 2 1

PRINTED IN THE UNITED STATES OF AMERICA

To Janice, Michael,
Joshua, and Jessica

Foreword

The field of hearing science is of a highly interdisciplinary nature. In order to have a good, broad understanding of the field it is necessary to have a more than superficial knowledge of (in alphabetical order) acoustics; audiology; auditory anatomy, physiology, and neurophysiology; communication theory; data processing; electroacoustics; experimental psychology; instrumentation; signal processing; statistics; and—of course—psychoacoustics. Hearing scientists with a broader vision also know something about acoustic phonetics, auditory development, cognition, speech perception, and related topics; since, after all, the ear is used largely for speech communication and the ear plays a crucial role in the early development of speech and language.

Since Leibnitz was the last man to know everything, it is not surprising that researchers in the field of hearing science have become progressively more specialized over the years. The process of knowing more and more about less and less represents progress of a sort; a dirac pulse of knowledge after all is no mean achievement. However, there are many dangers to overspecialization.

It is important for researchers to keep abreast of major new developments in related (and often seemingly unrelated) areas; and it is equally important for students to be exposed to a broad view of the field before the process of in-depth specialization takes hold. How can this be done? A good textbook providing a broad, unified treatment is a useful start.

Unfortunately, most textbooks in hearing science typically provide extensive coverage in the author's specific area of expertise and only scant coverage elsewhere. Another interestingly common type of book is that of an anthology of chapters by a diverse group of experts. Some of these anthologies provide excellent coverage of a range of topics but there are inevitable gaps. Further, the quality and level of coverage often fluctuate widely (if not ludicrously) between chapters. It takes a smart student to know which chapters to avoid.

One of the strengths of *Hearing: An Introduction to Psychological and Physiological Acoustics, Second Edition, Revised and Expanded* is that it provides broad coverage at a consistent level in terms that students of diverse backgrounds can understand. For the advanced undergraduate student or the postgraduate student in such disciplines as audiology and psychology, this book provides both an introduction and a broad overview of the field of hearing science that is decidedly lacking in contemporary treatments of the subject. It should be an extremely useful guide to these students, as well as to those researchers who wish to refresh their knowledge of the field beyond their areas of specialization. Herein lies another strength of the book in that it is up to date with respect to new developments in all aspects of the field of hearing science—and there have been many of late.

Dr. Gelfand appears to have taken Disraeli's dictum to heart: Wishing to read a good book (on hearing science), he wrote one.

Harry Levitt
Distinguished Professor
Speech and Hearing Sciences
Graduate School and University Center
of the City University of New York

Preface to the Second Edition

At least two aspects of hearing science make it an exciting area of study. One of these is its broad, interdisciplinary scope. The other, perhaps more enticing, attribute is that hearing science is vital and dynamic: The advances of continuing research not only provide new information to expand on the old but also cause us to rethink what was once well established. Thus, one should not be shocked to find that so much is new as well as that so much has changed since the first edition was written. Advances in our knowledge and understanding of frequency selectivity as well as in the extensive areas relating to cochlear microanatomy and micromechanics are two examples. New and even changed concepts in areas such as these make up one of the reasons that this second edition was undertaken.

The second motivation for writing this second edition was to address the comments and suggestions of the graduate students for whom this text is principally intended. These students' comments have had the following impact on this edition. Although the approach, structure, format, and the general (and often irregular) depth of coverage used in the first edition is maintained wherever possible, this second edition includes a new chapter that reviews basic physical concepts. Furthermore, the material from the earlier chapter "Hearing Theories and Sensory Action" has been redistributed into more appropriate locations.

This is a text meant for students with broadly different backgrounds and interests but is by no stretch of the imagination a "state-of-the-art" treatise. An important goal, therefore, was to provide suggestions for further study to those students whose interests lie in this direction. Hence, the practice of liberally referring the reader to other sources for further study is retained, and has been expanded as suggested by many.

My sincerest thanks are expressed to the numerous students who provided me with frank and invaluable feedback and direction. In this respect (and well as in many personal ones), I am especially indebted to the audiology graduate students at Queens College and to those in the Ph.D. Program in Speech and Hearing Scineces of the City University of New York.

The Preface to the First Edition is repeated here because its comments and acknowledgments are as much intended now as then. I am particularly indebted to my colleagues at Queens College and City University for their continuous examples of excellence and for their valued friendships.

At the risk of inadvertently omitting several, I would like to thank the following individuals for their influence and support: Arthur Booth-royd, Irving Hochberg, Renee Kaufman, John Lutolf, Maurice Miller, Neil Piper, Teresa Schwander, Carol Silverman, Joel Stark, Harris and Helen Topel, and Mark Weiss. It is not possible for me to exaggerate the personal feelings and special appreciation I reiterate here for Harry Levitt and Shlomo Silman, who know this without the need for printed superlatives.

Finally, my deepest gratitude goes to Janice, my wife and best friend, and to my children, Michael, Joshua, and Jessica, for their love, support, confidence, and unbelievable patience.

Stanley A. Gelfand

Preface to the First Edition

This book is concerned with the physiology and psychophysics of audition. Its intent is to introduce the new student to the sciences of hearing and to rekindle the interests of the experienced reader.

The hearing science student is often faced with the frustrating dilemma imposed by textbooks that are either too basic or too advanced. This problem is complicated by the widely divergent backgrounds of those who become interested in hearing. My intent was to provide a volume sufficiently detailed to be useful as a core text, yet not so dependent upon such prior knowledge that it would be beyond the grasp of most students. In order to accomplish this goal, I have tried to minimize the use of mathematical expressions (a difficult chore within the confines of the topic) and have placed qualitative concepts dealing with basic acoustics along with the text material rather than in a separate chapter. This assumes some prior knowledge of elementary physics, but the concepts needed are reiterated with the subject matter so that their application is facilitated.

In addition, the depth and breadth of topic coverage between chapters (and in some cases between sections of the same chapter) was varied based upon reactions to the material by a variety of students. This was done to maximize what the student may come away with as opposed to imposing an arbitrary standard of sophistication across the board. Of course, my own interests and biases have tainted the material by omission and commission in spite of honest attempts to keep these repressed. Thus, I freely admit to a purposefully irregular level of topic coverage for didactic purposes and apologize for the places where personal bias crept in.

It is doubtful that an introductory masters level or undergraduate course could cover all of the material in a single semester. It is more likely that this volume might be used as a core text for a two-term sequence dealing with psychological and physiological acoustics, along with appropriately selected readings from the research literature and state-of-the-art books. Suggested readings are provided in context throughout the text. However, most of the material has been used in a one semester "scan course." In either case, the student should find a sufficient number of citations for each topic to provide a firm foundation for further study.

Finally, the reader (particularly the beginning student) is reminded that the author of a textbook is merely one who has put material together. Bias finds its way into even descriptive text, and new findings occasionally disprove the "laws" of the past. This book is meant to be a first step; it is by no means the final word.

This work represents the contributions of many others. They share the responsibility for its fine points. The flaws are my own.

Special thanks are expressed to Dr. Maurice H. Miller for his suggestion that I prepare this book and for his constant assistance and confidence. I would also like to thank the reviewers of the manuscript for providing valuable comments and suggestions. Inestimable gratitude is expressed to my dear friend and colleague, Dr. Shlomo Silman, whose advice and confidence provided me with the motivation and drive to complete this work. My sincerest gratitude also goes to Dr. Harry Levitt, who so graciously agreed to write the foreword and who taught me to love hearing science.

The following individuals provided assistance and support in ways too varied and numerous to detail here: Marilyn Agin, Dr. Barbara Bohne, Dr. Joseph Danto, Jack Ficarra, Renee Kaufman, Harry Kubasek, Dr. Janice Leeds, Dr. David Lim, John Lutolf, Adrienne Rubinstein, Stanley Schwartz, Harris and Helen Topel, and especially Neil Piper.

Finally, my greatest appreciation is expressed to my wife, Janice, whose love and confidence kept me going, whose knowledge was invaluable, and who so willingly gave up weekends, holidays, and evenings so that I could write.

Stanley A. Gelfand

Contents

Contents

14 / SPEECH PERCEPTION   456

Speech Sounds: Production and Perception / Power of Speech Sounds / Speech Intelligibility / Dichotic Listening

1
Physical Concepts

This book is concerned with hearing, and what we hear is sound. Thus, both intuition and reason make it clear that a basic understanding of the nature of sound is prerequisite to an understanding of audition. The study of sound is *acoustics*. An understanding of acoustics, in turn, rests upon knowing several fundamental physical principles. This is so because acoustics is, after all, the physics of sound. We will therefore begin by reviewing a number of physical principles so that the following chapters can proceed without the constant need for the distracting insertions of basic definitions and concepts. The material in this chapter is intended to be a review of principles that were previously learned. Therefore, the review will be rapid and somewhat cursory, and the reader may wish to consult a physics or acoustics textbook for a broader coverage of these topics [1–7].

PHYSICAL QUANTITIES

Physical quantities may be thought of as being "basic" or "derived," and as either "scalars" or "vectors." The *basic* (or *base) quantities* of concern here are time, length (distance), and mass. The *derived quantities* are the result of various combinations of the base quantities (and other derived quantities), and include such phenomena as velocity, force, and work. If a quantity can be described completely in terms of just its magnitude (size) then it is a *scalar*. Length is a good example of scalar. On the other hand, a quantity is a *vector* if it needs to be described by *both* its *magnitude* and its *direction*. For example, if a body moves one meter from point x1 to point x2, then we say that it has been *displaced*. Here, the scalar quantity of length becomes the vector quantity of *displacement* when both magnitude and direction are involved. A derived quantity is a vector if any of its components is a vector. For example, force is a vector because it involves the components of mass (a scalar) and acceleration (a vector). The distinction between scalars and vectors is not just some esoteric concept. One must be able to distinguish between scalars and vectors because they are manipulated differently in calculations.

The base quantities may be more or less appreciated in terms of one's personal experience, and are expressed in terms of conventionally agreed upon *units*. These units are values that are measurable and repeatable. The unit of *time* (t) is the second (sec), the unit of *length* (l) is the *meter* (m), and the unit of *mass* (M) is the *kilogram* (kg). There is a common misconception that *mass* and *weight* are synonymous. This is actually untrue. Mass is related to the density of a body, which is the same for that body no matter where it is located. On the other hand, an object's weight is related to the force of gravity upon it, so that weight changes as a function of gravitational attraction. It is common knowledge that an object weighs more on earth than it would on the moon, and that it weighs more at sea level than it would in a high-flying airplane. In each of these cases, the mass of the body is the same in spite of the fact that its weight is different.

A brief word is appropriate at this stage regarding the availability of several different systems of units. When we express length in meters and mass in kilograms we are using the units of the International System (SI), or the *mks* (for meter-kilogram-second) *system*. An alternative scheme using smaller metric units coexists with mks, which is the *cgs system* (for centimeter-gram-second), as does the English system of weights and measures. Table 1.1 presents a number of the major basic and derived physical quantities we will deal with, their units, and conversion factors.*

Velocity (v) is the speed at which an object is moving, and is derived

---

*The reference value for 1 kg of mass is that of a cylinder of platinum-iridium alloy that is kept in the International Bureau of Weights and Measures in France. "Atomic" references are used for time and length. One second thus corresponds to the time needed to complete 9,192,631,700 cycles of the microwave radiation causing a change between the two lowest energy states in a cesium atom. One meter is 1,650,763.73 times the wavelength of orange-red light emitted by krypton-86 under certain conditions.

Table 1.1 Basic and Derived Physical Quantities, Units, and Conversion Factors

Quantity	Formula	SI units (mks)	Units (cgs)	Equivalent values
Time (t)	t	s	s	
Mass (M)	M	kg	g	1 kg = 1000 g
Displacement (x)	x	m	cm	1 m = 100 cm
Velocity (v)	v = x/t	m/s	cm/s	1 ms = 100 cm/s
Acceleration (a)	a = v/t $= x/t^2$	m/s^2	cm/s^2	$1\ m/s^2 = 100\ cm/s^2$
Force (F)	F = Ma $= Mv/t$	newton (N) $kg \cdot m/s^2$	dyne (d) $g \cdot cm/s^2$	$1\ N = 10^5$ dyne
Work (W)	W = Fx	joule $N \cdot m$	erg $d \cdot cm$	1 joule $= 10^7$ erg
Power (P)	P = W/t $= Fx/t$ $= Fv$	watt (w) joule/s	watt (w) erg/s	1 watt = 1 joule/s $= 10^7$ erg/s
Intensity (I)	I = P/area	w/m^2	w/cm^2	Reference values: $10^{-12}\ w/m^2$ $= 10^{-16}\ w/cm^2$
Pressure (p)	p = F/area	N/m^2	$dyne/cm^2$	Reference values: $2 \times 10^{-5}\ N/m^2$ $= 2 \times 10^{-4}\ dyne/cm^2$

from the basic quantities of displacement (which we have seen is a vector form of length) and time. On average, velocity is the distance traveled divided by the amount of time it takes to get from the starting point to the destination. Thus, if an object leaves point x1 at time t1 and arrives at x2 at time t2, then we can compute the average velocity as

$$v = (x2 - x1)/(t2 - t1) \qquad (1.1)$$

If we call (x2 − x1) displacement (x) and (t2 − t1) time (t), then, in general:

$$v = x/t = x \cdot t^{-1} \qquad (1.2)$$

Because displacement (x) is measured in meters and time (t) in seconds, velocity is expressed in meters per second (m/sec, or $m \cdot sec^{-1}$).

In contrast to average velocity as just defined, *instantaneous velocity* is used when we are concerned with the speed of a moving body at a *specific moment* in time. Instantaneous velocity reflects the speed at some point in time when the displacement and time between that point and the next one approaches zero. Therefore, instantaneous velocity is equal to the derivative of displacement with respect to time, written as

$$v = dx/dt \qquad (1.3)$$

As common experience verifies, a fixed speed is rarely maintained over time. Rather, an object may speed up or slow down over time. Such a change of velocity over time is *acceleration* (a). Suppose we are concerned with the average acceleration of a body moving between two points. The velocity of the body at the first point is v1 and the time as it passes that point is t1. Similarly, its velocity at the second point and the time when it passes this point are, respectively, v2 and t2. The average acceleration is the difference between these two velocities divided by the time interval involved:

$$a = (v2 - v1)/(t2 - t1) \qquad (1.4)$$

or, in general:

$$a = v/t = v \cdot t^{-1} \qquad (1.5)$$

If we recall that velocity corresponds to displacement divided by time (Eq. 1.2), we can substitute x/t for v, so that

$$a = \frac{x}{t/t} = \frac{x}{t^2} = x \cdot t^{-2} \qquad (1.6)$$

Therefore, acceleration is expressed in units of meters per second squared (m/sec^2, or m $\cdot$ sec^{-2}).

The acceleration of a body at a given moment is called its *instantaneous acceleration*, which is the derivative of velocity with respect to time, or

$$v = dv/dt \qquad (1.7)$$

Recalling that velocity is the first derivative of displacement (Eq. 1.3), and substituting, we find that acceleration is the second derivative of displacement:

$$a = d^2x/dt^2 \qquad (1.8)$$

Common experience and Newton's first law of motion tell us that if an object is not moving (at rest) then it will tend to remain at rest, and that if an object is moving in some direction at a given speed that it will tend to continue doing so. This phenomenon is *inertia*, which is the property of mass to continuing doing what is already doing. An outside influence is needed in order to make a stationery object move, or to change the speed or direction of a moving object. That is, a *force* (F) is needed to overcome the body's inertia. Because a change in speed is acceleration, we may say that force is that which causes a mass to be accelerated, i.e., to change its speed or direction. The amount of force is equal to the product of mass times acceleration (Newton's second law of motion):

$$F = Ma \qquad (1.9)$$

Recall that acceleration corresponds to velocity over time (Eq. 1.5). Substituting v/t for a reveals that force can also be defined in the form

$$F = Mv/t \qquad (1.10)$$

where Mv is the property of *momentum.* Stated in this manner, force is equal to momentum over time.

Because force is the product of mass and acceleration, the amount of force is measured in kg $\cdot$ m/sec^2. The unit of force is the *Newton* (N), which is the force needed to cause a 1 kg mass to be accelerated by 1 m/sec^2 (or, 1 N = 1 kg $\cdot$ m/sec^2). It would thus take a 2 N force to cause a 2 kg mass to be accelerated by 1 m/sec^2, or a 1 kg mass to be accelerated by 2 m/sec^2. Similarly, the force required to accelerate a 6 kg mass by 3 m/sec^2 would be 18 N. (The unit of force in cgs units is the dyne, where 1 dyne = 1 g $\cdot$ cm/sec^2; and 10^5 dynes = 1 N.)

Actually, many forces tend to act upon a given body at the same time. Therefore, the force referred to in Eqs. 1.9 and 1.10 is actually the *resultant or net* force, which is the net effect of all forces acting upon the object. The concept of net force is clarified by a few simple examples: If two forces are both pushing on a body in the same direction, then the net force would be the sum of these two forces. (For example, consider a force of 2 N that is pushing an object toward the north, and a second force of 5 N that is also pushing that object in the same direction. The net force would be 2 N + 5 N, or 7 N and the direction of acceleration would be to the north.) Alternatively, if two forces are pushing on the same body but in opposite directions, then the net force is the difference between the two, and the object will be accelerated in the direction of the greater force. (Suppose, for example, that a 2 N force is pushing an object toward the east and that a 5 N force is simultaneously pushing it toward the west. The net force would be 5 N − 2 N, or 3 N which would cause the body to accelerate toward the west.)

If two *equal* forces push in opposite directions, then net force would be zero, in which case there would be no change in the motion of the object. The latter situation is called *equilibrium*. Thus, under conditions of equilibrium, if a body is already moving it will continue in motion, and if it is already at rest it will remain still. This is, of course, what Newton's first law of motion tells us.

Experience, however, tells us that a moving object in the real world tends to slow down and will eventually come to a halt. This occurs, for example, when a driver shifts to "neutral" and allows his car to coast on a level roadway. Is this a violation of the laws of physics? Clearly, the answer is no. The reason is that in the real world a moving body is constantly in contact with other objects or mediums. The sliding of one body against the other constitutes a force opposing the motion called *friction* or *resistance*. For example, the coasting automobile is in contact with the surrounding air and the roadway; moreover, its internal parts are also moving on the other.

The opposing force of friction depends on two factors. Differing amounts of friction occur depending upon what is sliding on what. The magnitude of friction between two given materials is called the coefficient of friction. Although the details of this quantity are beyond current interest, it is easily understood that the coefficient of friction is greater for "rough" materials than for "smooth" or "slick" ones.

The second factor affecting the force of friction is easily demonstrated by an experiment the reader can do by rubbing the palms of his hands back and forth on one another. First rub slowly and then rapidly. Not surprisingly, the rubbing will produce heat. The temperature rise is due to the conversion of the mechanical energy into heat as a result of the friction, and will be addressed again in another context. For the moment, we will accept the amount of heat as an indicator of the amount of friction. Note that the hands become hotter when they are rubbed together more rapidly. Thus, the amount of friction is not only due to the coefficient of friction (R) between the materials involved (here, the palms of the hands), but also to the velocity (v) of the motion. Stated as a formula, the force of friction (F) is thus

$$F = Rv \qquad (1.11)$$

A compressed spring will bounce back to its original shape once released. This property of a deformed object to return to its original form is called *elasticity*. The more elastic or stiff an object, the more readily it returns to its original form after being deformed. Suppose one is trying to compress a coil spring. It becomes increasingly more difficult to continue squeezing the spring as it becomes more and more compressed.

Stated differently, the more the spring is being deformed, the more it opposes the applied force. The force which opposes the deformation of a spring-like material is called the *restoring force.*

As the example just suggested, the restoring force depends on two factors, the *elastic modulus* of the object's material and the degree to which the object is displaced. An elastic modulus is the ratio of stress to strain. *Stress* (s) is the ratio of the applied force (F) to the area (A) of an elastic object over which it is exerted, or

$$s = F/A \qquad (1.12)$$

The resulting relative displacement or change in dimensions of the material subjected to the stress is called *strain.* Of particular interest is Young's modulus, which is the ratio of compressive stress to compressive strain. Hooke's law states that stress and strain are proportional within the elastic limits of the material, which is equivalent to stating that a material's elastic modulus is a constant within these limits. Thus, the restoring force (F) of an elastic material which opposes an applied force is

$$F = Sx \qquad (1.13)$$

where S is the stiffness constant of the material and x is the amount of displacement.

The concept of "work" in physics is decidedly more specific than its general meaning in daily life. In the physical sense, *work* (W) is done when the application of a force to a body results in its displacement. The amount of work is therefore the product of the force applied and the resultant displacement, or

$$W = Fx \qquad (1.14)$$

Thus, work can be accomplished only when there is displacement: If the displacement is zero, then the product of force and displacement will also be zero no matter how great the force. Work is quantified in Newton-meters (N·m); and the unit of work is the *joule* (J). Specifically, 1 J is equal to 1 N·m.

The capability to do work is called *energy.* The energy of an object in motion is called *kinetic energy,* and the energy of a body at rest is its *potential energy.* Total energy is the body's kinetic energy plus its potential energy. Work corresponds to the change in the body's kinetic energy. The energy is not consumed, but rather is converted from one form to the other. Consider, for example, a pendulum that is swinging back and forth. Its kinetic energy is greatest when it is moving the fastest, which is when it passes through the midpoint of its swing. On the other hand, its potential energy is greatest at the instant that it reaches the extreme of its swing, when its speed is zero.

We are concerned not only with the amount of work, but also how fast it is being accomplished. The rate at which work is done is *power* (P), and is equal to work divided by time,

$$P = W/t \qquad \text{(Eq. 1.15)}$$

or joules per second (J/sec). The *watt* (W) is the unit of power, and 1 W is equal to 1 J/sec (or 1 J·sec-1).

Recalling that W = Fx (Eq. 1.14), then Eq. 1.15 may be rewritten as

$$P = Fx/t \qquad (1.16)$$

If we now substitute v for x/t (Eq. 1.2), we find that

$$P = Fv \qquad (1.17)$$

Thus, power is also equal to the product of force and velocity.

The amount of power per unit of area is called *intensity*. Formally,

$$I = P/A \qquad (1.18)$$

where I is intensity, P is power and A is area. Therefore, intensity is measured in watts per square meter (w/m^2) in SI units, or as watts per square centimeter (w/cm^2) in cgs units. Because of the difference in the scale of the area units in the mks and cgs systems, we find that 10^{-12} w/m^2 corresponds to 10^{-16} w/cm^2. This apparently peculiar choice of equivalent values is being provided because they represent the amount of intensity required to just barely hear a sound.

An understanding of intensity will be better appreciated if one considers the following. Using for the moment the common knowledge idea of what sound is, imagine that a sound source is a tiny pulsating sphere. This point source of sound will produce a sound wave that will radiate outward in every direction, so that the propagating wave may be conceived of as a sphere of ever-increasing size. Thus, as distance from the point source increases, the power of the sound will have to be divided over the ever-expanding surface. Suppose now that we measure how much power registers on a one-unit area on this surface at various distances from the source. As the overall size of the sphere is getting larger with distance from the source, so this one-unit sample must represent an ever-decreasing proportion of the total surface area. Therefore, less power "falls" onto the same area as the distance from the source increases. It follows that the magnitude of the sound appreciated by a listener would become less and less with increasing distance from a sound source.

Just as power divided by area yields intensity, so force (F) divided by area yields a value called *pressure* (p):

$$p = F/A \qquad\qquad (1.19)$$

so that pressure is measured in N/m^2 (or in dynes/cm^2). As for intensity, the softest audible sound can also be expressed in terms of its pressure, for which 2×10^{-5} N/m^2 and 2×10^{-4} dynes/cm^2 are equivalent values.

HARMONIC MOTION AND SOUND

What is sound? It is convenient to answer this question with a formally stated sweeping generality. For example, one might say that sound is a form of vibration that propagates through a medium (such as air) in the form of a wave. Although this statement is correct and straightforward, it can also be uncomfortably vague and perplexing. This is so because it assumes a knowledge of definitions and concepts which are used in a very precise way, but which are familiar to most people only as "gut-level" generalities. As a result, we must address the underlying concepts and develop a functional vocabulary of physical terms which will not only make the general definition of sound meaningful, but will also allow the reader to appreciate its nature.

Vibration is the to-and-fro motion of a body, which could be anything from a guitar string to the floorboards under the family refrigerator, or a molecule of air. Moreover, the motion may have a very simply pattern as produced by a tuning fork, or an extremely complex one such as what one might hear at lunch time in an elementary school cafeteria. Even though few sounds are as simple as that produced by a vibrating tuning fork, such an example provides what is needed to understand the nature of sound.

Figure 1.1 shows an artist's conceptualization of a vibrating tuning fork at different moments of its vibration pattern. The heavy arrow facing the prong to the reader's right in Fig. 1.1a represents the effect of applying an initial force to the fork, such as by striking it against a hard surface. The progression of the pictures in the figure from (a) through (e) represents the movements of the prongs as time proceeds from the moment that the outside force is applied.

Even though both prongs vibrate as mirror images of one another, it is convenient to consider just one of them for the time being. Figure 1.2 highlights the right prong's motion after being struck. Point C (center) is

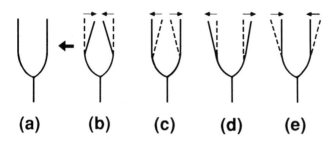

(a)   (b)   (c)   (d)   (e)

Figure 1.1   Striking a tuning fork (indicated by the heavy arrow) results in a pattern of movement that repeats itself over time. One complete cycle of these movements is represented from frames (a) through (e). Note that the two prongs move as mirror images of one another.

simply the position of the prong at rest. Upon being hit (as in Fig. 1.1a) the prong is pushed as shown by arrow 1 to point L (left). The prong then bounces back (arrow 2), picking up speed along the way. Instead of stopping at the center (C), the rapidly moving prong overshoots this point. It now continues rightward (arrow 3), slowing down along the way until it comes to a halt at point R (right). It now reverses direction and begins moving leftward (arrow 4) at an ever-increasing speed, so that it again overshoots the center. Now, again following arrow 1, the prong slows down until it reaches a halt at L, where it reverses direction and repeats the process.

The course of events just described is the result of applying a force to an object having the properties of elasticity and inerta (mass). The initial force to the tuning fork displaces the prong. Because the tuning fork possesses the property of elasticity, the deformation caused by the applied force is opposed by a *restoring force* in the opposite direction. In the case of the single prong in Fig. 1.2, the initial force toward the left is opposed by a restoring force toward the right. As the prong is pushed further to the left, the magnitude of the restoring force increases relative to the initially applied force. As a result, the prong's movement is slowed down, brought to a halt at point L, and reversed in direction. Now, under the influence of its elasticity, the prong starts moving rightward. Here, we must consider the mass of the prong.

As the restoring force brings the prong back toward its resting position (C), the inertial force of its mass causes it to increase in speed, or accelerate. When the prong passes through the resting position it is actually moving fastest. Here, inertia does not permit the moving mass (prong) to simply stop, so instead it overshoots the center and continues

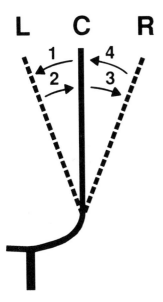

Figure 1.2   Movements toward the right (R) and left (L) of the center (C) resting position of a single tuning fork prong. The numbers and arrows refer to the text.

its rightward movement under the force of its inertia. However, prong's movement is now resulting in deformation of the metal again once it passes through the resting position. Elasticity therefore comes into play with the build-up of an opposing (now leftward) restoring force. As before, the restoring force eventually equals the applied (now inertial) force, thus halting the fork's displacement at point R and reversing the direction of its movement. Here, the course of events described above again come into play (except that the direction is leftward), with the prong building up speed again and overshooting the center (C) position as a result of inertia. The process will continue over and over again until it dies out over time, seemingly "of its own accord."

Clearly, the dying out of the tuning fork's vibrations does not occur by some mystical influence. On the contrary, it is due to yet another physical phenomenon called *resistance*. The vibrating prong is always in contact with the air around it. As a result, there will be *friction* between the vibrating metal and the surrounding air particles. The friction causes some of the mechanical energy involved in the movement of the tuning fork to be converted into heat. The energy which has been converted into heat by friction is no longer available to support the to-and-fro

movements of the tuning fork. Hence, the oscillations die out as continuing friction causes more and more of the energy to be converted into
heat. This reduction in the size of the oscillations due to resistance is
called *damping*.

The events and forces just described are summarized in Fig. 1.3,
where the tuning fork's motion is represented by the curve. This curve
represents the displacement to the right and left of the center (resting)
position as the distance above and below the horizontal line, respectively. Horizontal distance from left to right represents the progression
of time. The initial dotted line represents its initial displacement due to
the applied force. The elastic restoring forces and inertial forces of the
prong's mass are represented by arrows. Finally, damping is shown by
the reduction in the displacement of the curve from center as time goes
on.

The type of vibratition just described is called *simple harmonic motion*

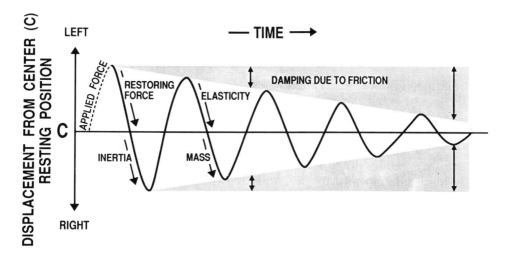

Figure 1.3 Conceptualized diagram graphing the to-and-fro movements of the
tuning fork prong in Fig. 1.2. Vertical distance represents the displacement of the
prong from its center (C) or resting position. The dotted line represents the initial
displacement of the prong as a result of some applied force. Arrows indicate the
effects of restoring forces due to the fork's elasticity, and the inertia due to its
mass. The damping effect due to resistance (or friction) is shown by the decreasing displacement of the curve as time progresses, and is highlighted by the
shaded triangles (and double-headed arrows) above and below the curve.

(SHM) because the to-and-fro movements repeat themselves at the same rate over and over again. We will discuss the nature of SHM in greater detail below with respect to the motion of air particles in the sound wave.

The tuning fork serves as a sound source by transferring its vibration to the motion of the surrounding air particles (see Fig. 1.4). (We will again concentrate on the activity to the right of the fork, remembering that a mirror image of this pattern occurs to the left.) The rightward motion of the tuning fork prong displaces air molecules to its right in the same direction as the prong's motion. These molecules are thus displaced to the right of their resting positions, thereby being forced closer and closer to the particles to their own right. In other words, the air pressure has been increased above its resting (ambient or atmospheric) pressure because the molecules are being compressed. This state is clearly identified by the term *compression*. The amount of compression

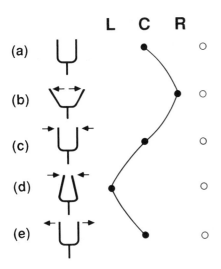

Figure 1.4   Transmittal of the vibratory pattern from a tuning fork to the surrounding air particles. Frames represent various phases of the tuning fork's vibratory cycle. In each frame, the filled circle represents an air particle next to the prong as well as its position, and the unfilled circle shows an air molecule adjacent to the first one. The latter particle is shown only in its resting position for illustrative purposes. Letters above the filled circle highlight the relative positions of the oscillating air particle (C, center (resting); L, leftward; R, rightward). The line connecting the particle's positions going from frame (a) through (e) reveals a cycle of simple harmonic motion.

(air pressure) increases as the tuning fork continues displacing the air molecules rightward, and reaches a maximum positive pressure when the prong and air molecules attain their greatest rightward amplitude.

The prong will now reverse direction, overshoot its resting position, and then proceed to its extreme leftward position. The compressed air molecules will also reverse direction along with the prong. The reversal occurs because air is an elastic medium, so that the rightwardly compressed particles undergo a leftward restoring force. The rebounding air molecules accelerate due to mass effects, overshoot their resting position, and continue to an extreme leftward position. The amount of compression decreases as the molecules travel leftward, and falls to zero at the moment when the molecules pass through their resting positions.

As the air molecules move left of their ambient positions, they are now at an increasingly greater distance from the molecules to their right than when they were in their resting positions. Consequently, the air pressure is reduced below atmospheric pressure. This state is the opposite of compression, and is called *rarefaction*. The air particles are maximally rarefied so that the pressure is maximally negative when the molecules reach the leftmost position. Now, the restoring force yields a rightward movement of the air molecules, which is enhanced by the push of the tuning fork prong that has also reversed direction. The air molecules now accelerate rightward, overshoot their resting positions (where rarefaction and negative pressure are zero), and continue rightward. Hence, the SHM of the tuning fork has been transmitted to the surrounding air, so that the air molecules are now also under simple harmonic motion.

Consider now one of the air molecules set into SHM by the influence of the tuning fork. This air molecule will vibrate back and forth in the same direction as that of the vibrating prong. When this molecule moves rightward, it will cause a similar displacement of the particle to its own right. Thus, the SHM of the first air molecule is transmitted to the one next to it. The second one similarly initiates vibration of the one to its right, and so forth down the line.

In other words, each molecule moves to-and-fro around its own resting point, and causes successive molecules to vibrate back and forth around their own resting points, as shown schematically by the arrows marked "individual particles" in Fig. 1.5. Notice in the figure that each molecule stays in its own general location and moves to-and-fro about this average position; and that it is the vibratory pattern which is transmitted.

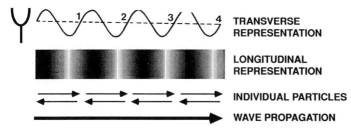

Figure 1.5   Various representations of a sinusoidal wave illustrating points made in the text. Four complete cycles are noted by the numbers.

This propagation of vibratory motion from particle to particle constitutes the sound wave. This wave appears as alternating compressions and rarefactions radiating from the sound source as the particles transmit their motions outward, and is represented in Fig. 1.5.

The distance covered by one cycle of a propagating wave is called its *wavelength* (λ). If we begin where a given molecule is at the point of maximum positive displacement (compression), then the wavelength would be the distance to the next molecule which is also at its point of maximum compression. This is the distance between any two successive positive peaks in the figure. (Needless to say, such a measurement would be equally correct if made between identical points on any two successive replications of the wave.) The wavelength of a sound is inversely proportional to its frequency, as follows:

$$\lambda = c/f \qquad (1.20)$$

where f is frequency and c is a constant representing the speed of sound. (The speed of sound in air approximates 344 meters per second at a temperature of 20 degrees C.) Similarly, frequency can be derived if one knows the wavelength, as:

$$f = c/\lambda \qquad (1.21)$$

Figure 1.5 reveals that the to-and-fro motions of each air molecule is in the same direction that the overall wave is propagating. This kind of wave which characterizes sound is a *longitudinal wave*. In contrast to longitudinal waves, most people are more familiar with *transverse waves*, such as those that develop on the water's surface when a pebble is dropped into a still pool. The latter are called transverse waves because the water particles vibrate up and down around their resting positions at right angles (transverse) to the horizontal propagation of the surface waves out from the spot where the pebble hit the water.

   Even though sound waves are longitudinal, it is more convenient to show them diagrammatically as though they were transverse, as in upper part of Fig. 1.5. Here, the dashed horizontal baseline represents the particle's resting position (ambient pressure), distance above the baseline denotes compression (positive pressure), and distance below the baseline shows rarefaction (negative pressure). The passage of time is represented by the distance from left to right. Beginning at the resting position, the air molecule is represented as having gone through one *cycle* (or complete repetition) of SHM at point 1, two cycles at point 2, three complete cycles at point 3, and four cycles at point 4.

   The curves in Fig. 1.5 reveal that the waveform of SHM is a sinusoidal function, and is thus called a *sinusoidal (or sine) wave*. Figure 1.6 elucidates this concept and also indicates a number of the characteristics of sine waves. The center of the figure shows one complete cycle of SHM, going from points a through i. The circles around the sine wave correspond to the various points on the wave, as indicated by corresponding letters. Circle (a) corresponds to point a on the curve, which

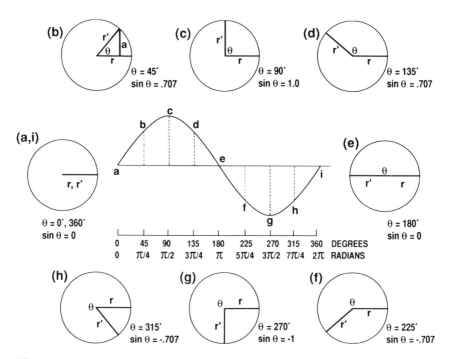

Figure 1.6   The nature of sinusoidal motion (see text).

falls on the baseline. This point corresponds to the particle's resting position.

Circle (a) shows a horizontal radius (r) drawn from the center to the circumference on the right. Imagine as well a second radius (r') that will rotate around the circle in a counter-clockwise direction. The two radii lines are superimposed in circle *a*, so that the angle between them is 0°. There is clearly no distance between these two superimposed lines. This situation corresponds to point a on the sine wave at the center of the figure. Hence, point a may be said to have an angle of 0°, and no displacement from the origin. This concept may appear quite vague at first, but will become clear as the second radius (r') rotates around the circle.

Let us assume that radius r' is rotating center-clockwise at a *fixed speed*. When r' has rotated 45°, it arrives in the position shown in circle (b). Here, r' is at an angle (θ) of 45° to r. We will call this angle the *phase angle*, which simply reflects the degree of rotation around the circle, or the number of degrees into the sine wave at the corresponding point b. We now drop a vertical line from the point where r' intersects the circle down to r. We label this line d, representing the vertical distance between r and the point were r' intersects the circle. The length of this line corresponds to the displacement of point b from the baseline of the sine wave (dotted line at b). We now see that point b on the sine wave is 45° into the cycle of SHM, at which the displacement of the air particle from its resting position is represented by the height of the point above the baseline. It should now be clear that the sine wave is related to the degrees of rotation around a circle. The sine wave's shape corresponds to the sine of θ as r' rotates around the circle, which is simply equal to d/r'.

The positive peak of the sine wave at point c corresponds to circle (c), in which r' has rotated to the straight up position. It is now at a 90° angle to r, and the distance (d) down to the horizontal radius (r) is greatest. Here, we have completed a quarter of the wave and an arc equal to a quarter the circumference of the circle. Notice now that further counter-clockwise rotation of r' results in decreasing the distance (d) down to the horizontal, as shown in circle (d) and by the displacement of point d from the baseline of the sine wave. Note also that θ is now 135°. Here, the air particle has reversed direction and is now moving back toward the resting position. When the particle reaches the resting position (point e), it is again at no displacement. The zero displacement condition is shown in circle (e) by the fact that r and r' constitute a single horizontal line (diameter). Alternatively stated, r and r' intersect the circle's circumference at points that are 180° apart. Here, we have com-

pleted half of the cycle of SHM, and the phase angle is 180° and the
displacement from the baseline is again zero.

Continuing rotation of r′ places its intersection with the circumference in the lower left quadrant of the circle, as in circle (f). Now, θ is 225°,
and the particle has overshot and is moving away from its resting position in the negative (rarefaction) direction. The vertical displacement
from the baseline is now downward or negative, indicating rarefaction.
The negative peak of the wave occurs at 270°, where displacement is
maximum in the negative direction [point and circle (g)].

Circle (h) and point h show that the negative displacement has become smaller as the rotating radius passes 315° around the circle. The air
particle has reversed direction again and is now moving toward its original position. At point i, the air particle has one again returned to its
resting position, where displacement is again zero. This situation corresponds to having completed a 360° rotation, so that r and r′ are once
again superimposed. Thus, 360° corresponds to 0°, and circle i is one in
the same with circle (a). We have now completed one full cycle.

Recall that r′ has been rotating at a fixed speed. It therefore follows
that the number of degrees traversed in a given amount of time is determined by how fast r′ is moving. If one complete rotation takes 1 sec,
then 360° is covered each second. It clearly follows that if 360° takes one
sec, then 180° takes 0.5 sec, 90° takes 0.25 sec, 225° takes 0.75 sec, etc. It
should now be apparent that the phase angle reflects the elapsed time
from the onset of rotation. Recall from Fig. 1.6 that the waveform shows
how particle displacement varies as a function of time. We may also
speak of the horizontal axis in terms of phase, or the equivalent of the
number of degrees of rotation around a circle. Hence, the *phase* of the
wave at each of the labeled points in Fig. 1.6 would be: 0° at a, 45° at b,
90° at c, 135° at d, 180° at e, 225° at f, 270° at g, 315° at h, and 360° at i.
With an appreciation of phase, it should be apparent that each set of
otherwise identical waves in Fig. 1.7 differs with respect to phase: (a)
wave 2 is offset from wave 1 by 45°; (b) wave 3 and 4 are apart in phase
by 90°; and (c) waves 5 and 6 are 180° out of phase.

We may now proceed to define a number of other fundamental
aspects of sound waves. A *cycle* has already been defined as one complete repetition of the wave. Thus, four cycles of a sinusoidal wave were
shown in Fig. 1.5 because it depicts four complete repetitions of the
waveform. Because the waveform is repeated over time, this sound is
said to be *periodic*. In contrast, a waveform that does not repeat itself over
time would be called *aperiodic*.

The amount of time that it takes to complete one cycle is called its
period, denoted by the symbol t (for time). For example, a periodic wave

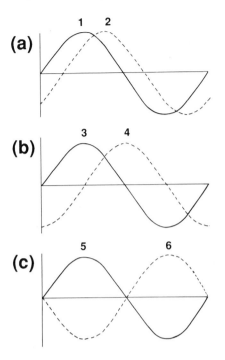

(a)

(b)

(c)

Figure 1.7   Pairs of sinusoidal waves of identical frequency differing in phase by (a) 45°, (b) 90°, and (c) 180°. The numbers serve only to identify the individual waves.

that repeats itself every millisecond is said to have a period of 1 msec, or t = 1 msec or 0.001 sec). The periods of the waveforms considered in hearing science are overwhelmingly less than one second, typically in the milliseconds and even microseconds. However, there are instances when longer periods are encountered.

The number of times a waveform repeats itself per unit of time is its *frequency* (f). The standard unit of time is the second; thus, frequency is the number of times that a wave repeats itself in a second, or the number of cycles per second (cps). By convention, the unit of cycles per second is the *Hertz* (Hz). Thus, a wave that is repeated 1000 times per second has a frequency of 1000 Hz, and the frequency of a wave that repeats at 2500 cycles per second is 2500 Hz.

If period is the time it takes to complete one cycle, and frequency is the number of cycles that occur each second, then it follows that period and frequency are intimately related. Consider a sine wave that is repeated 1000 times per second. By definition it has a frequency of 1000

Hz. Now, if exactly 1000 cycles take exactly 1 sec, then each cycle must clearly have a duration of 1 msec, or 1/1000 sec. Similarly, each cycle of a 250 Hz tone must last 1/250 sec, or a period of 2.5 msec. Formally, then, frequency is the reciprocal of period, and period is the reciprocal of frequency:

$$f = 1/t \qquad \text{(Eq. 1.22)}$$

and

$$t = 1/f \qquad \text{(Eq. 1.23)}$$

It has already been noted that the oscillating air particle is moving back and forth around its resting or average position. In other words, the air particle's displacement changes over the course of each cycle. The magnitude of the air particle's displacement is called *amplitude*. Figure 1.8 illustrates a difference in the amplitude of a sinusoid, and contrasts this with a change in its frequency. In both frames of the figure, the tone represented by the solid curve has a greater amplitude than the one portrayed by the dashed line. This is shown by the greater vertical distance from the baseline (displacement) at any point along the horizon-

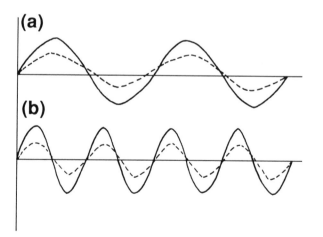

Figure 1.8 Within each frame (a and b), the sinusoidal wave depicted by the solid curve has the same frequency but greater amplitude as that represented by the dashed curve. The curves in frame (b) have twice the frequency as those shown in frame (a). The abscissa is time and the ordinate is amplitude, unlabeled for simplicity.

tal axis (time). (Exceptions occur at those times when both curves have zero amplitudes.)

At any given moment, the particle may be at its extreme positive or negative displacement from the resting position in one direction or the other, or it may be somewhere between these two extremes (including being *at* the resting position, where displacement is zero). Because each of these displacements is a momentary glimpse which holds true only for that instant, the magnitude of a signal at a given instant is aptly called its *instantaneous amplitude.*

Because the instantaneous amplitude changes from moment to moment, we also need to be able to describe the magnitude of a wave in more general terms. The overall displacement from the negative to positive peak yields the signal's *peak-to-peak amplitude,* while the magnitude from baseline to a peak is called the wave's *peak amplitude.* Of course, the actual magnitude is no more often at the peak than it is an any other phase of the sine wave. Thus, although peak amplitudes do have uses, we most often are interested in a kind of "average" amplitude that more reasonably reflects the magnitude of a wave throughout its cycles. The simple average of the sinusoid's positive and negative instantaneous amplitudes cannot be used because this number will always be equal to zero. The practical alternative is to use the *root-mean-square* (rms) *amplitude.* This value is generally and simply provided by measuring equipment, but it conceptually involves the following calculations: First the values of all positive and negative displacements are squared, so that all resulting values are positive numbers (and zero for those values that fall right on the resting position). The mean of all these values is obtained, and the rms value is finally obtained by taking the square root of this mean. The rms amplitude of a signal is numerically equal to 0.707 times the peak amplitude (or 0.354 times the peak-to-peak amplitude). As a practical matter, we do not deal directly with the air particle's displacement, but rather express a sound's magnitude in terms intensity or pressure. Let us therefore now briefly review the manner in which a sound's magnitude is specified in the hearing sciences.

DECIBEL NOTATION

The range of magnitudes we concern ourselves with in hearing is enormous. As we shall discuss in Chap. 9, the sound pressure of the loudest sound that we can tolerate is on the order of 10 million times greater than that of the softest audible sound. One can immediately imagine the cumbersome taks that would be involved if we were to deal with such an immense range of numbers on a linear scale. The problems involved with and related to such a wide range of values make it desirable to transform the absolute physical magnitudes into another form, called *decibels* (dB), which make the values both palatable and rationally meaningful.

One may conceive of the decibel as basically involving two characteristics, namely ratios and logarithms. First, the value of a quantity is expressed in relation to some meaningful baseline value in the form of a ratio. Because it makes sense to use the softest sound one can hear as our baseline, we use the intensity or pressure of the softest audible sound as our reference value.

As introduced earier, this reference intensity is 10^{-12} w/m², and the corresponding reference sound pressure is 2×10^{-5} N/m².* The appropriate reference value becomes the denominator of our ratio and the absolute intensity (or pressure) of the sound in question becomes the numerator. Thus, instead of talking about a sound having an absolute intensity of 10^{-10} w/m², we express this its intensity relatively in terms of how it relates to our reference, as the ratio: $(10^{-10}$ w/m²$) / (10^{-12}$ w/m²$)$. This intensity ratio reduces to simply 10^2. This ratio is replaced with its common logarithm. The reason is that the linear distance between numbers having the same ratio relationship between them (say, 2:1) becomes wider when the absolute magnitudes of the numbers gets larger. For example, the distance between the numbers in each of the following pairs increases appreciably as the size of the numbers becomes larger, even though they all involve the same 2:1 ratio: 1–2, 10–20, 100–200, and 1000–2000. The logarithmic conversion is used because equal ratios are represented as equal distances on a logarithmic scale.

The decibel is a relative entity. This, of course, means that the decibel in and of itself is a dimensionless quantity, and is meaningless without knowledge of the reference value, which constitutes the denominator of the ratio. Because of this, it is necessary to make the reference value explicit when a sound is expressed in decibel form. This is accomplished by stating that the magnitude of the sound is whatever number of decibels with respect to the reference quantity. Moreover, it is common practice to add the word "level" to the original quantity

---

*Recall also that the corresponding references values in cgs units are 10^{-16} w/cm² for sound intensity and 2×10^{-4} dynes/cm² for sound pressure.

when dealing with dB values. Intensity expressed in dB is called intensity level (IL) and sound pressure in dB is called sound pressure level (SPL). The reference values indicated above are generally assumed when decibels are expressed as dB IL (or dB SPL). For example, one might say that the intensity level of a sound is "50 dB re: 10^{-12} w/m²" or "50 dB IL."

The general formula for the decibel is expressed in terms of power, as

$$dB = 10 \log (P/P_o) \tag{1.24}$$

where P is the power of the sound being measured and P_o is the reference power to which the former is being compared. Acoustical measurements are, however, typically made in terms of intensity or sound pressure. The applicable formula for decibels of intensity level is thus:

$$IL = 10 \log (I/I_o) \tag{1.25}$$

where I is the intensity (in w/m²) of the sound in question, and I_o is the reference intensity, or 10^{-12} w/m². Continuing with the example introduced above, where the value of I is 10^{-10} w/m, we thus find that

$$IL = 10 \log \left(\frac{10^{-10}\text{w/m}^2}{10^{-12}\text{w/m}^2}\right)$$
$$= 10 \log 10^2 = 10 \times 2$$
$$= 20 \text{ dB re: } 10^{-12} \text{ w/m}^2.$$

In other words, an intensity of 10^{-10} w/m² corresponds to an intensity level of 20 dB (re: 10^{-12} w/m²), or 20 dB IL.

Sound intensity measurements are important and useful, and are preferred in certain situations. (See Rasmussen [8] for a timely review of this topic.) However, most acoustical measurements involved in hearing are made in terms of sound pressure, and are thus expressed in decibels of sound pressure level. Intensity is proportional to pressure squared:

$$I \propto p^2 \tag{1.26}$$

or

$$p \propto I^{1/2} \tag{1.27}$$

Therefore, converting the dB IL formula into the equivalent equation for dB SPL involves replacing the intensity values with the squares of the corresponding pressure values. Therefore

$$SPL = 10 \log (p^2/p_o^2) \tag{1.28}$$

where p is the measured sound pressure and p_o is the reference sound pressure (2×10^{-5} N/m²). This formula may be simplified to

$$SPL = 10 \log (p/p_o)^2 \qquad (1.29)$$

Recall that the logarithm of a number squared corresponds to two time the log of that number ($\log x^2 = 2 \cdot \log x$). Consequently, the square may be removed to result in

$$SPL = 2 \times 10 \log (p/p_o) \qquad (1.30)$$

Therefore, the simplified formula for decibels of SPL becomes:

$$SPL = 20 \log (p/p_o) \qquad (1.31)$$

where the value of 20 (instead of 10) is due to having removed the square from the earlier described version of the formula.*

By way of example, a sound pressure of 2×10^{-4} N/m² corresponds to a SPL of 20 dB (re: 2×10^{-5} N/m²), which may be calculated as follows:

$$\begin{aligned}
SPL &= 20 \log \left(\frac{2 \times 10^{-4}\,\text{N/m}^2}{2 \times 10^{-5}\,\text{N/m}^2}\right) \\
&= 20 \log 10^1 = 20 \times 1 \\
&= 20\,\text{dB} \qquad\qquad \text{re: } 2 \times 10^{-5}\,\text{N/m}^2
\end{aligned}$$

What would happen if the intensity (or pressure) in question is same as the reference intensity (or pressure)? In other words, what is the dB value of the reference itself? In terms of intensity, the answer to this question may be found by simply using 10^{-12} w/m² as both the numerator (I) and denominator (I_o) in the dB formula; thus

$$IL = 10 \log \left(\frac{10^{-12}\,\text{w/m}^2}{10^{-12}\,\text{w/m}^2}\right) \qquad (1.32)$$

Because anything divided by itself equals 1, and the logarithm of 1 is 0, this equation reduces to:

$$\begin{aligned}
IL &= 10 \log 1 = 10 \times 0 \\
&= 0\,\text{dB} \qquad\qquad \text{re: } 10^{-12}\,\text{w/m}^2
\end{aligned}$$

---

*One cannot take the intensity ratio from the IL formula and simply insert it into the SPL formula, or vice versa. The square root of the intensity ratio yields the corresponding pressure ratio, which may then be placed into the SPL equation. Failure to use the proper terms will result in an erroneous doubling of the value in dB SPL.

Hence, 0 dB IL is the intensity level of the reference intensity. Just as 0 dB IL indicates the intensity level of the reference intensity, so 0 dB SPL similarly implies that the measured sound pressure corresponds to that of the reference

$$\text{SPL} = 20 \log \left(\frac{2 \times 10^{-5} \text{ N/m}^2}{2 \times 10^{-5} \text{ N/m}^2} \right) \tag{1.33}$$

Just as we have seen in the previous example, this equation is solved simply as follows:

$$\text{SPL} = 20 \log 1 = 20 \times 0$$
$$= 0 \text{ dB} \qquad \text{re: } 2 \times 10^{-5} \text{ N/m}^2$$

In other words, 0 dB SPL indicates that the pressure of the sound in question corresponds to the reference sound pressure of 2×10^{-5} N/m^2. This important point is that 0 dB does *not* mean "no sound." Rather, 0 dB implies that the quantity being measured is equal to the reference quantity. Negative decibel values indicate that the measured magnitude is smaller than the reference quantity.

COMPLEX WAVES

Thus far we have dealt only with sinusoids, those sounds which include only one frequency. When two or more pure tones are combined, the result is called a complex wave. Figure 1.9 shows what occurs when two sinusoids being combined have exactly *the same frequencies and ampli-tudes*. In Fig. 1.9a, the first and second sinusoids (labeled 1 and 2) are *in phase* with each other. Here, the two waves are equal to one another in terms of (instantaneous) displacement at every moment in time. The resulting wave (labeled R) has twice the displacement of the two compo-nents, but is otherwise identical to them. This finding illustrates the central concept involved in combining waves: The amplitudes of the two waves are algebraically added to each other at every point along the horizontal (time) axis. In the case of two identical, in-phase sinusoids, the resultant wave becomes twice as big at each point along the time axis, and remains zero where the two waves cross the baseline. The latter occurs because the amplitudes of the two waves at these moments are zero (0 + 0 = 0). For readily apparent reasons, this case is often called reinforcement.

Figure 1.9c shows what happens when we combine two otherwise identical sinusoids which are *180° out of phase* with each other. This is, of

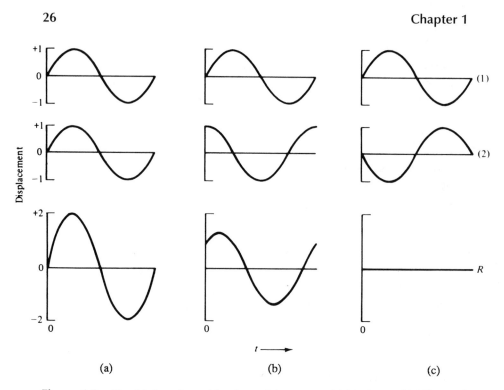

Figure 1.9 Combining sinusoids of equal frequency (a) in-phase; (b) 90° out of phase, and (c) 180° out of phase. (See text.) [From Arnold M. Small [9], Acoustics, in *Normal Aspects of Speech, Hearing, and Language* (Fred D. Minifie, Thomas J. Hixon, and Frederick Willams ,eds.), © 1973, p. 16. Reprinted by permission of Prentice-Hall, Inc.]

course, the opposite of the relationship depicted in Fig. 1.9a. Here, wave 1 is equal and opposite to wave 2 at every moment in time. Algebraic addition under these circumstances causes the resulting displacement to equal zero at all points along the horizontal (time) axis. The result will be complete *cancellation*.

If the two otherwise identical sinusoids are out of phase by any other value than 180°, then the shape of the resulting wave will depend upon how their two displacements compare at each moment in time. Two sinusoids are shown 90° out of phase in Fig. 1.9b. The result of algebraically adding their magnitudes on a point-by-point basis is shown below the two original waves. In general, combining two identical sinusoids having the same frequency which are out of phase (except 180°) results in a sinusoid with the same frequency, but which is different in its phase and amplitude.

What happens when we combine sinusoids that differ in frequency? The mechanism for combining waves of dissimilar frequencies is really the same as what applies for those having the same frequency: *Any* two or more waves are combined by algebraically summing their instantaneous displacements on a point-by-point basis along the horizontal (time) axis, regardless of their individual frequencies and amplitudes or their phase relationships. However, the combination of waves having unequal frequencies will not yield a sinusoidal result. Instead, the result will depend upon the specifics of the sounds being combined.

Consider the three sinusoids depicted on the left-hand side of Fig. 1.10, labeled f1, f2, and f3. Note that two cycles of f1 are completed in the same time as four cycles of f2 or six cycles of f3. Thus, frequency of f2 is two times that of f1; and the frequency of f3 is three times f1. The actual fequencies of f1, f2, and f3 could be any values meeting the described conditions; e.g., 100, 200, and 300 Hz; 1000, 2000, and 3000 Hz, or 20, 40, and 60 Hz, etc. Because f2 and f3 are integral multiples of f1, we say that they are harmonics of f1. Hence, f1, f2, and f2 constitute an harmonic series. The lowest frequency of this series is called the fundamental frequency. Otherwise stated, harmonics are whole-number multiples of the fundamental frequency; and the fundamental is the largest whole-number common denominator its harmonics.* Clearly, the harmonics are separated from one another by amounts equal to the fundamental frequency.

The right-hand side of Fig. 1.10 shows what happens when f1, f2, and f3 are combined in various combinations. Notice that the combining of two or more sinusoidal waves differing in frequency generates a resultant wave that is no longer sinusoidal in character. Note, however, that the combined waveforms shown in this figure are still periodic. In other words, even though these combined waveforms are no longer sinusoidal, they still retain the characteristic of repeating themselves at regular intervals over time. Moreover, notice at all three waves (f1 + f2, f1 + f3, and f1 + f2 + f3) repeat themselves with the same period as f1;

---

*By convention, "fundamental frequency" (typically specified as f_0) is usually also called the "first harmonic" in the physical sciences (i.e., the value of the first harmonic is $1 \times f_0$). Confusion arises because others use "first harmonic" to mean the first component above the fundamental (i.e., by "first harmonic," they mean $2 \times f_0$). We will therefore be specifying the lowest component frequency as f1, at least for purposes of the current discussion. The idea is to avoid confusion by temporarily avoiding the "0" subscript; and instead to use the number "1" to mean the *first* component (the first harmonic) which is also the *lowest* one (the fundamental).

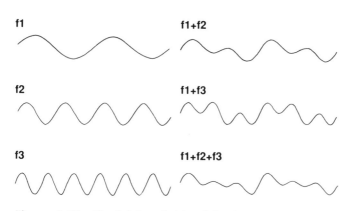

Figure 1.10 The left-hand side of the figure shows three sinusoidal waves of frequencies f1, f2 and f3. The frequency of f2 is twice that of f1; and f3 is three times the frequency of f1. Thus, f2 and f3 are harmonics of f1. The right hand side of the figure depicts the waveforms of the complex periodic waves that result from the in-phase addition of f1 + f2, f1 + f3, and f1 + f2 + f3. The frequency of f1 is the fundamental frequency of each of these complex periodic waves.

which is the lowest component in each case. These are examples of complex periodic waves, so called because they are composed of more than one component and because they repeat themselves at regular time intervals. The lowest frequency component of a comples periodic wave is called its fundamental frequency. Hence, f1 is the fundamental frequency of each of the complex periodic waves in Fig. 1.10. The period of the fundamental frequency constitutes the rate at which the complex periodic wave repeats itself. In other words, the time needed for one cycle of a complex periodic wave is the same as the period of its fundamental frequency.

The example shown in Fig. 1.11 involves combining only odd harmonics (f1, f3, . . .) whose amplitudes become smaller with increasing frequency. The resulting complex periodic waveform becomes progressively squared-off as the number of odd harmonics is increased, eventually resulting in the aptly named "square wave" shown at the bottom of the figure.

The combination of components which are not harmonically related results in a complex waveform which does not repeat itself over time. Such sounds are thus called *aperiodic*. In the extreme case, consider a wave which is completely random. An artist's conceptualization of two separate glimpses of a random waveform is shown in Figs. 1.12a and b. The point of the two pictures is that the waveform is quite different from

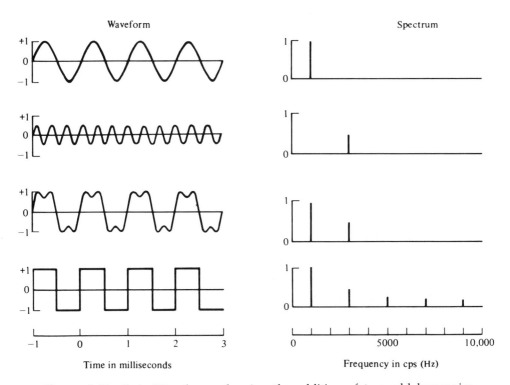

Waveform   Spectrum

Time in milliseconds   Frequency in cps (Hz)

Figure 1.11 Left: Waveforms showing the addition of two odd harmonics (from the top, f1 and f3), which if continued would eventually result in a square wave (bottom). Right: Discrete frequency spectra corresponding to the waveforms at the left. [From Arnold M. Small [9], Acoustics, in *Normal Aspects of Speech, Hearing, and Language* Fred D. Minifie, Thomas J. Hixon, and Frederick Williams, eds.), © 1973, p. 19. Reprinted by permission of Prentice-Hall, Inc.]

moment to moment. Over the long run, such a wave would contain all possible frequencies, and all of them would have the same average amplitudes. The sound described by such waveforms is called random, or Gaussian, noise. Because all possible frequencies are equally represented, they are also called white noise on analogy to white light. Abrupt sounds that are extremely short in duration must also be aperiodic because they are not repeated over time. Such sounds are called transients. The waveform of a transient is shown in Fig. 1.12c.

Because the wave-form shows amplitude as a function of time, the frequency of a pure tone and the fundamental frequency of a complex periodic tone can be determined only indirectly by examining such a representation, and then only if the time scale is explicit. Moreover, one

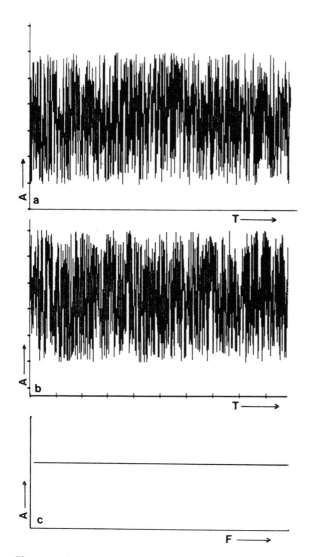

Figure 1.12 Artist's conceptualizations of the waveforms of (a, b) white (random) noise as it might appear at two different times; (c) a transient; and (d) continuous spectrum of white noise or a transient.

cannot determine the frequency content of a complex sound by looking at its waveform. In fact, dramatically different waveforms result from the combination of the same component frequencies if their phase relationships are changed. Another means of presenting the material is therefore needed when one is primarily interested in information about frequency. This information is portrayed by the *spectrum*, which shows amplitude as a function of frequency. In effect, we are involved here with the issue of going between the time domain (shown by the waveform) and the frequency domain (shown by the spectrum). The underlying mathematical relationships are provided by Fourier's theorem, which basically says that a complex sound can be analyzed into its constituent sinusoidal components. The process by which one may break down the complex sound into its component parts is called Fourier analysis. Fourier analysis enables one to plot the spectrum of a complex sound.

The spectra of several periodic waves are shown in the right side of Fig. 1.11, and the spectrum of white noise is shown in Fig. 1.12d. The upper two spectra in Fig. 1.11 correspond respectively to the waveforms of the sinusoids to their left. The top wave is that of a 1000 Hz tone. This information is shown on the associated spectrum as a single (discrete) vertical line drawn at the point along the abscissa corresponding to 1000 Hz. The height of the line indicates the amplitude of the wave. The second waveform in the figure is for a 3000 Hz tone which has a lower amplitude that does the 1000 Hz tone shown above it. The corresponding spectrum shows this as a single vertical line drawn at the 3000 Hz location along the abscissa. Its lower height (compared to the 1000 Hz spectrum above) reveals the lower amplitude of this tone.

The third waveform in Fig. 1.11 depicts the complex periodic wave that results when the 1000 and 3000 Hz tones are combined. To the right of this waveform is its spectrum. This spectrum shows two discrete vertical lines, one each at the 1000 and 3000 Hz locations, with the amplitudes of the two components shown by their respective heights. Finally, the bottom waveform and spectrum in the figure are those for a square wave. As one would expect from the above description of square waves, its spectrum is composed of many discrete vertical lines, one each at the frequencies corresponding to odd multiples of the lowest (fundamental) component, with their heights decreasing as frequency increases.

To summarize, the spectrum of a periodic wave shows a vertical line at the frequency of each sinusoidal component of that wave; and the amplitude of each component is shown by the height of its corresponding line. Consequently, the spectrum of a periodic sound is referred to as a *discrete* spectrum. As should be apparent, the phase relationships among the various components is lost when a sound is represented by its spectrum.

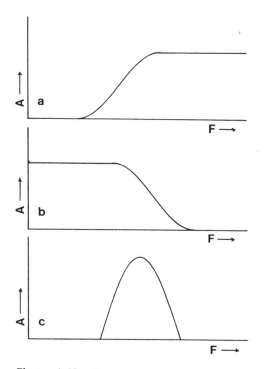

Figure 1.13 Continuous spectra of aperiodic sounds with (a) greater amplitude in the high frequencies (high-pass filter); (b) greater amplitude in the low frequencies (low-pass filter); and (c) a concentration of energy within a given band of frequencies (band-pass filter).

Figure 1.12d shows the spectrum of white noise. Because white noise contains all conceivable frequencies, it would be a fruitless exercise to even try to draw individual (discrete) vertical lines at each of its component frequencies. The same point applies to the three spectra depicted in Fig. 1.13. We therefore draw a continuous line over the tops of where all of these vertical lines would have been, so that the spectrum of an aperiodic sound is referred to as a *continuous* spectrum. In the case of white noise, this is a straight horizontal line, saying in effect that all frequencies are represented at equal amplitudes. Similarly, Fig. 1.13 shows the continuous spectra of aperiodic sounds which contain (a) greater amplitude in the higher frequencies, (b) greater amplitude in the lower frequencies, and (c) a concentration of energy within a particular range (band) of frequencies. These three spectra correspond to the characteristics of high-pass, low-pass and band-pass filters, respectively.

STANDING WAVES

Let us consider two situations. In the first situation, imagine the sound waves propagating rightward and leftward from a vibrating tuning fork placed in the center of a small room. These sound waves will hit and be reflected from the walls, so that now there will also be reflected waves propagating in the opposite directions in addition to the original waves. (Considering for the moment only the right wall for simplicity, we can envision a rightward-going original wave and a leftward-going reflected wave.) The other situation involves plucking the center of a guitar string that is tied tautly at both ends. Here, the waves initiated by the pluck move outward toward each fixed end of the string, from which a reflected wave propagates in the opposite direction.

To reiterate, in both cases just described there are continuous original and continuous reflected waves moving toward one another. The reflected waves are equal in frequency to the original ones, and both the reflected and original waves are of course propagating at the same speed. Now, recall from prior discussion that two waves will interact with one another such that their instantaneous displacements add algebraically. Thus, the net displacement (of the air particles in the room or of the string) at any moment which occurs at any point (in the room or along the string) will be due to how the superimposed waves interact. It turns out that the resultant wave produced by this interaction constitutes a pattern which actually stands still even though it is derived from component waves which themselves are propagating. Hence, the points of maximum displacement (peaks of the waves) and no displacement (baseline crossings of the waves) will always occur at fixed locations in the room or along the string. This phenomenon is called a quite descriptively called a *standing wave*.

Because the vibration pattern of the string is easily visualized, we will refer only to the string example for the remainder of the discussion, although these points apply similarly to the room example as well. The locations of no (zero) displacement in the standing wave pattern are called nodes, and the places of maximum displacement are thus called antinodes. Even brief consideration will reveal that the displacement must be zero at the two ends of the string (where they are tied and thus cannot move).* Hence, nodes must occur at the two ends of the string. It follows that if there is a node at each end of the string, then there must be an antinode at the center of the string, halfway between the two

---

*This corresponds to the hard walls of the room, which prevent the air molecules from being displaced.

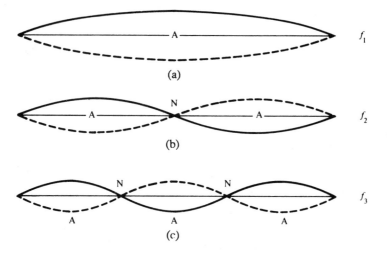

Figure 1.14 Modes of vibration (see text). [From Arnold M. Small [9], Acoustics, in *Normal Aspects of Speech, Hearing, and Language* (Fred D. Minifie, Thomas J. Hixon, and Frederick Williams, eds.), © 1973, p. 39. Reprinted by permission of Prentice-Hall, Inc.]

nodes. (This should not be suprising because we already know that the zero displacements (0 and 180° phase) and maximum displacements (90 and 270°) alternate for any cycle of a sinusoid.)

This standing wave pattern is depicted in Fig. 1.14a. Some thought will confirm that the arrangement just described (node at each end, antinode at the center) constitutes the longest possible standing wave pattern that can occur for any given string. We will call it the first *mode* of vibration. The figure also highlights the fact that this standing wave pattern comprises exactly half (0 to 180°) of a cycle. Consequently its length corresponds to exactly one-half of a wavelength (λ). Its length therefore is equal to one-half of the wavelength ($\lambda/2$) of some frequency. This frequency, in turn, may be determined by applying Eq. 1.21 (which states that $f = c/\lambda$). By substitution, the frequency of the string's first mode of vibration would be $c/2L$ (where L is the length of the string, and c is the appropriate speed of the wave for that string*). It should now be apparent that the first mode of vibration correponds to the fundamental frequency.

---

*The speed of a wave along a vibrating string is not the same as for air. Instead, we would be dealing with the speed of a transverse wave along a string, which is the square root of the ratio of the string's tension (T) to its mass (M). Hence, the formula would be $f = 1/2L \cdot \sqrt{T/M}$

The standing wave just described is not the only one which can occur for the string, but rather is the longest one. Other standing waves may develop as well as long as they meet the requirement that nodes occur at the two tied ends of the string. Several other examples are shown in Fig. 1.14, which reveals that each of these standing wave patterns must divide the string into parts which are exactly equal in length to one another. Thus, there will be standing wave patterns which divide the string into exact halves, thirds, fourths, fifths, etc. These are the second, third, fourth, fifth, etc. modes of vibration. In turn, they produce frequencies which are exact multiples (harmonics) of the fundamental frequency.

Suppose we were to set the air inside of a tube into vibration by, for example, blowing across the open end of the tube. If we were to do this experiment for several tubes, we would find that the shorter tubes made higher pitches sounds than do the longer ones. We would also find that the same tube would produce a higher pitch when open at both ends than when it is open at only one end. The frequency(ies) at which a body or medium vibrates is referred to as its natural or resonant frequency(ies).

In the case of a column of air vibrating in a tube open at both ends, the greatest pressure and the least particle displacement can occur in the center of the tube, while the greatest displacement and thus lowest pressure can occur at the two open ends (Fig. 1.15a). This is analogous to the vibration of the string. One may understand this in the sense that going from one end of the tube to the other involves going from a pressure node to an antinode to a node (or from displacement antinode to note to antinode), or 180 degrees of a cycle. This pattern is related to the out-of-phase reflection of the wave at the two ends of the tube, so that the pattern is duplicated when the length of the tube is covered twice. Hence, the lowest (fundamental) frequency capable of covering the tube exactly twice in one cycle must have a wavelength twice the length of the tube. Thus, the lowest resonant frequency (f1) of a tube open at both ends is the frequency whose wavelength is twice the length of the tube, or $f1 = c/2L$. Harmonics will occur at each multiple of this fundamental frequency.

Air vibration in a tube closed at one end is most restricted at the closed end, where pressure must thus be greatest and displacement the least (Fig. 1.15b). (Reflections at the closed end occur without phase reversal.) Thus, in terms of displacement, there must be a node at the closed end and an antinode at the open end. This means that the length of the tube corresponds to a quarter of a wavelength, so that the lowest resonant frequency (f1) of a tube closed at one end and open at the other is the one whose wavelength is four times the length of the tube, or $f1 = c/4L$. Since a

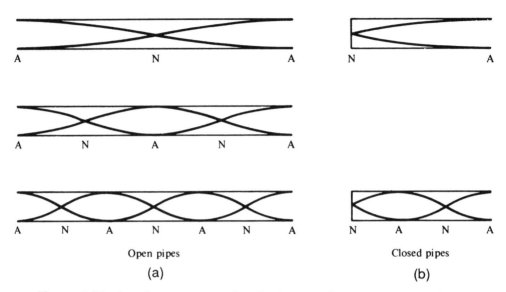

Open pipes   Closed pipes
(a)   (b)

Figure 1.15 Standing waves produced (a) in a tube open at one end (½-wavelength resonator) and (b) in a tube open at one end and closed at the other (¼-wavelength resonator). Nodes indicated by Ns, antinodes by As. (From Arnold M. Small [9], Acoustics, in *Normal Aspects of Speech, Hearing, and Language* [Fred D. Minifie, Thomas J. Hixon, and Frederick Williams eds.) © 1973, p. 47. Reprinted by permission of Prentice-Hall, Inc.]

node can occur at only one end, such a tube produces only the fundamental and its odd harmonics (e.g., f1, f3, f5, f7, etc.).*

IMPEDANCE

Impedance is the opposition to the flow of energy through a system. Some knowledge of impedance thus helps one to understand how a system transmits energy, and why it is more responsive to some frequencies than it is to others. We may generally define impedance (Z), in ohms, as the ratio of force to velocity:

$$Z = F/v \qquad (1.34)$$

---

*As a matter of perspective, one might note that the outer ear canal and the vocal tract approximate quarter-wavelength resonators; while the constriction in the mouth created by the tongue in the production of the /s/ sound approximates a half-wavelength resonator.

Therefore, the greater the amount of force needed to result in a given amount of velocity, the greater the impedance of the system.

We may also consider impedance in terms of its components. These are shown in the form of a mechanical representation of impedance in Fig. 1.16a. Here, we see that impedance Z is the interaction of resistance R, positive reactance Xm, and negative reactance Xs. These components are respectively related to friction, mass, and stiffness. Friction is represented in the figure by the ridged surface across which the block (mass) is moved. Friction causes a portion of the energy applied to the system to be converted into heat; this dissipation of energy into heat is termed resistance. Resistance is not related to frequency, and occurs in phase with the applied force. It is shown on the x-axis in Fig. 1.16c.

Reactance is the storage, as opposed to the dissipation, of energy by the system. Mass (positive) reactance Xm is associated with the mass of the system (shown by the block in the figure). Since all mass has the

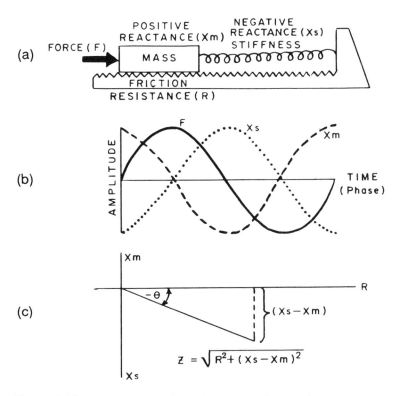

Figure 1.16 Impedance and its components (see text).

property of inertia, the application of a force F to the mass M causes the mass to accelerate according to the formula F = MA (where A is acceleration). If the force is applied sinusoidally, then the mass reactance is related to frequency as Xm = M2πf, where f is frequency. Thus, the magnitude of Xm is directly proportional to frequency (the higher the frequency the greater the mass reactance). Since acceleration precedes force by a quarter-cycle, Xm will lead the applied force in phase by 90° (Fig. 1.16b). This is why Xm is termed positive reactance, and its value is shown in the positive direction on the y-axis (Fig. 1.16c).

Stiffness (negative) reactance Xs is represented by the spring in Fig. 1.16a. We will represent the spring's stiffness as S. Applying a force compresses (displaces) the spring according to the formula F = S · X, where X is the amount of displacement. When the stimulus is applied sinusoidally, Xs is related to frequency as Xs = S/2πf. In other words, the amount of stiffness reactance is inversely proportional to frequency (Xs goes down as frequency goes up). Since displacement follows force by a quarter-cycle, Xs lags behind the applied force in phase by 90° (Fig. 1.16b). It is thus called negative reactance and is plotted downward on the y-axis (Fig. 1.16c).

Since the stiffness and mass components are 180° out of phase (Fig. 1.16b), a system's net reactance is equal to the difference between them (Xs − Xm). This relation is shown in Fig. 1.16c for the condition where Xs exceeds Xm, which is the case for the normal ear. Notice that the overall impedance Z results from the interaction between the resistance R and the net reactance. The negative phase angle −Θ in the figure shows that the net reactance of negative. The relationship between impedance, resistance, and reactance is thus:

$$Z = \sqrt{R^2 + (Xs - Xm)^2} \qquad (1.35)$$

Looking at the effect of frequency, we find that

$$Z = \sqrt{R^2 + (S/\omega - M\omega)^2} \qquad (1.36)$$

where ω represents 2πf. The implication is that frequency counts. Since Xm is proportional to frequency while Xs is inversely proportional to frequency, they should be equal at some frequency. This is the system's resonant frequency, at which the reactance components cancel each other out, leaving only the resistance component.

The amount of resistance, which is associated with how rapidly damping occurs, determines the sharpness the tuning around the resonant frequency. The less the resistance, the more narrowly tuned the resonance is; and the more the resistance, the broader the responsiveness of the system around the resonant frequency.

REFERENCES

1. L. L. Beranek, *Acoustics*, American Institute of Physics, New York, 1986.
2. P. Hewitt, *Conceptual Physics*, Little, Brown and Co., Boston, 1974.
3. L. E. Kinsler, A. R. Frey, A. B. Coppens, and J. B. Sanders, *Fundamentals of Acoustics*, 3rd Ed., Wiley, New York, 1982.
4. A. P. G. Peterson and E. E. Gross, *Handbook of Noise Measurement*, 7th Ed., General Radio, Concord, Massachusetts, 1972.
5. J. R. Pierce and E. E. David, Jr., *Man's World of Sound*, Doubleday, Garden City, New York, 1958.
6. F. W. Sears, M. W. Zemansky, and H. D. Young, *University Physics*, 6th Ed., Addison-Wesley, New York, 1982.
7. W. A. van Bergeijk, J. R. Pierce, and E. E. David, Jr., *Waves and the Ear*, Doubleday, Garden City, New York, 1960.
8. G. Rasmussen, Intensity—its measurement and uses, *Sound and Vibration 23* (3), 12–21 (1989).
9. A. M. Small, Acoustics, in, *Normal Aspects of Speech, Hearing, and Language* (F. D. Minifie, T. J. Hixon, and F. Williams, eds.), Prentice-Hall, Englewood Cliffs, New Jersey, 1973, pp. 11–72.

2

Anatomy

GROSS ANATOMY AND OVERVIEW

The auditory system comprises the ears and their connections to and within the central nervous system. From the standpoint of physical layout, the auditory system may be divided into the outer, middle, and inner ears; the auditory nerve; and the central auditory pathways.

This section provides a very brief and simplified overview of the auditory system, in the hope that a brief glance at the forest will help the student avoid being blinded by the trees.

The major divisions of the ear are shown in Fig. 2.1, and their relative positions within the head are given in Fig. 2.2. The outer ear is made up of the pinna (auricle) and ear canal (external auditory meatus). The eardrum (tympanic membrane) separates the outer and middle ears, and is generally considered to be part of the latter. The middle ear also includes the tympanic (middle ear) cavity; the ossicular chain with its associated muscles, tendons, and ligaments; and the Eustachian (auditory) tube. The inner ear begins at the oval window. It includes the sensory organs of hearing (the cochlea) and of balance (the semicircular canals, utricle, and saccule). While the balance system is certainly important, the concern here is hearing, and accordingly the balance apparatus is mentioned only in so far as it is directly associated with the auditory system.

The inner ear, beyond the oval window, is composed of the vestibule, the cochlea, and the vestibular apparatus. A membranous duct is

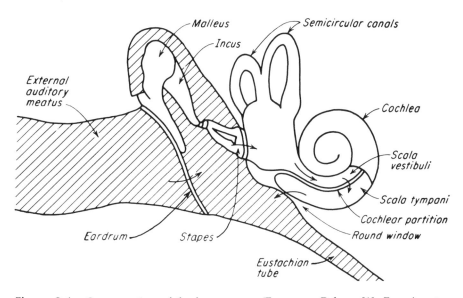

Figure 2.1 Cross-section of the human ear. (From von Bekesy [1], *Experiments in Hearing*, © 1960 by McGraw-Hill. Used with permission of McGraw-Hill Book Company.)

continuous throughout these. In the cochlea, it separates the perilymph-filled scala vestibuli and scala tympani above and below from the endolymph-filled scala media between them. The scala media contains the organ of Corti, whose hair cells are the sensory receptors for hearing. When stimulated, the hair cells initiate activity in the auditory nerve fibers with which they are in contact. The auditory nerve leaves the inner ear through the internal auditory canal (internal auditory meatus), enters the brain at the angle of the pons and cerebellum, and terminates in the brainstem at the cochlear nuclei. We are now in the central auditory system.

TEMPORAL BONE

The ear is contained within the temporal bone. Knowledge of the major landmarks of this bone is thus important in understanding the anatomy and spatial orientation of the ear. The right and left temporal bones are two of the thirty-two bones that make up the skull. Eight of these bones (including the two temporal bones) contribute to the cranium, and the remainder form the facial skeleton. Figure 2.3 gives a lateral (side) view

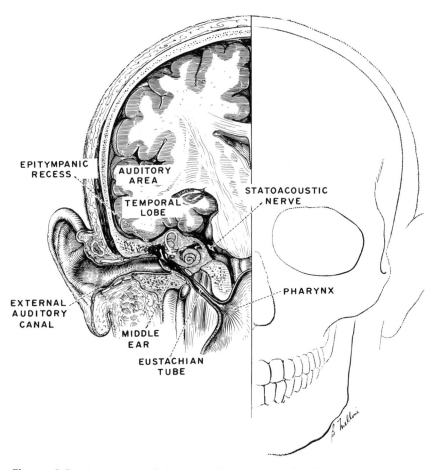

Figure 2.2 Structures of the ear relative to the head. (Courtesy of Abbott Laboratories.)

of the skull, emphasizing the temporal bone. The temporal bone forms the inferior portion of the side of the skull. It is bordered by the mandible, zygomatic, parietal, sphenoid, and occipital bones. The temporal bone itself is generally divided into five anatomical divisions: the squamous, mastoid, petrous, and tympanic portions, and the anteroinferiorly protruding styloid process (Fig. 2.4).

The squamous portion is the fan-shaped part of the temporal bone.

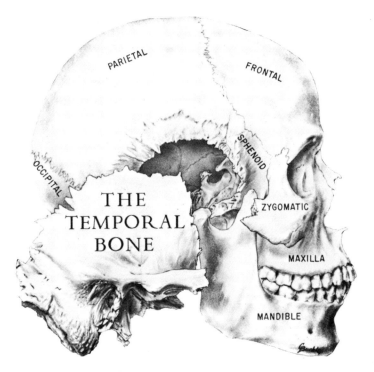

Figure 2.3   Lateral view of the skull emphasizing the position of the temporal bone. [From Anson and Donaldson [2], *The Surgical Anatomy of the Temporal Bone and Ear,* © 1967 by W. B. Saunders (with permission).]

It is quite thin, often to the point of being translucent. Its inferior surface forms the roof and part of the posterior wall of the ear canal. The zygomatic process protrudes forward from the squamous portion to meet the zygomatic bone. The fan-shaped squamous plate is also in contact with the sphenoid bone anteriorly and with the parietal bone superiorly and posteriorly. The mandible attaches to the temporal bone just anterior to the ear canal, near the base of the zygomatic process, forming the temporomandibular joint.

The mastoid portion lies behind and below the squamous, and forms the posterior aspect of the temporal bone. The mastoid portion attaches to the parietal bone superiorly and to the occipital bone posteriorly. It projects downward to form the mastoid process, which appears as a somewhat cone-shaped extension below the base of the skull. The

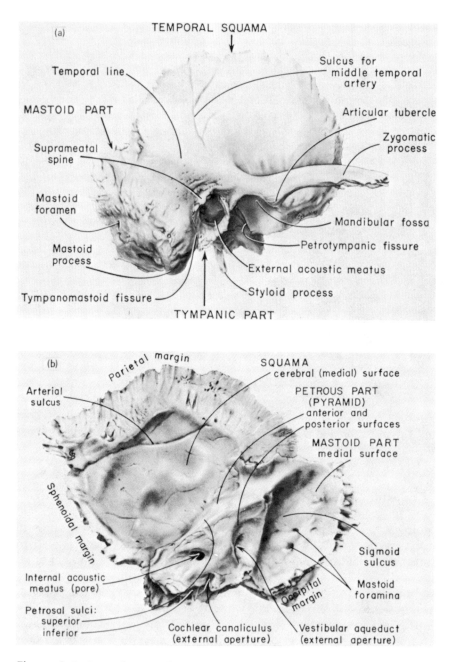

Figure 2.4 Lateral (a) and medial (b) aspects of the temporal bone. [From Anson and Donaldson [2], *The Surgical Anatomy of the Temporal Bone and Ear,* © 1967 by W. B. Saunders (with permission).]

mastoid process contains interconnecting air cells of variable size, shape, and number. Continuous with these air cells is a cavity known as the tympanic antrum, which lies anterosuperior to the mastoid process. The antrum also connects with the epitympanic recess (attic) of the middle ear via the aditus ad antrum. The antrum is bordered inferiorly by the mastoid process, superiorly by a thin bony plat called the tegmen tympanum, medially by the wall of the lateral semicircular canal, and laterally by the squamous.

The tympanic portion forms the floor and the anterior and inferoposterior walls of the ear canal. It is bordered by the squamous portion above, the petrous portion below, and the mastoid process posteriorly. The lower part of the tympanic portion partially covers the styloid process, a thin, cylinder-like anteroinferior projection from the base of the temporal bone. The styloid process, which varies in length from as little as 5 mm to as much as ~ 50 mm, is generally considered to be a separate portion of the temporal bone. While it does not contribute to the hearing mechanism, the styloid process is important as a connecting point for several muscles involved in speech production.

The petrous portion houses the sensory organs of hearing and balance, and contains the internal auditory canal. It is medially directed and is fused at its base to the tympanic and squamous portions. The mastoid lies posterior to the petrous portion, and in fact develops from it postnatally. The details of the petrous portion are equivalent to those of the inner ear, discussed below.

OUTER AND MIDDLE EAR

Pinna

The pinna (auricle) is the external appendage of the ear. It is an irregularly shaped ovoid of highly variable size, which folds over the side of the head posteriorly, superiorly, and inferiorly. It is basically composed of skin-covered elastic cartilage, although it contains some grossly undifferentiated muscles which are of a completely vestigial nature in man. The pinna has a number of extrinsic muscles as well, which are also essentially vestigial in humans.

The landmarks of the pinna are shown in Fig. 2.5. Most of its perimeter is demarcated by a ridgelike rim called the helix. If we first follow the helix posteriorly from the top of the ear, we see that it curves widely back and down to end in the earlobe (lobule) at the bottom of the pinna. Unlike the rest of the pinna, the lobule does not have any cartilage. Starting again from the apex of the helix, we see that it proceeds anteri-

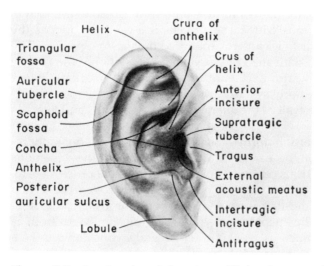

Figure 2.5 Landmarks of the pinna. [From Anson and Donaldson [2], *The Surgical Anatomy of the Temporal Bone and Ear*, © 1967 by W. B. Saunders (with permission).]

orly and downward, and then turns posteriorly in a rather sharp angle to form the crus (limb) of the helix—an almost horizontal shelf at about the center of the pinna. The scaphoid fossa is a depression lying between the posterior portion of the helix posteriorly and a structure called the antihelix anteriorly.

The antihelix is a ridge which runs essentially parallel to the posterior helix. Its upper end bifurcates to form two crura, a rather wide superoposterior crus and a narrower anterior crus which ends under the angle where the helix curves backward. A triangular depression is thus formed by the two crura of the antihelix and the anterior part of the helix, and is called the triangular fossa. From the crura, the antihelix curves downward and then forward, and ends in a moundlike widening, the antitragus. Opposite and anterior to the antitragus is a backwardfolding ridge called the tragus. The inferoanterior acute angle formed by the tragus and antitragus is called the intertragal incisure. The tragus, the antitragus, and the crus of the helix border a relatively large and cup-shaped depression called the concha. Sebaceous glands are present in the skin of the concha, as well as in the ear canal. At the bottom of the concha, protected by the tragus, is the entrance to the ear canal.

Ear Canal

The ear canal (external auditory meatus) leads from the concha to the eardrum, and varies in both size and shape. The outer portion of the canal, about one-third of its length, is cartilagenous; the remaining two-thirds is bony. The canal is by no means straight; rather it is quite irregular in its course. It takes on a somewhat S-shaped form medially. It curves first anterosuperiorly, then posterosuperiorly, and finally antero-inferiorly. It is for this reason that the pinna must be pulled up and back in order for one to see the eardrum.

The ear canal has a diameter of about 0.7 cm at its entrance, with an average horizontal diameter of 0.65 cm and a mean vertical diameter of 0.9 cm [3]. As would be expected from its irregular course, the length of the canal is also not uniform. Instead, it is approximately 2.5 cm long posterosuperiorly and 3.1 cm long inferoanteriorly [4]. Also contributing to the greater length of the lower part of the canal is the oblique orientation of the eardrum as it sits in its annulus at the end of the canal.

The canal is lined with tight-fitting skin that is thicker in the cartilagenous segment than in the bony part. Ceruminous (wax) and sebaceous (oil) glands are plentiful in the cartilagenous segment, and are also found on the posterior and superior walls of the bony canal. The wax and oil lubricate the canal and help to keep it free of debris and foreign objects. Tiny hairs similarly contribute to the protection of the ear from invasion.

Eardrum

The canal terminates at the eardrum (tympanic membrane), which tilts laterally at the top so as to sit in its annulus at an angle of about 55° to the ear canal (see Fig. 2.1). The membrane is quite thin and translucent, with an average thickness of approximately 0.074 mm [4]. It is elliptical in shape, with a vertical diameter of about 0.9–1.0 cm and a horizontal cross section of approximately 0.8–0.9 cm. The eardrum is concave outward, and the peak of this broad cone is known as the umbo. This inward displacement is associated with the drum's attachment to the manubrium of the malleus, the tip of which corresponds to the umbo (Fig. 2.6). In contact with the drum, the malleus continues upward in a direction corresponding to the one-o'clock position in the right ear and the eleven-o'clock position in the left. The malleal prominence of the malleus is formed by the lateral process of the malleus, from which run the malleal folds which divide the drum into the pars flaccida (Shrapnell's membrane) above and the pars tensa below.

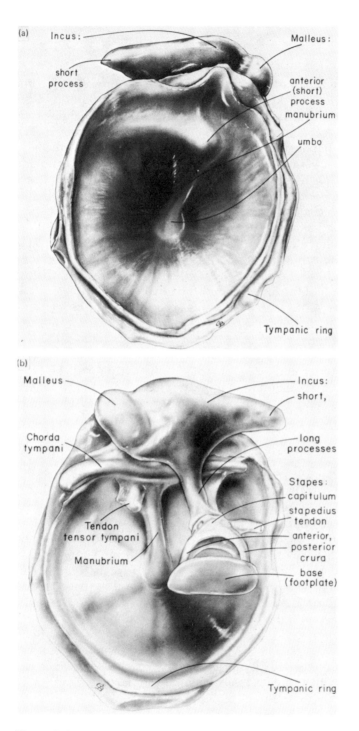

Figure 2.6 Lateral (a) and medial (b) aspects of the tympanic membrane and its connections to the ossicular chain. [From Anson and Donaldson [2], *The Surgical Anatomy of the Temporal Bone and Ear*, © 1967 by W. B. Saunders (with permission).]

The eardrum is made up of four layers. The outermost layer is continuous with the skin of the ear canal, and the most medial layer is continuous with the mucous membrane of the middle ear. The pars flaccida is composed solely of these two layers. The pars tensa has two additional layers: a layer of radial fibers just medial to the skin layer, and a layer of nonradial fibers between the radial and mucous membrane layers.

Tympanic Cavity

The middle ear cavity (tympanum) may be thought of schematically as a six-sided box. The lateral wall is the eardrum, and opposite to it the promontory of the basal cochlear turn forms the medial wall. Figure 2.7 shows such a conceptualization of the right middle ear, looking in to-

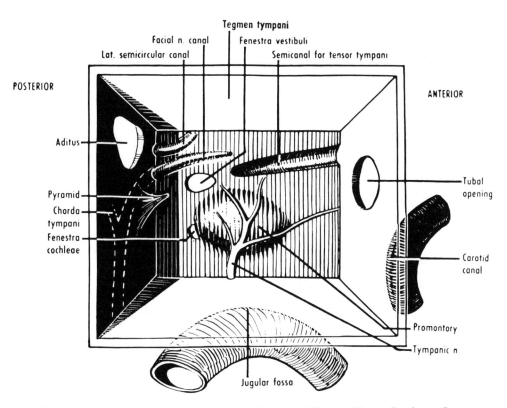

Figure 2.7 Schematic representation of the middle ear. [From Gardner, Gray, and O'Rahilly [5], *Anatomy*, 4th Ed., © 1975 by W. B. Saunders (with permission).]

ward the medial wall as though the eardrum (lateral wall) were removed. The roof is formed by the tegmen tympani, which separates the middle ear from the middle cranial fossa above. The floor of the tympanum separates it from the jugular bulb. In the anterior wall is the opening to the Eustachian tube, and above it the canal for the tensor tympani muscle. The canal of the internal carotid artery lies behind the anterior wall, posteroinferior to the tubal opening. The posterior wall contains the aditus ad antrum through which the upper portion of the middle ear (epitympanic recess) communicates with the mastoid antrum. The posterior wall also contains the fossa incudis, a recess that receives the short process of the incus; and the pyramidal eminence which houses the stapedial muscle. The stapedial tendon exists from the pyramidal prominence at its apex.

Returning to the medial wall, we see that the oval window is located posterosuperiorly to the promontory, while the round window is posteroinferior to the latter. Superior to the oval window lies the facial canal prominence, with the cochleariform process on its anterior aspect. The tendon of the tensor tympani muscle bends around the cochleariform process to proceed laterally to the malleus.

The Eustachian (auditory) tube serves to equalize the air pressure on both sides of the eardrum, and to allow for drainage of the middle ear by serving as a portal to the nasopharynx. It is about 37 mm in length, and courses medially, down, and forward to exit into the nasopharynx via a prominence called the torus tubarius. The lateral third of the tube is bony, while the remainder is elastic cartilage. The two sections of the tube form an angle of about 160° extending down to the nasopharynx. The meeting of the bony and cartilaginous portions is called the isthmus, and at this point the lumen of the tube may be as little as 1.0–1.5 mm in diameter compared to about 3.0–6.0 mm at the normally open port into the middle ear. The cartilaginous part is normally closed, and opens in response to swallowing, yawning, sneezing, or shouting. This reflexive opening of the Eustachian tube is caused by action of the tensor palatini muscle, which uncurls the normally closed hook-shaped cartilages that make up this part of the tube.

Ossicular Chain

Sound energy impinging upon the eardrum is conducted to the inner ear by way of the malleus, incus, and stapes (the ossicular chain), which are the smallest bones in the body. These are shown individually, their details highlighted, in Fig. 2.8. The ossicles are shown in place in Fig. 2.6b, and more schematically in Fig. 2.9. As revealed in Fig. 2.9, they are

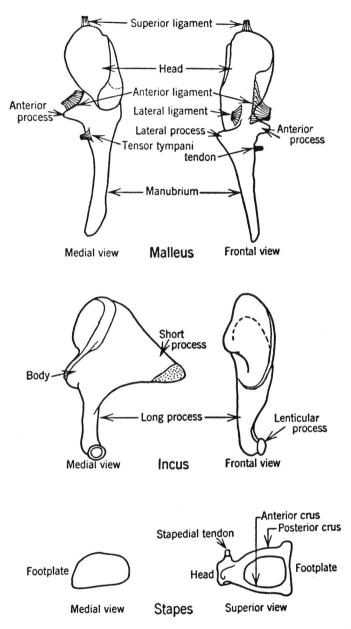

Figure 2.8   Individual ossicles. (From Ernest Glen Wever and Merle Lawrence, *Physiological Acoustics*, © 1982 by Princeton University Press. Reprinted by permission of Princeton University Press.)

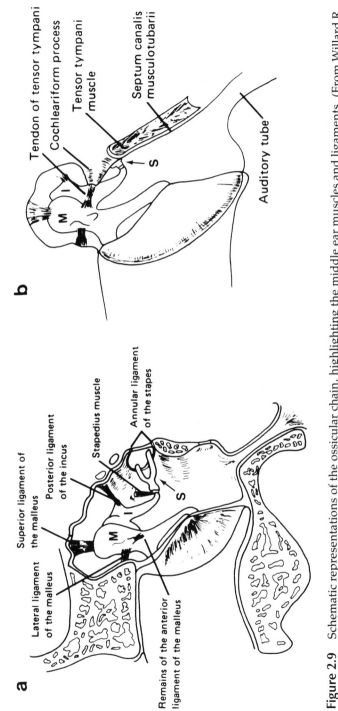

Figure 2.9 Schematic representations of the ossicular chain, highlighting the middle ear muscles and ligaments. (From Willard R. Zemlin [6], *Speech and Hearing Science*, 3rd Ed., © 1988. Reprinted by permission of Prentice-Hall, Inc.)

suspended in the middle ear by a series of ligaments, by the tendons of the two intratympanic muscles, and by the attachments of the malleus to the eardrum and of the stapes to the oval window.

The malleus is commonly called the hammer, although it more closely resembles a mace. It is the largest of the ossicles, being about 8.0–9.0 mm long and weighing approximately 25 mg. The head of the malleus is located in the epitympanic space, to which it is connected by its superior ligament. Laterally, the manubrium (handle) is embedded between the mucous membrane and fibrous layers of the eardrum. The anterior process of the malleus projects anteriorly from the top of the manubrium just below the neck. It attaches to the tympanic notch by its anterior ligament, which forms the axis of mallear movement. The malleus is connected to the tensor tympani muscle via a tendon which inserts at the top of the manubrium.

The incus bears a closer resemblance to a tooth with two roots than to the more commonly associated anvil. It weighs approximately 30 mg, and has a length of about 5.0 mm along its short process and about 7.0 mm along its long process. Its body is connected to the posteromedial aspect of the mallear head within the epitympanic recess. The connection is by a saddle joint, which was originally thought to move by a cog-like mechanism when the malleus was displaced inward [7]. However, subsequent research has demonstrated that these two bones move as a unit rather than relative to one another [3]. The short process of the incus connects via its posterior ligaments to the fossa incudis on the posterior wall of the tympanic cavity. Its long process runs inferiorly, parallel to the manubrium. The end of the long process then bends medially to articulate with the head of the stapes in a true ball-and-socket joint.

The stapes (stirrup) is the smallest of the ossicles. It is about 3.5 mm high, and the footplate is about 3.0 mm long by 1.4 mm wide. It weighs on the order of 3.0–4.0 mg. The head of the stapes connects to the footplate via two crura. The anterior crus is straighter, thinner, and shorter than the posterior crus. The footplate, which encases the very fine stapedial membrane, is attached to the oval window by the annular ligament. The stapedius tendon inserts on the posterior surface of the neck of the stapes, and connects the bone to the stapedius muscle.

Intratympanic Muscles

The middle ear contains two muscles, the tensor tympani and the stapedius (Fig. 2.9). The stapedius muscle is the smallest muscle in the body, with an average length of 6.3 mm and a mean cross-sectional area of 4.9 mm^2 [3]. The muscle is completely encased within the pyramidal eminence on the posterior wall of the tympanic cavity, and takes origin from the walls of its own canal. Its tendon exits through the apex of the pyramid and courses horizontally to insert on the posterior aspect of the neck of the stapes. Contraction of the stapedius muscle thus pulls the stapes posteriorly. The stapedius is innervated by the stapedial branch of the seventh cranial (facial) nerve.

The tensor tympani muscle has an average length of 25 mm and a mean cross-sectional area of approximately 5.85 mm^2 [3]. The tensor tympani occupies an osseous semicanal on the anterior wall of the tympanum, just superior to the Eustachian tube, from which it is separated by a thin bony shelf. The muscle takes origin from the cartilage of the auditory tube, from the walls of its own canal, and from the part of the sphenoid bone adjacent to the canal. Emerging from the canal, the tendon of the tensor tympani hooks around the cochleariform process, and inserts on the top of the manubrium of the malleus. Contraction of the tensor tympani thus pulls the malleus anteromedially—at a right angle to the uninterrupted motion of the ossicles. The tensor tympani muscle is innervated by the tensor tympani branch of the otic ganglion of the fifth cranial (trigeminal) nerve.

Both intratympanic muscles are completely encased within bony canals, and attach to the ossicular chain by way of their respective tendons. Bekesy [8] pointed out that this situation reduces the effects that muscular contractions might have upon the transmission of sound through the middle ear system. Contraction of either muscle increases the stiffness of the ossicular chain as well as of the eardrum. The stapedius muscle pulls posteriorly whereas the tensor tympani pulls anteromedially, so that they might initially be thought to be antagonists. However, the effect of these muscles is to lessen the amount of energy conducted by the ossicular chain, and they thus function as synergists with respect to hearing.

Of particular interest is the acoustic reflex—the response of the intratympanic muscles to intense sounds. It is generally accepted that the acoustic reflex *in man* is due mainly, if not exclusively, to contraction of the stapedius; the tensor responds only to extremely intense sounds, as part of a startle response.

The acoustic reflex arc has been described in detail [9,10]. The afferent (sensory) branch of the arc is the auditory nerve, terminating in the ventral cochlear nucleus, which communicates with the superior olivary complex on both sides (via the trapezoid body). These bilateral connections permit a reflex response in both ears even when only one ear is stimulated. The efferent (motor) pathway of the arc proceeds from the medial accessory nucleus of the superior olivary complex on each side to the nuclei of the facial nerve for the stapedius reflex, and to the nuclei of the trigeminal nerve to cause tensor tympani contraction.

INNER EAR

Osseous Labyrinth

The inner ear structures are contained within a system of spaces and canals, the osseous labyrinth (Fig. 2.10), in the petrous portion of the temporal bone. These spaces and canals are grossly divided into three sections: the vestibule, the cochlea, and the semicircular canals. The oval window accepts the stapedial footplate and opens medially into the vestibule, which is about 4.0 mm in diameter and somewhat ovoid in shape. The snail-shaped cochlea lies anterior and slightly inferior to the vestibule, and is approximately 5.0 mm high and 9.0 mm in diameter at its base. Posterior to the vestibule are the three semicircular canals, lying at right angles to one another, each about 1.0 mm in diameter.

Membranous Labyrinth and Inner Ear Fluids

The general shape of the bony labyrinth is followed by the enclosed membranous labyrinth (Fig. 2.11), which contains the end organs of

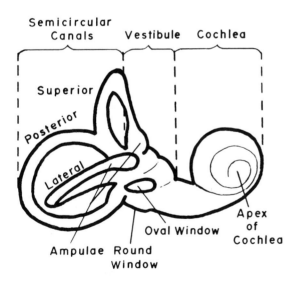

Figure 2.10   The osseous labyrinth.

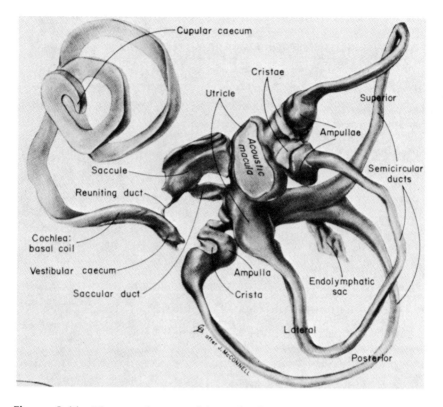

Figure 2.11 The membranous labyrinth. [From Donaldson and Miller [4], "Anatomy of the ear," in *Otolaryngology*, Vol. 1 (Paparella and Schumrick, eds.), © 1973, W. B. Saunders (with permission).]

hearing and balance. The space between the bony walls of the osseous labyrinth and the membranous labyrinth is filled with perilymphatic fluid (perilymph). The membranous labyrinth itself is mostly filled with endolymphatic fluid (endolymph), but the cochlear hair cells are actually bathed in a third fluid, cortilymph, which will be discussed below.

Lawrence [11] enumerated four functions of the inner ear fluids. First, they deliver nutrients to the inner-ear cells which are not in direct contact with the blood (and also remove waste). Second, they provide the chemical environment needed for the transfer of energy from a vibratory stimulus to a neural signal. Third, the fluids are the medium which carries the vibratory stimulus from the footplate to the sensory structures along the cochlear partition. Finally, the distribution of pressure in the inner ear system is controlled by the cochlear fluids, although this last function is still debated. The inner ear fluids are themselves quite interesting, although their study is difficult because they are found in such small amounts. For example, Lawrence reported that the total volumes of these fluids in man are only 78.3 mm^3 of perilymph and the miniscule amount of 2.76 mm^3 of endolymph.

Perilymph is chemically similar to other extracellular fluids. Smith et al. [12] found that guinea pig perilymph has a very high concentration of sodium and a very low concentration of potassium, as does cerebrospinal fluid and blood serum. Interestingly, they found that endolymph has just the opposite concentrations: It is high in potassium but low in sodium. It has the distinction of being the only extracellular fluid in the body which is high in potassium, with the possible exception of some parotid gland secretions [13]. The relative sodium and potassium concentrations in guinea pigs also appear to hold true for man [13,14].

Perilymph appears to be a filtrate formed under capillary pressure from the vessels of the spiral ligament above the insertion of Reissner's membrane in the scala vestibuli [11]. It is probably resorbed by the spiral ligament within the scala tympani near the basilar membrane [15]. Although the stria vascularis plays an important part in the production of endolymph, the precise origin of this fluid is not fully understood. The endolymph seems to flow slowly toward the endolymphatic duct and sac (see below), since occlusion of this duct results in a buildup of endolymph in lab animals [16]. In addition, an exchange of sodium and potassium ions radially between the endolymph and the stria vascularis, and across Reissner's membrane, maintains the appropriate ion balance in the endolymph. This exchange, along with the resting potentials associated with these ions, probably makes possible the energy conversion process in the organ of Corti.

Since endolymph contains a high concentration of potassium similar to that of intracellular fluids, it is a poor environment for the function of the hair cells and the unmyelinated fibers of the auditory nerve within the organ of Corti. The tunnel of Corti and other spaces of the organ are filled with a third fluid, cortilymph, which is high in sodium, and which is effectively isolated from the endolymph by the reticular lamina [17,18]. The blood vessels beneath the basilar membrane appear to be the source of cortilymph. Although both corilymph and perilymph are high in sodium, it is unlikely that they are the same: Perilymph is toxic to the hair cells, and the two fluids have different sources.

Returning to the structures of the inner ear, the vestibule contains two balance organs which are concerned with linear acceleration and gravity effects. These organs are the utricle and saccule. The semicircular canals, located behind the vestibule, widen anteriorly into five saclike structures, which open into the somewhat elongated utricle. These widenings are the ampullae, and they contain the sensory receptors for rotational acceleration. (The interested reader is referred to any of the fine books in the References section for a detailed discussion of the balance system.) The most important connection between the areas of hearing and balance is the ductus reuniens, which joins the membranous labyrinth between the cochlea and the utricle.

The cochlear aqueduct leads from the vicinity of the round window in the scala tympani to the subarachnoid space medial to the dura of the cranium. Although the aqueduct leads from the perilymph-filled scala to the cerebrospinal-fluid-filled subarachnoid space, it is barely if at all patent in man. Thus, it is doubtful that there is any real interchange between these two fluid systems. The endolymphatic duct leads from the membranous labyrinth within the vestibule to the endolymphatic sac. The sac is located partially between the layers of the dura in the posterior cranial fossa and partly in a niche in the posterior aspect of the petrous portion of the temporal bone. Both the cochlear aqueduct and the endolymphatic duct and sac have been implicated in the regulation of hydraulic pressure in the inner ear.

Cochlea

The human cochlea is about 35 mm long, and forms a somewhat coneshaped spiral with 2¾ turns. It is widest at the base, where the diameter is approximately 9.0 mm, and tapers toward the apex. It is about 5.0 mm high. The modiolus is the core which forms the axis of the spiral (Fig. 2.12). Through it course the auditory nerve and the blood vessels that supply the cochlea.

It is easier to visualize the cochlea by imagining the spiral uncoiled, as in Fig. 2.13. In this figure, the base of the cochlea is shown at the left and the apex at the right. We see three chambers: the scala media, scala vestibuli, and scala tympani. The scala media is self-contained and separates the other two. The scalae vestibuli and tympani, on the other hand, communicate with one another at the apex of the cochlea, through an opening called the helicotrema. The scala media is enclosed within the membranous labyrinth and contains endolymph, while the other two contain perilymph. The scala vestibuli is in contact with the stapes at the oval window, while the scala tympani has a membrane-covered contact

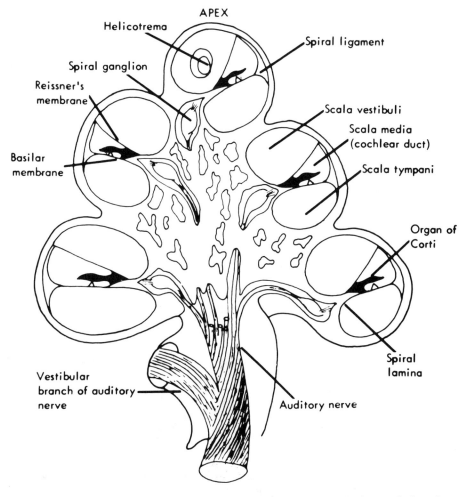

Figure 2.12 Schematic cross-section of the cochlea through the modiolus also showing the auditory nerve. (From Willard R. Zemlin [6], *Speech and Hearing Science*, 3rd Ed. © 1988. Reprinted by permission of Prentice-Hall, Inc.)

with the middle ear at the round window. The scala media is separated from the scala vestibuli above by Reissner's membrane, and from the scala tympani below by the basilar membrane. Bekesy [1] reported that the basilar membrane is approximately 32 mm long, and that it tapers from about 0.5 mm wide at the apex to about 0.1 mm wide near the stapes at its base. Furthermore, it is thicker at the base than at the apex.

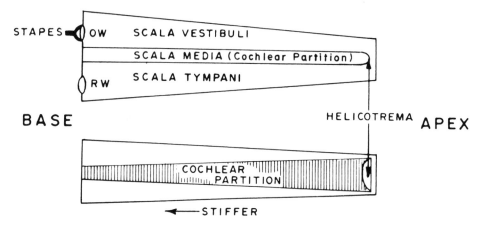

Figure 2.13 Schematic representation of the uncoiled cochlea (OW, oval window; RW, round window).

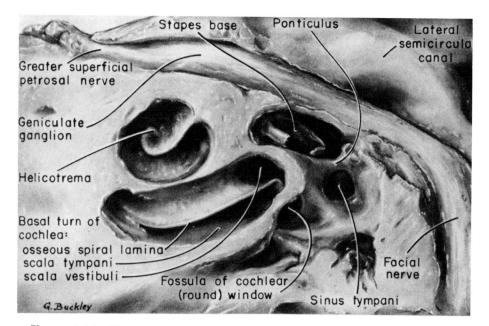

Figure 2.14 The osseous spiral lamina, scala vestibuli, scala tympani, and helicotrema. [From Anson and Donaldson [2], *The Surgical Anatomy of the Temporal Bone and Ear*, © 1967, by W. B. Saunders (with permission).]

The scala media is connected to the bony shelf on the inner wall of the cochlear spiral—the osseous spiral lamina. The osseous spiral lamina is clearly visible in Fig. 2.14, separating the scala vestibuli above from the scala tympani below. This figure also shows the orientation of the helicotrema at the apical turn, and the relationship between the round window and the scala tympani at the base of the cochlea. The scala media is attached to the outer wall of the cochlea by the spiral ligament, a fibrous connective tissue.

The structures of the scala media are shown schematically in Fig. 2.15. Looking first at the osseous spiral lamina on the inner wall, we see that this bony shelf is actually composed of two plates, separated by a space through which pass fibers of the auditory nerve. These fibers enter via openings called the habenula perforata. Resting on the osseous spiral lamina is a thickened band of periosteum, the limbus. Reissner's mem-

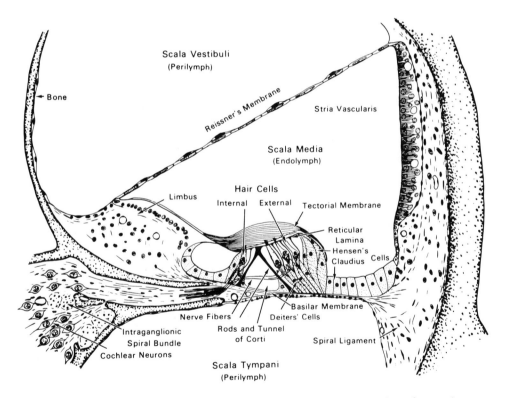

Figure 2.15 Cross section of the organ of Corti. (From Davis [24], with permission.)

brane extends from the top of the inner aspect of the limbus to the outer wall of the canal. The side of the limbus facing the organ of Corti is concave outward. The tectorial membrane is attached to the limbus at the upper lip of this concave part, forming a space called the internal spiral sulcus. The basilar membrane extends from the lower lip of the limbus to the spiral ligament at the outer wall of the duct. The spiral ligament itself has been described in considerable detail [19–21]; and is involved in the metabolic activities of the inner ear in addition to its role as a crucial supporting structure.

The basilar membrane has two sections. The inner section extends from the osseous spiral lamina to the outer pillars, and is relatively thin. The remainder is thicker and extends to the spiral ligament. These two sections are called the zona arcuata and the zona pectinata, respectively. Sitting on the basilar membrane is the end organ of hearing—the organ of Corti. The width, thickness, and orientation of the basilar membrane and the organ of Corti on it vary along the coure of the cochlear duct [22]. Fig. 2.16 shows how these dimentions vary at the basal, middle, and apical regions of the chinchilla cochlea.

The organ of Corti runs longitudinally along the basilar membrane. Grossly, it is made up of a single row of inner hair cells (IHCs), three rows of outer hair cells (OHCs) (though as many as four or five rows have been reported in the apical turn), various supporting cells, and the pillar cells forming the tunnel of Corti. The tunnel pillars contributes considerably to the rigidity of the zona arcuada of the basilar membrane [23]. This tunnel separates the IHCs and OHCs. Each of the approximately 3500 IHCs is supported by a phalangeal cell which holds the rounded base of the IHC as in a cup. There are about 12,000 OHCs, shaped like test tubes, which are supported by Deiters' cells. Between the inner and outer hair cells (HCs) are the tilted and rather conspicuous pillars (rods) or Corti, which come together at their tops to enclose the triangular tunnel of Corti. Fibers of the eighth cranial (auditory) nerve traverse the tunnel to contact the OHCs. Just lateral to Deiters' cells are several rows of tall, supporting cells called Hensen's cells. Lateral to these are the columnar cells of Claudius, which continue laterally to the spiral ligament and the stria vascularis.

The reticular lamina is made up of the tops of the hair cells (cuticular plates, see below) along with the upward-extending processes of the phalangeal and Deiters' cells. The distinctive surface pattern of the reticular lamina is shown in Fig. 2.17. The pillar cells maintain a strong structural attachment between the reticular lamina above and the basilar membrane below, and thus the reticular lamina provides a source of support for the hair cells at their upper surfaces. This relationship is

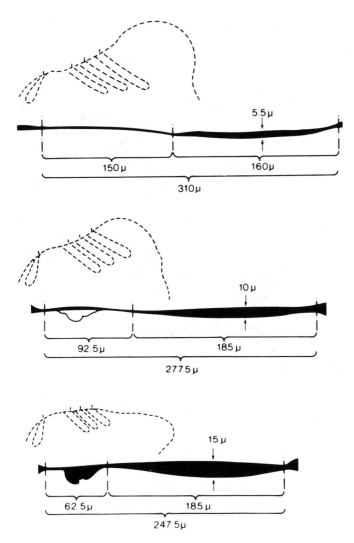

Figure 2.16 The dimentions and relationships of the basilar membrane and organ of Corti in the apical (top drawing), middle (center drawing) and basal (bottom) turns of the chinchilla cochlea. (From Lim [22], with permission of *J. Acoust. Soc. Am.*)

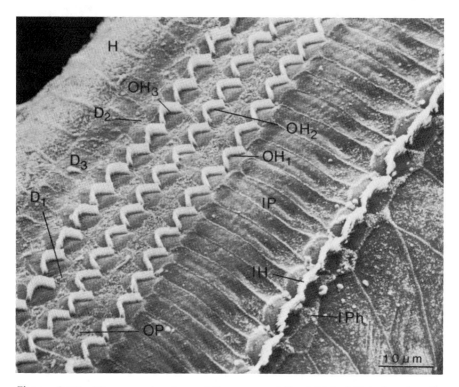

Figure 2.17 The upper surface of the organ of Corti (chinchilla) showing the stereocilia of the inner and outer HCs protruding through the reticular lamina. The outside aspect (toward the spiral ligament) is at the left and the medial side (toward the modiolus) is at the right. Landmarks indicated are the Hensen's cells (H), three rows of Deiters' cells (D 1–3) and outer hair cells (OHC 1–3), outer (OP) and inner (IP) pillar cells, inner hair cells (IH), and inner phalangeal cells (IPh). (From Lim [26], with permission of *Hearing Research.*)

exemplified in Fig. 2.18, showing the OHCs and Deiters' cells in the reticular lamina, as well as the stereocilia of the HCs protruding through the lamina. The reticular lamina effectively isolates the structures and spaces of the organ of Corti from the endolymph-filled portions of the scala media [25].

The tectorial membrane extends from the upper lip of the limbus medially, courses over the hair cells, and connects laterally to the Hensen's (and perhaps to the most lateral Deiters') cells by a border (or

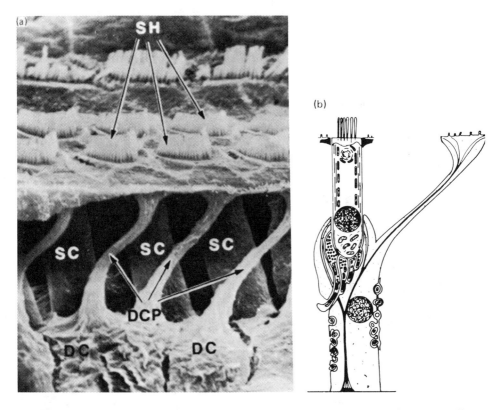

Figure 2.18 Scanning electron micrograph (a) and diagram (b) of Deiters' cells and the reticular lamina. (From Bourne and Danielli [67], by permission of Academic Press.)

marginal. Its relationship to the rest of the organ of Corti is depicted in Fig. 2.19. Its connection to the limbus is a strong and robust one; however, the attachment of the tectorial membrane to the cells of Hensen is quite fragile. The undersurface of the main body of the tectorial membrane (fibrous layer) is marked by Hensen's stripe located above the inner hair cells.

The tectorial membrane is frequently described as being ribbon-like in appearance, although the drawing in Fig. 2.19 makes it clear that such descriptions are grossly oversimplified. Its consistency is amorphous and often referred to as gelatinous, being largely made up of fibers.

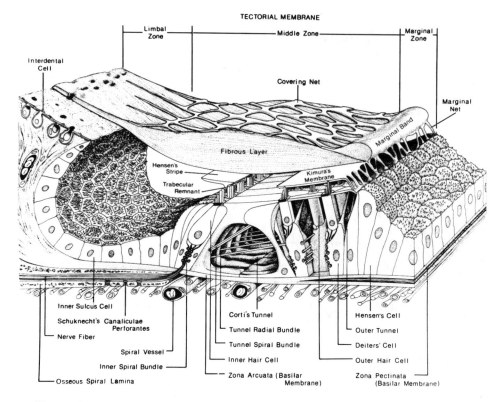

Figure 2.19   The tectorial membrane in relation to the other structures of the organ of Corti. (From Lim [22], with permission of *J. Acoust. Soc. Am.*)

Recent findings have shown that these fibers are composed of collagen II [27]. Collagen II accounts for the considerable tensile strength of the membrane, shown by Zwislocki et al. [29]. Data by Bekesy [1] and more recent physical findings by Frommer [28] and Zwislocki, et al. [29] have revealed that the tectorial membrane is rather compliant. Thus, it is unlikely that it moves around the fulcrum formed at the limbus as a stiff unit. Zwislocki, et al. have clearly portrayed its most likely natural movement to resemble that of a rubber band as opposed to the motion of a stiff book cover. Such a mode of motion is not in complete agreement with the generally encountered concept that the hair cells are sheared between the stiff beams formed by the reticular lamina and tectorial membrane during their upward deflection (see Chap. 4). Comprehensive discussions of the tectorial membrane in all its many aspects may be found in reviews by Steel [30,31] and Lim [26].

Hair Cells

As already mentioned, it is generally accepted that there are roughly 12,000 outer hairs cells and 3500 inner hair cells distributed along a cochlear length approximating 35 mm in man. Recent work [32,33] has verified these generalizations, and has also established the density of HCs, or number of these per millimeter of cochlear length. For example, Ulehlova et al. [32] reported that average human HC densities are about 86 IHCs/mm and 343 OHCs/mm. However, these studies have also established that there is considerable intersubject variability in cell counts, cochlear length, and, consequently, in the density of HCs from cochlea to cochlea.

The inner and outer hair cells were shown in relation to the cross-section of the organ of Corti in Fig. 2.15. A closer look at these cells is provided in Figs. 2.20 and 2.21. The structures and organization of the inner and outher HCs have been described in great detail [22,26]. Their structures and orientation in the organ of Corti reflect their long-established function as the receptors which transduce the mechanical signal carried to them into electrochemical activity to be transmitted to the nervous system. Yet, the contrasting structures and associations of the inner and outer HCs reflect considerable functional differences between them. These differences have become apparent only relatively recently, and they impact upon numerous aspects of cochlear processes. In fact, the accumulating knowledge of inner and outer HC roles and interactions is bringing together a great deal of data about the cochlea, which were previously elusive and apparently paradoxical, into a cohesive understanding of cochlear functioning (see Chap. 5).

Although the flask-shaped IHCs and tube-shaped OHCs have many cytoarchitectural aspects in common, there are certain differences that have great implications for functional distinctions between the two types of cells. The IHCs contain an extensive system of tubulovessicular endoplasmic reticulum, Golgi apparatus and mitochondria. The concentrations of mitochondria and Golgi apparatus suggest a high level of metabolic activity which may be related to the transduction of mechanical to electrochemical energy. Its endoplasmic reticulum system has only one subsurface cistern layer, and is far less developed than what we shall observe in the OHCs.

The OHCs contain a highly organized endoplasmic reticulum system that includes extensive subsurface, apical and subsynaptic cisterns, and the Hensen's body. That this system is reminiscent of the sarcoplasmic reticulum of muscle has been noted for some time [35]. Moreover, the subsurface cisterns are connected to the cell membrane of the

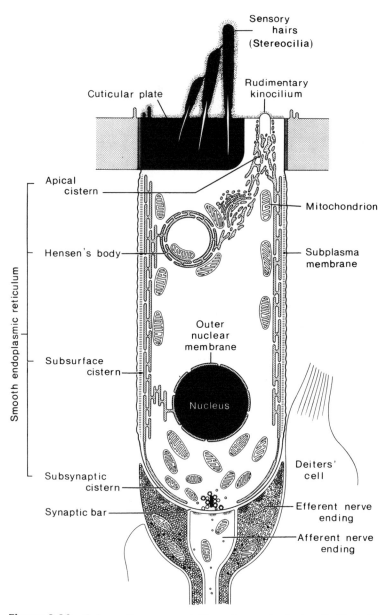

Figure 2.20 Schematic representation of an outer hair cell. Note the extensive cistern system, and that the cell makes direct contact with efferent as well as afferent nerve endings. Note also the cross-links between the stereocilia. (Used with permission from Lim, D. J.: Effects of noise and ototoxic drugs at the cellular level in the cochlea: A review, *Am. J. Otolaryngol. 7*, 73–99. 1986.)

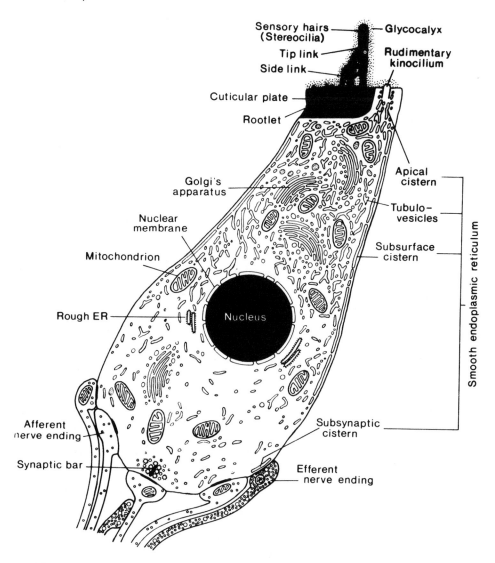

Figure 2.21 Schematic representation of an inner hair cell. See text. (Used with permission from Lim, D. J.: Effects of noise and ototoxic drugs at the cellular level in the cochlea: A review. *Am. J. Otolaryngol. 7,* 73–99, 1986.)

OHC by pillars, representing a further similarity to muscle [36]. In addition to the structural similarities to muscle, it is well established that OHCs contain contractile proteins in their cell bodies and cell membranes (actin, myosin, tubulin), stereocilia (actin, fibrin), and cuticular plates (actin, α-actin, fibrin, myosin, and tropomyosin) [36–41].

The upper surface of each HC contains a thickening called the cuticular plate which is topped by stereocilia, and a noncuticular area that contains the basal body of a rudimentary kinocilium. Fig. 2.22 shows

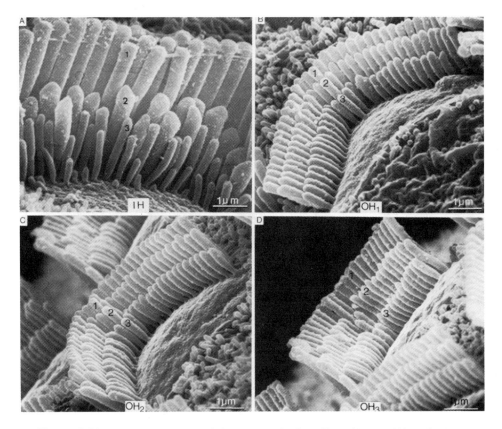

Figure 2.22   Close up views of the stereocilia bundles of inner (A) and outer (B–D) hair cells demonstrating the decreasing cilia heights from row to row (numbered 1 to 3). (From Lim [26], with permission of *Hearing Research*.)

close-up views of the stereocilia bundles from all three rows of OHCs and also for IHCs. The figure highlights the tapering of stereocilia heights from row to row on each HC. It is firmly established that at least the tallest stereocilia of the OHCs are firmly attached to the undersurface of the tectorial membrane; however, it appears that the IHC stereocilia are not attached to Hensen's stripe, or are that this attachment is tenuous if it does exist. Discussions of this controversy may be found in several recent reviews [26,30,31].

There are as many as about 150 stereocilia on each OHC. These are arranged in a "W"-shaped pattern on each OHC, with the base of the W facing away from the modiolus. The legs of the "W" form an obtuse angle (about 120 degrees) on OHCs in the basal turn and an acute angle (roughly 60°) on cells in the apical turn. These stereocilia increase from about 58 at the cochlear apex to 150 at the base [42]. The stereocilia taper toward the base, as shown in Fig. 2.20. It has been established that when the stereocilia are displaced, they remain stiff, bending at the tapered base in response to physical stimulation [43–46].

Each IHC has roughly 50–70 stereocilia. These are thicker (greater in diameter) than those on the OHCs [22]. The IHC stereocilia bundle is most often described as being essentially straight, although Lim [26] has pointed out that it approximates a very wide W shape. Their number do not appear to change appreciably along the length of the cochlea [26].

The structures and interrelationships of the cuticular plate and stereocilia have been described by several researchers [47–52]. The stereocilia are composed of bundles of actin filaments which are extensively cross-linked, and the cuticular plate into which the stereocilia rootlets are planted is similarly made up of a mosaic of cross-linked actin filaments. The filaments of the stereocilia rootlets extend into the cuticular plate, where fine cross-bridges also interconnect the rootlet and cuticular plate filaments. Figure 2.23 shows this relationship schematically. These structures underlie the stiffness of the stereocilia. Comprehensive reviews dealing with these structures have been written by Hirokawa [51] and Tilney and Tilney [52].

The height (length) of the stereocilia has been found to vary systematically along the length of the cochleas of a wide variety of species [22,53–55], including humans [56]. Specifically, the length of the stereocilia has been found to increase going from the base (high-frequency end) to the apex (low-frenquency end) of the cochlea. In man, Wright [56] found that the longest IHC stereocilia increased linearly from about 4–5 μm near to the base to approximately 7–8 μm near the apex. He

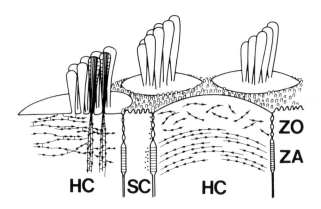

Figure 2.23   The stereocilia and cuticular plate are made up of a complex arrangement of cross-bridged actin filaments. Note in particular the extension of the stereocilia rootlet filaments into the cuticular plate in the left-most hair cell. Also note the tapering toward the base of each stereocilium. (HC, hair cell; SC, supporting cell; ZO, tight junction; ZA, intermediate junction). (Used with permission from Hirokawa and Tilney [50].)

found that OHC stereocilia length also increased with distance up the cochlear, although there was more variability and the relationship was not linear.*

A particularly interesting aspect of the HC stereocilia may be seen in Fig. 2.20. Looking back to this figure, one may notice that the stereocilia are joined by tiny lines. These lines represent filaments that serve as cross-links among the stereocilia. These cross-links occur in both inner and outer HCs in laboratory animals [43–45,62,63], and also occur in humans [64]. (Recently, cross-links have also been found between the

---

*The importance of the gradation of stereocilia height can be appreciated when one considers reptiles like the alligator lizard whose cochleas do not have tectorial membranes. The alligator lizard's cochlear anatomy and stereocilia have been described in detail [57–59]. However, the principal point here is that these animals' hair cells are tuned to different frequencies on the basis of stereocilia length [53,60,61]. That is, longer cilia are mechanically tuned to lower frequencies and shorter ones to higher frequencies. The interested reader should consult these papers for a full discussion of the topic, which clearly goes beyond the current scope. However, one may note that a possible interaction of the stereocilia the tectorial membrane has been used to explain the inconsistencies between the tuning of the alligator lizard's free-standing stereocilia and those of animals with a tectorial membrane [59,60].

stereocilia of adjacent inner hair cells [65].) Three configurations of cross-links occur between the stereocilia of both inner and outer HCs (Figs. 2.24–2.27): Side-to-side cross-links join stereocilia, which are juxtaposed within the same row. Row-to-row cross-links go from stereocilia in one row to adjacent ones in the next row. Finally, tip-to-side, or upward-pointing, cross-links go from the tip of stereocilia in a shorter row to the side of the stereocilia in the adjacent taller row.

The stria vascularis contains a rich network of capillaries, and is attached to the spiral ligament on the lateral wall of the scala media. The stria vascularis has three layers, composed of characteristic cell types. Its hexagonal, marginal epithelial cells are rich in mitochondria and have several microvilli on the endolymphatic surface. The more irregular intermediate cells have a smaller number of mitochondria, and have projections into the marginal layer. The long, flat basal cells form the deepest layer, in contact with the spiral ligament, and are adjacent to and often

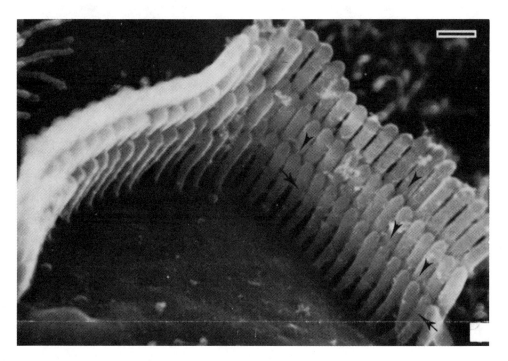

Figure 2.24 Side-to-side (arrows) and tip-to-side (upward-pointing) cross-links on OHCs. (From Furness and Hackney [66], with permission of *Hearing Research*.)

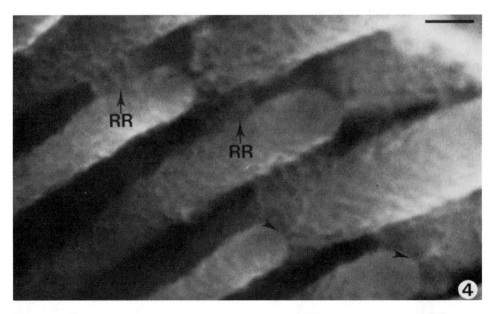

Figure 2.25   Row-to-row cross-links (RR) on OHCs. (From Furness and Hackney [66], with permission of *Hearing Research*.)

surround the capillaries. Considerable metabolic activity is suggested by the generous supply of mitochondria in these cells; and the structure of the stria vascularis is consistent with a secretory or absorptive function. However, it is doubtful that the stria vascularis is actually the blood supply of the organ of Corti, as will be discussed below. It appears that its function is that of an ion transport and control structure, producing the ion concentrations in the endolymph that enable energy transformation to occur; it also possibly controls certain inorganic substances and water for the same purpose [11].

Blood Supply to the Cochlea

The arterial supply to the cochlea, the cochlear artery, is derived from the internal auditory artery, which is a branch of the basilar artery. Venous drainage of the cochlea is into the internal auditory vein. The vascular supply of the cochlea is shown schematically in Fig. 2.28 [11]. The system involves one branch supplying (1) the spiral ligament above the point of attachment of Reissner's membrane, (2) the capillary network within the stria vascularis, (3) the spiral prominence, and (4) the terminal

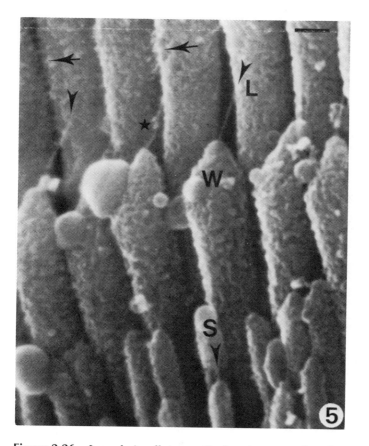

Figure 2.26 Inner hair cell stereocilia showing examples of side-to-side (arrows) and tip-to-side (arrowheads) cross links, which may be relatively long (L) or short (S). (From Furness and Hackney [66], with permission of *Hearing Research*.)

branches that descend to collecting venules; and also a second branch feeding (5) the limbus and (6) a plexus under the basilar membrane.

The cochlear blood supply is intriguing since there is no direct contact between its structures and the vascular system. This is complicated by the fact that in addition to the vascularized stria vascularis and spiral eminence, whose proximity to the endolymph makes them intuitively good candidates for supplying the organ of Corti, there is also a capillary bed under the basilar membrane. To determine the source of nutritive support to the HCs, Lawrence [25] interrupted the blood supply of the

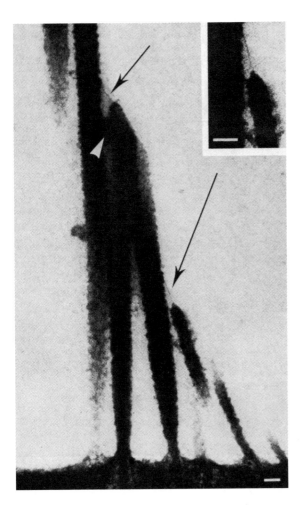

Figure 2.27 Tip-to-side cross-links (arrows) on an OHC, similar to what is shown schematically in Fig. 2.20 The white arrowhead shows a row-to-row link. Insert: close-up of an upward-pointing cross-links. (From Pickles, Comis and Osborne [62], with permission of *Hearing Research.*)

vessels entering the spiral ligament in one group of guinea pigs, and the supply to the basilar membrane vessels in a second group. Interruption of the basilar blood supply caused HC degeneration without affecting the stria vascularis or spiral eminence. Interrupting the blood supply of the latter structures resulted in their own destruction but had no such effect upon the organ of Corti. It thus appears that the blood supply of the organ of Corti is the basilar membrane vessels, most likely acting via

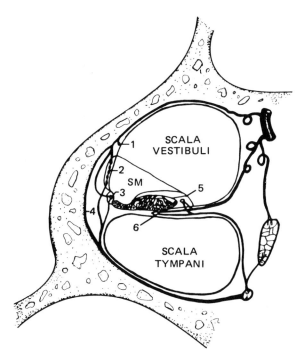

Figure 2.28   Cochlear blood supply (SM, scala media). [From Lawrence [11], Inner ear physiology, in *Otolaryngology*, Vol. 1 (Paparella and Schumrick. eds.), © 1973 by W. B. Saunders (with permission).]

the cortilymph. On the other hand, the stria vascularis and spiral eminence probably maintain the ionic character of the endolymph.

INNERVATION

The sensory hair cells of the cochlea interact with the nervous system by way of the auditory (cochlear) branch of the eighth cranial or stato-acoustic nerve. The auditory nerve was probably first described in the 1500s by Falloppia. However, its structure and connections have only become well defined during the twentieth century, and the details of its anatomy and physiology are still the subject of active research.

There are roughly 30,000 neurons in the human auditory nerve and approximately 50,000 or more cochlear neurons in the cat [68,69]. These neurons are primarily afferents which carry sensory information up from the hair cells, but also include efferents which descend from the brainstem to the cochlea. The efferent fibers of the auditory nerve represent the terminal portion of the olivocochlear bundle, described later in this chapter. The cell bodies of the afferent auditory neurons constitute the spiral ganglia, residing in Rosenthal's canal in the modiolus. These neurons may be myelinated or unmyelinated before exiting through the habenula perforata, but all auditory nerve fibers are unmyelinated once they enter the organ of Corti. A general perspective of the connections of the auditory nerve through the cochlear spirals was shown in Fig. 2.12 above. Figure 2.29 provides a closer perspective of how the auditory nerve and spiral ganglia relate to a cross-section of the cochlear duct.

Most sensory neurons are bipolar, so called because the cell body is located part way along the axon (Fig. 2.30) Auditory neurons are of this general type. More specifically, the cells of the spiral ganglia are composed of at least two distinctive types (Fig. 2.31). Studying the cat,

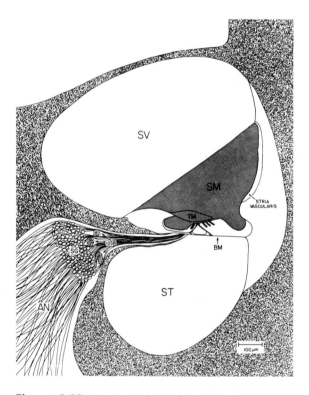

Figure 2.29   Relationship of the auditory nerve to a cross-section of the cochlear duct (cat). (AN, auditory nerve; SG, spiral ganglion; IGSB, intraganglionic spiral bundle primarily composed of efferents; TM, tectorial membrane; BM, basilar membrane; SV, SM, ST, scalae vestibuli, media and tympani, respectively. (From Kiang et al [70], with permission of *Hearing Research*.)

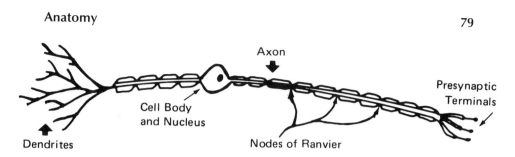

Figure 2.30 A typical bipolar sensory neuron.

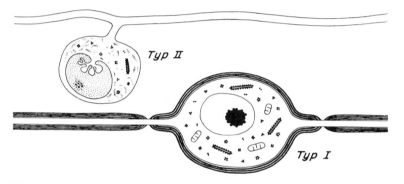

Figure 2.31 Examples of Type I (lower) and Type II (upper) auditory neurons. [From Spoendlin [73], The afferent innervation of the cochlea, in *Evoked Electrical Activity in the Auditory Nervous System* (R. F. Naunton and C. Fernandez, eds.), © 1978 by Academic Press.]

Spoendlin [71,72] demonstrated that approximately 95% of these cells are relatively large, myelinated, bipolar neurons. Spoendlin classified these cells as Type I neurons. In contrast, he found that roughly 5% of these spiral ganglion cells were relatively small, unmyelinated, and tended to be pseudo-monopolar in structure. These were coded Type II neurons.

Upon existing the habenula perforata into the organ of Corti, the now unmyelinated fibers follow different routes to distribute themselves asymmetrically between the inner and outer hair cells [72,73], as shown schematically in Fig. 3.32.* About 95% of these fibers are *radial fibers*, which course directly out to innervate the IHCs. The remaining 5%

---

*Although most of the work described here on cochlear innervation patterns has been done on cats, the same distributions of nerve fibers and hair cells has also been reported for guinea pigs [75] and for humans [76].

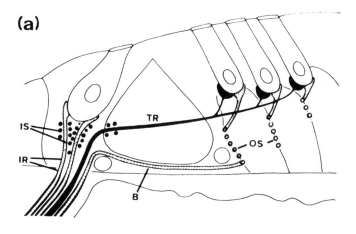

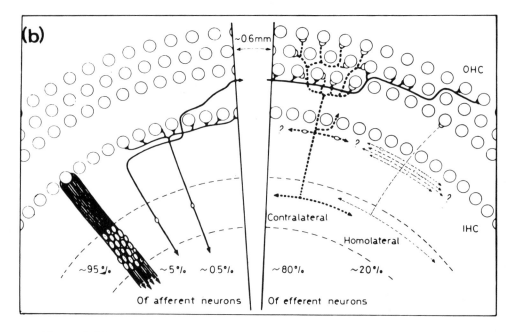

Figure 2.32 (a) Afferent and efferent innervation of the organ of Corti. Afferents gray and efferents black; IS, inner fibers; IR, inner radial fibers; TR, tunnel radial fibers; B, basilar fibers; OS, outer spiral fibers. (b) Arrangement of nerve fibers to the inner and outer hair cells. (From Spoendlin [86], with permission.)

consist of 2,500 to 3,000 fibers that cross the tunnel of Corti as basal fibers, and then turn to follow a route of about 0.6 mm toward the base as the *outer spiral bundle*. These outer spiral fibers then make their way up between the Deiters' cells to synapse with the OHCs.

The outer spiral bundle gives off collaterals so that each neural fiber innervates roughly 10 OHCs, and each OHC receives collaterals from several neurons [87]. Each IHC receives roughly 20 radial fibers in an exclusive relationship. Liberman [77] demonstrated that a given IHC makes contact with three types of radial fibers, differing in terms of their average diameters, cellular characteristics, and spontaneous firing rates (see Chap. 5). Moreover, these three types of radial fibers attach to the IHC at characteristic locations, as shown in Fig. 2.33. The thickest fibers (having the highest spontaneous rates) always attach on the surface of the IHC which is toward the OHCs. The thinnest and medium thickness fibers (having low and medium spontaneous rates, respectively) attach to the IHC on the surface facing toward the modiolus.

Spoendlin [72,73] suggested that the radial and outer spiral fibers within the organ of Corti were, respectively, the continuations of the Types I and II spiral ganglion cells. However, it was not possible to establish this relationship as a matter of fact at that time. In 1982, Liberman [77] described how the course of single auditory neurons can be traced after marking them with horseradish peroxidase (HRP). He found that all 56 of the Type I auditory neurons he labeled with intracellular injections of HRP could be traced to radial fibers going to IHCs. Kiang et al. [79] injected HRP into the auditory nerve within the internal auditory canal. They were then able to trace the courses of fifty radial and eleven outer spiral fibers. Their HRP labeling studies confirmed Spoendlin's conjectures that the large calibre (over 2 μm), bipolar Type I cells continue as radial fibers in the organ of Corti; and that the small calibre (under 1 μm), pseudomonopolar Type II cells correspond to the outer spiral fibers. Figure 2.34a shows a conceptualized example of the courses followed by the two types of cells; and Figs. 2.34b and 2.34c show the differences between the two types of cells seen in the spiral ganglia.

The central connections of the Type I neurons are firmly established [e.g., 80–82]. Even though some studies failed to find effective connections of the Type II at the cochlear nucleus [81–83]; others have clearly demonstrated that these cells do in fact project to the cochlear nucleus level [e.g., 84,85]. Hence, it appears that both types of spiral ganglion cells project into the cochlear nuclei. In any case, the differences between the physical characteristics of Type I and II neurons, as well as the fact that they innervate distinct classes of hair cells in a manner that is

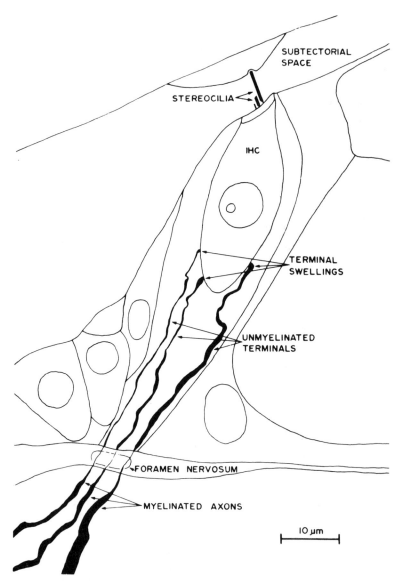

Figure 2.33   The thickest radial fibers attach to the IHC surface facing the OHCs, whereas the thinnest and medium thickness fibers attach on the surface toward the modiolus. (From Liberman and Simmons [78], with permission of *J. Acoust. Soc. Am.*)

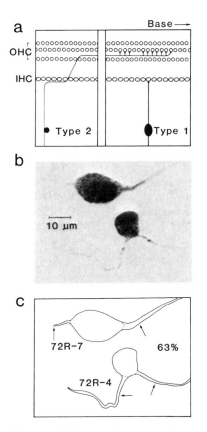

Figure 2.34 (a) Conceptualized examples of the innervation patterns of a Type I/radial cell to an IHC and a Type II/outer spiral cell to an OHC. (b) Photomicrographs of typical Type I (upper) and Type II (lower) neurons. (c) Line drawings of the two cells pictured in (b). Note the differences in shape between the bipolar Type I and pseudomonopolar Type II cells. (From Kiang et al [79], with permission of *Science*.)

dramatically different in pattern and shear numbers, suggests that very different roles are played by the two sets of neurons and hair cells. Moreover, it is safe to infer that all of the data based on intracellular recordings from auditory neurons to date, as those described in Chap. 5, are derived from Type I cells.

Figures 2.32 and 2.35 show the two different types of fibers that have been identified, differing in their endings [88,89]. These are (1) cells with smaller nonvesiculated endings, which are afferent (ascending sensory neurons and (2) cells with larger vesiculated endings, which are derived from the efferent (descending) neurons of the olivocochlear bundle (see below). The vesiculated endings contain acetylcholine. Various studies found degeneration of these vesiculated units when parts of the descending olivocochlear bundle were cut [90,91]. However, there was no degeneration of the nonvesiculated afferent neurons. The endings of the efferent fibers are in direct contact with the OHCs, whereas they terminate on the afferent neural fibers of the IHCs rather than on these sensory cells themselves (Fig. 2.35). This suggests that the efferents act directly upon the OHCs (*pre*synaptically), but that they act upon the associated afferent fibers of the IHCs (*post*synaptically). The density of efferent fibers is substantially greater for the OHCs than for the IHCs. Furthermore, there is greater efferent innervation for the OHCs at the base of the cochlea than at the apex; and this innervation of the OHCs also tapers from the first row through the third.

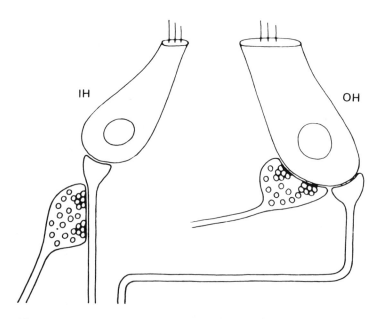

Figure 2.35   Relationship between afferent and efferent fibers and the inner (IH) and outer (OH) cells. (From Spoendlin [86], with permission.)

CENTRAL AUDITORY PATHWAYS

Afferent Pathways

The auditory (or cochlear) nerve appears as a twisted trunk, its core made up of fibers derived from the apex of the cochlea and its outer layers coming from more basal regions. The nerve leaves the inner ear via the internal auditory meatus, and enters the brain at the lateral aspect of the lower pons. Thus, the fibers of the auditory nerve constitute the first-order neurons of the ascending central auditory pathways.

The number of nerve fibers associated with the auditory system increases dramatically at the various way stations from the auditory nerve and the cortex. Chow [92] estimated that these fibers increase in number from roughly 30,000 first-order neurons to approximately 10 million at the auditory cortex in the rhesus monkey.

Upon entering the brainstem, the first-order neurons of the auditory nerve synapse with cell bodies in the dorsal and ventral cochlear nuclei (Fig. 2.36). Specifically, neurons arising from the more basal areas of the cochlea terminate in the dorsal portion of the dorsal cochlear nucleus (DCN); and the ventral cochlear nucleus (VCN) and the ventral portion of the DCN receive neurons originating in the more apical parts of the cochlea. Several studies [94,95] have shown that degeneration of the cochlear nuclei follows lesions of the cochlea. These place- or frequency-related connections are covered in the discussion of tonotopic organization in Chap. 6.

Second-order neurons arise from the cochlear nuclei. The trapezoid body is formed from the ventral acoustic stria, which arises from the VCN. The fibers of the trapezoid body decussate—cross to the opposite side—to synapse with the nuclei of the contralateral superior olivary complex (SOC) or to ascend in the lateral lemniscus. Other fibers of the trapezoid body terminate at the SOC on the ipsilateral side, and at the trapezoid nuclei. The dorsal part of the VCN gives rise to the intermediate acoustic stria, which contralateralizes to ascend in the lateral lemniscus of the opposite side. The dorsal acoustic stria is made up of fibers from the DCN, which cross to the opposite side and ascend in the contralateral lateral lemniscus.

The superior olivary complex contains a lateral principal nucleus that approximates an S in shape, and a medial accessory nucleus. Fibers from the VCN on both sides mainly synapse with the medial accessory nucleus; the medial accessory nucleus in turn is the source of third-order neutrons which ascend via the lateral lemniscus on the same side. Thus, the SOC receives a *bilateral* representation (at least

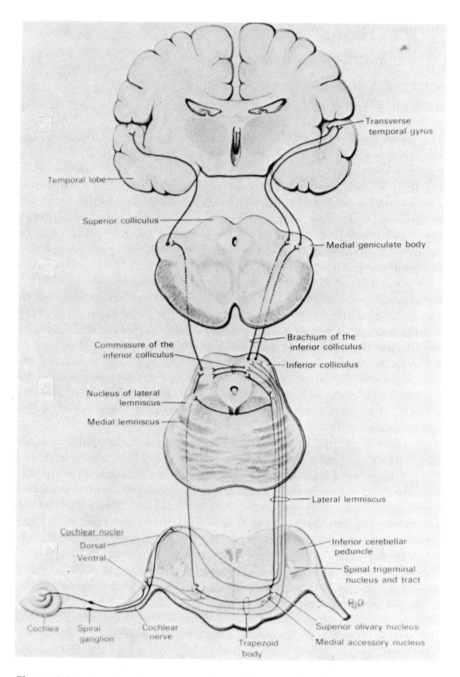

Figure 2.36 Schematic representation of the central auditory pathways. (From M. B. Carpenter [93], *Core Text of Neuroanatomy*, 2nd Ed., © 1978 by The Williams & Wilkins Co.)

from the VCN), and the lateral lemniscus includes fibers from the SOC as well as from the trapezoid body and acoustic stria. While fibers from the cochlear nuclei of one side ascend directly up the opposite lateral lemniscus, it appears that there are no fibers from the homolateral cochlear nuclei [96].

Also ascending within the lateral lemniscus are fibers arising from the several nuclei of the lateral lemniscus itself. Although the nuclei of the lateral lemniscus have classically been viewed as dorsal and ventral, recent evidence [97] has revealed a third nucleus which appears to be a continuation of the nuclei stemming from the SOC. Furthermore, the ventral nucleus, and to a slightly lesser extent the dorsal nucleus, are highly variable; they are in fact even quite variable between the right and left sides of the same subject. Communication between the lateral lemnisci of the two sides is via the commissural fibers of Probst, which appear to involve, at least primarily, the dorsal nuclei.

The majority of the ascending fibers synapse with the nuclear mass in the inferior colliculus (IC) at the level of the midbrain. There is also communication between the colliculi of the two sides via the commissure of the inferior colliculus. Several fibers may pass the IC and follow a direct course to the medial geniculate body (MGB) of the thalamus. The pathway from the IC to the MGB goes by way of the brachium of the inferior colliculus. This pathway does not appear to contain neuron bodies in the human adult, and is made up of fibers from the IC as well as of the fibers that bypass the colliculus as they ascend to the MGB [98]. Fibers ascending from the IC terminate primarily in the par principalis of the MGB.

The medial geniculate body is the last subcortical way station, and all ascending pathways to the auditory cortex synapse here. The MGB has three principal regions, including the ventral, medial and dorsal divisions; but is also often divided into two, the par principalis and a ventral nucleus. The human MGB is categorized into ventral, medial and dorsal divisions which have structures that are largely similar to those of other mammals [99]. One might note that besides the routes already mentioned, there is also some evidence that the MGB might receive direct projections from the cochlear nucleus in the chimpanzee, even though these not seen in the cat [100]. The interested reader should refer to a recent review by Winer [99] for an extensive review of the organization of the human MGB.

The medial geniculate body is the last subcortical way station, and all ascending pathways to the auditory cortex synapse here. The MGB has two main parts, the par principalis and a ventral nucleus. Fibers ascending from the IC terminate primarily in the par principalis.

The auditory (geniculotemporal) radiations project from the MGB to the transverse temporal gyrus on the temporal cortex of the same side. Also referred to as Heschl's gyrus, this cortical area corresponds to areas 41 and 42 of Brodmann's classification system (Fig. 2.37). Area 41 is the primary auditory cortex. Area 41, which consists of the middle portion of the anterior and part of the posterior temporal gyri, is actually obscured from view within the central sulcus. Area 42, which is an auditory association area, is adjacent to area 41 on parts of the posterior transverse and superior temporal gyri.

Experiments on monkeys [102,103] indicate that the primary auditory cortex communicates with the auditory association cortex by way of short neural fibers. The auditory association area in turn gives rise to generous projections to other parts of the brain, such as the temporoparietal cortex. There appears to be interhemispheric communication between the auditory association cortices of each side via the corpus callosum but the interhemispheric connections between the primary au-

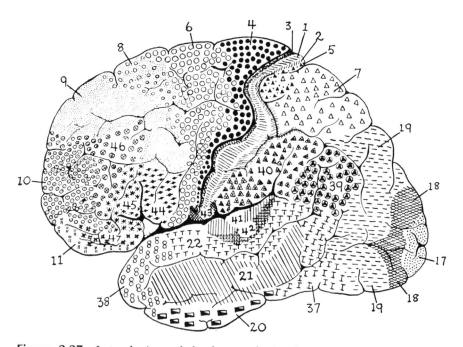

Figure 2.37 Lateral view of the human brain showing Brodmann's areas. (From M. B. Carpenter [101], *Human Neuroanatomy*, 7th Ed., © 1976 by The Williams & Wilkins Co.,)

ditory areas on both sides are not as homotopically related. Interhemispheric projection between the auditory areas of the two temporal lobes
appears to be greater for the medial than for the lateral parts of these
areas.

Efferent Pathways

As described above, descending efferent fibers enter the inner ear and
make contact with the OHCs directly, and with the IHCs indirectly via
synapses with their associated afferent fibers. These fibers are the
cochlear terminations of the olivocochlear bundle (OCB). The OCB has
been described in considerable detail [104–113] since it was originally
characterized in 1946 by Rasmussen [114].*

The general organization of the olivocochlear pathway system is
depicted in Fig. 2.38. It is made up of neurons derived from the regions
of the medial and lateral superior olives (MSO and LSO) on both sides.
They enter the inner ear along with the vestibular nerve, and then distribute themselves to the inner and outer hair cells.

The figure shows that we are really dealing with two efferent systems rather than one. About half of the very roughly 1600 efferents are
made up of fibers derived from the vicinity of the lateral superior olive.
These unmyelinated, small diameter fibers project to the ipsilateral
cochlea, where they synapse with the afferents of the *inner* hair cells. (A
comparably small number of myelinated fibers from the ipsilateral medial superior olive go to outer hair cells on the same side.) This pathway
constitutes the uncrossed olivocochlear bundle (UOCB). The second system involves large-diameter, myelinated neurons originating from the
vicinity of the medial superior olive. These cross the midline of the
brainstem at the level of the fourth ventricle and eventually terminate
directly upon the *outer* hair cells on the opposite side. A few unmyelinated fibers from the lateral superior olivary area also cross the midline,
going to the contralateral inner hair cells. This pathway is the crossed
olivocochlear bundle (COCB). Thus, the COCB primarily entails the
medial system to the OHCs whereas the UOCB is principally the lateral
system terminating on the afferents of the IHCs, implying potentially
different functions (see Chap. 6).

In addition to the COCB, and UOCB, other efferent connections
have been demonstrated coming from the inferior colliculus, the nuclei

---

*For this reason, it is often referred to as Rasmussen's bundle.

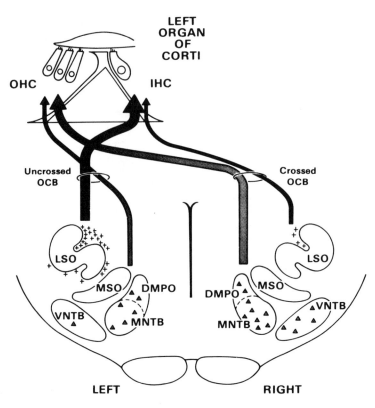

Figure 2.38 Schematic representation of the crossed and uncrossed olivo-cochlear bundles. As suggested by the wider lines, the crossed OCB goes mainly from the MSO to the contralateral OHCs, and the uncrossed OCB goes mainly from the LSO to the ipsilateral IHCs. OCB, olivocochlear bundle; LSO, lateral superior olive; MSO, medial superior olive; DMPO, dorsal perolivary nucleus; MNTB, medial nucleus of trapezoid body; VNTB, ventral nucleus of trapezoid body; triangles, large OCB neurons; crosses, small OCB neurons. [Adapted from Warr [105], The olivocochlear bundle: Its origins and terminations in the cat, in *Evoked Electrical Activity in the Auditory Nervous System* (R. F. Naunton and C. Fernandex, eds.), © 1978 by Academic Press.]

of the lateral lemniscus, and possibly the cerebellum [115–118]; as well as descending fibers that may also provide cortical control over lower centers including, for example, corticofugal pathways to the inferior colliculus [119,120] and to the medial geniculate [121–123].

REFERENCES

1. G. Bekesy, *Experiments in Hearing*, McGraw-Hill, New York, 1960.
2. B. J. Anson and J. A. Donaldson, *The Surgical Anatomy of the Temporal Bone and the Ear*, Saunders, Philadelphia, 1967.
3. E. G. Wever and M. Lawrence, *Physiological Acoustics*, Princeton Univ. Press, Princeton, New Jersey, 1982.
4. J. A. Donaldson and J. M. Miller, Anatomy of the ear, in *Otolaryngology* (M. M. Paparella and D. A. Shumrick, eds.), Vol. 1: *Basic Sciences and Related Disciplines*, Saunders, Philadelphia, 1973, pp. 75–110.
5. E. Gardner, D. J. Gray, and R. O'Rahilly, *Anatomy*, 4th ed., Saunders, Philadelphia, 1975.
6. W. R. Zemlin, *Speech and Hearing Science, Third Edition*, Prentice-Hall, Englewood Cliffs, N.J., 1988.
7. H. Helmholtz, Die Mechanik der Gehörknöchelchen und des Trommelfells, *Pflüg. Arch. ges. Physiol. I*, 1–60 (1868).
8. G. Bekesy, Zur Physik des Mittelohres und über das Hören bei fehlerhaftem Trommelfell, *Akust, Zeitschr. i*, 13–23 (1936).
9. O. Jepsen. Middle-ear muscle reflexes in man, in *Modern Developments in Audiology*, (J. Jerger, ed.), Academic, New York, 1963, pp. 194–239.
10. E. Borg, On the neuronal organization of the acoustic middle ear reflex: A physiological and anatomical study, *Brain Res. 49*, 101–123 (1973).
11. M. Lawrence, Inner ear physiology, in *Otolaryngology* (M. M. Paparella and D. A. Shumrick, eds.), Vol. 1: *Basic Sciences and Related Disciplines*, Saunders, Philadelphia, 1973, pp. 275–298.
12. C. A. Smith, O. H. Lowry, and M-L Wu, The electrolytes of the labyrinthine fluids, *Laryngoscope 64*, 141–153 (1954).
13. S. Rauch and A. Köstlin, Aspects chemiques de l'endolymphe et de la perilymphe, *Pract. Ontol. 20*, 287–291 (1958).
14. S. Rauch, Biochemische Studien zum Hörvorgang, *Pract. Otol. 25*, 81–88 (1963).
15. I. Kirakae, Y. Nomura, M. Nagakura, Y. Matsuba, and S. Sugiura, A consideration on the circulation of perilymph, *Ann. Otol. 70*, 337–343 (1961).
16. R. Kimura, Experimental blockage of the endolymphatic duct and sac and its effect on the inner ear of the guinea pig, *Ann. Otol. 76*, 664–687 (1967).
17. H. Engström and J. Wersäll, Is there a special nutritive cellular system around the organ of Corti? *Ann. Otol. 62*, 507–512 (1953).
18. H. Engström, The cortilymph, the third lymph of the inner ear, *Acta Morphol. Neerl. Scand. 3*, 195–204 (1960).
19. T. Takahashi, and R. S. Kimura, The ultrastructure of the spiral ligament in the Rhesus monkey, *Acta Otol. 69*, 46–60 (1970).
20. C. Morera, A. Dal Sasso, and S. Iurato, Submicroscopic structure of the spiral ligament in man, *Rev. Laryngol. 101*, 73–85 (1980).
21. M. M. Henson, O. W. Henson, Jr., and D. B. Jenkins, The attachment of the spiral ligament to the cochlear wall: Anchoring cells and the creation of tension, *Hearing Res. 16*, 231–242 (1984).

22. D. J. Lim, Cochlear anatomy related to cochlear microphonics. A review, *J. Acoust. Soc. Am. 67*, 1686–1695 (1980).

23. C. E. Miller, Structural implications of basilar membrane compliance measurements, *J. Acoust. Soc. Am. 77*, 1465–1474 (1985).

24. H. Davis, Advances in the neurophysiology and neuroanatomy of the cochlea, *J. Acoust. Soc. Amer. 34*, 1377–1385 (1962).

25. M. Lawrence, Effects of interference with terminal blood supply on the organ of Corti, *Laryngoscope 76*, 1318–1337 (1966).

26. D. J. Lim, Functional structure of the organ of corti: a review, *Hearing Res. 22*, 117–146 (1986).

27. I. Thalmann, G. Thallinger, T. H. Comegys, E. C. Crouch, N. Barret, and R. Thalmann, Composition and supramolecular organization of the tectorial membrane, *Laryngoscope 97*, 357–367 (1987).

28. G. H. Frommer, Observations of the organ of Corti under in vivo-like conditions, *Acta Otol. 94*, 451–460 (1982).

29. J. J. Zwislocki, S. C. Chamberlain, and N. B. Slepecky, Tectorial membrane 1: Static mechanical properties in vivo, *Hearing Res. 33*, 207–222 (1988).

30. K. P. Steel, The tectorial membrane of mammals, *Hearing Res. 9*, 327–359 (1983).

31. K. P. Steel, Composition and properties of mammalian tectorial membrane. In *Auditory Biochemistry* (D. G. Drescher, ed.), Thomas, Springfield, Illinois, 1985, pp. 351–365.

32. L. Ulehlova, L. Voldrich, and R. Janisch, Correlative study of sensory cell density and cochlear length in humans, *Hearing Res. 28*, 149–151 (1987).

33. A. Wright, A. Davis, G. Bredberg, L. Ulehlova, and H. Spencer, Hair cell distributions in the normal human cochlea, *Acta Otol., Suppl. 444*, 1–48 (1987).

34. D. J. Lim, Effects of noise and ototoxic drugs at the cellular level in cochlea: A review, *Am. J. Otol. 7*, 73–99 (1986).

35. D. J. Lim and W. Melnick, Acoustic damage of the cochlea: A scanning and transmission electron microscope observation, *Arch. Otol. 94*, 294–305 (1971).

36. A. Flock, B. Flock, and M. Ulfendahl, Mechanisms of movement in outer hair cells and a possible structural basis, *Arch. Otorhinolaryngol. 243*, 83–90 (1986).

37. A. Flock, Contractile proteins in hair cells, *Hearing Res. 2*, 411–412 (1980).

38. A. Flock, A. Bretscher, and K. Weber, Immunohistochemical localization of several cytoskeletal proteins in inner ear sensory and supporting cells, *Hearing Res. 7*, 75–89 (1982).

39. H. P. Zenner, Cytoskeletal and muscle like elements in cochlear hair cells, *Arch. Otorhinolaryngol, 230*, 82–92 (1980).

40. D. Drenckhahn, J. Kellner, H. G. Mannherz, U. Groschel-Steward, J. Kendrick-Jones, and J. Scholey, Absence of myosin-like immuno-reactivity in stereocilia of cochlear hair cells, *Nature 300*, 531–532 (1982).

41. N. Slepecky, M. Ulfendahl, and A. Flock, Effects of caffeine and tetracaine

on outer hair cell shortening suggest intracellular calcium involvement, *Hearing Res. 32,* 11–32 (1988).

42. A. Wright, Scanning electron microscopy of the human cochlea—the organ of Corti, *Arch. Otorhinolargyngol. 230,* 11–19 (1981).
43. A. Flock, B. Flock, and E. Murray, Studies on the sensory hairs of receptor cells in the inner ear, *Acta Otol. 83,* 85–91 (1977).
44. A. Flock, and D. Strelioff, Studies on hair cells in isolated coils from the guinea pig cochlea, *Hearing Res. 15,* 11–18 (1984).
45. D. Strelioff, and A. Flock, Stiffness of sensory-cell hair bundles in the isolated guinea pig cochlea, *Hearing Res. 15,* 19–28 (1984).
46. A. C. Crawford, and R. Fettiplace, The mechanical properties of ciliary bundles of turtle cochlear hair cells, *J. Physiol. 364,* 359–379 (1985).
47. A. Flock, and H. C. Cheung, Actin filaments in sensory hairs of inner ear receptor cells *J. Cell Biol. 75,* 339–343 (1977).
48. L. G. Tilney, D. J. DeRosier, and M. J. Mulroy, The organization of actin filaments in the skeleton of cochlear hair cells, *J. Cell Biol. 86,* 244–259 (1980).
49. A. Flock, H. C. Cheung, and G. Utter, Three sets of actin filaments in sensory hairs of the inner ear: Identification and functional organization determined by gel electrophoresis, immunofluorescence, and electron microscopy, *J. Neurocytol. 10,* 133–147 (1981).
50. N. Hirokawa and L. G. Tilney, Interactions between actin filaments and between actin filaments and membranes in quick-frozen and deeply etched hair cells of the chick ear. *J. Cell Biol. 95,* 249–261 (1982).
51. N. Hirokawa, Cytoskeletal architecture of the chicken hair cells revealed with the quick-freeze, deep-etch technique, *Hearing Res. 22,* 41–54 (1986).
52. L. G. Tilney and M. S. Tilney, Functional organization of the cytoskeleton, *Hearing Res. 22,* 55–77 (1986).
53. T. F. Weiss, M. J. Mulroy, R. G. Turner, and C. L. Pike, Tuning of single fibers in the cochlear nerve of the alligator lizards: Relation to receptor morphology, *Brain Res. 115,* 71–90 (1976).
54. L. G. Tilney and J. C. Saunders, Actin filaments, stereocilia, and hair cells of bird cochlea. I. Length, number, width, and distribution of stereocilia of each hair cell are related to the position of the hair cell on the cochlea, *J. Cell Biol. 96,* 807–821 (1983).
55. J. C. Saunders, M. E. Schneider, and S. P. Dear, The structure and function of actin in hair cells, *J. Acoust. Soc. Am. 78,* 299–311 (1985).
56. A. Wright, Dimensions of the cochlear stereocilia in man and the guinea pig, *Hearing Res. 13,* 89–98 (1984).
57. M. J. Mulroy, Cochlear anatomy of the alligator lizard, *Brain Behav. and Evol. 10,* 69–87 (1974).
58. M. J. Mulroy and T. G. Oblack, Cochlear nerve of the alligator lizard, *J. Comp. Neurol. 233,* 463–472 (1984).
59. M. J. Mulroy, and R. S. Williams, Auditory stereocilia in the alligator lizard, *Hearing Res. 25,* 11–21 (1987).

60. L. S. Frishkopf and D. J. DeRosier, Mechanical tuning of free-standing stereociliary bundles and frequency analysis in the alligator lizard, *Hearing Res. 12*, 393–404 (1983).

61. T. Holton and A. J. Hudspeth, A micromechanical contribution to cochlear tuning and tonotopic organization, *Science 222*, 508–510 (1983).

62. J. O. Pickles, S. D. Comis, and M. P. Osborne, Cross-links between stereocilia in the guinea-pig organ of Corti, and their possible relation to sensory transduction, *Hearing Res. 15*, 103–112 (1984).

63. D. N. Furness, and C. M. Hackney, Cross-links between stereocilia in the guinea pig cochlea, *Hearing Res. 18*, 177–188 (1985).

64. P. H. Rhys Evans, S. D. Comis, M. P. Osborne, J. O. Pickles, and D. J. R. Jefferies, Cross-links between stereocilia in the human organ of Corti, *J. Laryngol. Otol. 99*, 11–20 (1985).

65. C. M. Hackney and D. N. Furness, Stereociliary cross-links between adjacent inner hair cells, *Hearing Res. 34*, 207–212 (1988).

66. D. N. Furness and C. M. Hackney, High-resolution scanning-electron microscopy of stereocilia using the osmium-thiocarbohydrazide coating technique, *Hearing Res. 21*, 243–249 (1986).

67. G. Bourne and J. Danielli, eds., *International Review of Cytology*, Vol. III, Academic Press, New York, 1958.

68. G. Rasmussen, Studies of the VIIIth cranial nerve of man, *Laryngoscope 50*, 67–83 (1940).

69. J. M. Harrison and M. E. Howe, Anatomy of the afferent auditory nervous system of mammals, in *Handbook of Sensory Physiology V5/1* (W. D. Keidel and W. D. Neff, eds.), Springer, Berlin, 1974, pp. 283–336.

70. N. Y. S. Kiang, M. C. Liberman, W. F. Sewell, and J. J. Guinan, Single unit clues to cochlear mechanisms, *Hearing Res. 22*, 171–182 (1986).

71. H. Spoendlin, Innervation of the organ of Corti of the cat, *Acta Otol. 67*, 239–254 (1969).

72. H. Spoendlin, Degeneration behavior in the cochlear nerve, *Arch Klin. Exp. Ohren. Nasen. Kehlkopfheilkd 200*, 275–291 (1971).

73. H. Spoendlin, The afferent innervation of the cochlea, in *Evoked Electrical Activity in the Auditory Nervous System* (R. F. Naunton and C. Fernandez, eds.) Academic Press, London, 1978, pp. 21–41.

74. H. Spoendlin, *The Organization of the Cochlear Receptor*, Karger, Basel, 1966.

75. D. Morrison, R. A. Schindler, and J. Wersäll, Quantitative analysis of the afferent innervation of the organ of Corti in guinea pig, *Acta Otol. 79*, 11–23 (1975).

76. Y. Nomura, Nerve fibers in the human organ of Corti, *Acta Otol. 82*, 317–324 (1976).

77. M. C. Liberman, Single-neuron labeling in the cat auditory nerve, *Science 216*, 1239–1241 (1982).

78. L. M. Liberman and D. D. Simmons, Applications of neural labeling to the study of the peripheral auditory system, *J. Acoust. Soc. Am. 78*, 312–319 (1985).

79. N. Y. S. Kiang, J. M. Rho, C. C. Northrop, M. C. Liberman, and D. K. Ryugo, Hair-cell innervation by spiral ganglion cells in adult cats, *Science 217*, 175–177 (1982).

80. D. M. Fekete, E. M. Rouiller, M. C. Liberman, and D. K. Ryugo, The central projections of intracellularly labelled auditory nerve fibers in cats, *J. Comp. Neurol. 229*, 432–450 (1984).

81. H. Spoendlin, Differentiation of cochlear afferent neurons, *Acta Otol. 91*, 451–456 (1981).

82. H. Spoendlin, Innervation of the outer hair cell system, *Am J. Otol. 3*, 274–278 (1982).

83. H. Spoendlin, Neural connection of the outer hair-cell system, *Acta Otol. 87*, 381–387 (1979).

84. P. A. Leak-Jones and R. L. Snyder, Uptake transport of horseradish peroxidase by cochlear spiral ganglion neurons, *Hearing Res. 8*, 199–223 (1982).

85. M. A. Ruggero, P. A. Santi, and N. C. Rich, Type II cochlear ganglion cells in the chinchilla, *Hearing Res. 8*, 339–356 (1982).

86. H. Spoendlin, Neuroanatomical basis of cochlear coding mechanisms, *Audiology 14*, 383–407 (1975).

87. H. Engström, H. W. Ades, and A. Andersson, *Structural Pattern of the Organ of Corti*, Almqvist & Wiksell, Stockholm, 1966.

88. H. Engstrom, On the double innervation of the inner ear sensory epithelia, *Acta Otol. 49*, 109–118 (1958).

89. C. A. Smith and F. Sl Sjöstrand, Structure of the nerve endings of the guinea pig cochlea by serial sections, *J. Ultrasound Res. 5*, 523–556 (1961).

90. C. A. Smith and G. L. Rasmussen, Recent observations on the olivo-cochlear bundle, *Ann. Otol. 72*, 489–506 (1963).

91. H. Spoendlin and R. R. Gacek, Electromicroscopic study of the efferent and afferent innervation of the organ of Corti, *Ann. Otol. 72*, 660–686 (1963).

92. K. Chow, Numerical estimates of the auditory central nervous system of the monkey, *J. Comp. Neurol. 95*, 159–175 (1951).

93. M. B. Carpenter, *Core Text of Neuroanatomy*, 2nd Ed., Williams and Wilkins, Baltimore, 1978.

94. T. P. S. Powell and W. M. Cowan, An experimental study of the projection of the cochlea, *J. Anat. 96*, 269–284 (1962).

95. N. Moskowitz and J. C. Liu, Central projections of the spiral ganglion of the squirrel monkey, *J. Comp. Neurol. 144*, 335–344 (1972).

96. W. T. Barnes, H. W. Magoun, and S. W. Ranson, The ascending auditory projection in the brainstem of the monkey, *J. Comp. Neurol. 79*, 129–152 (1943).

97. J. A. Ferraro and J. Minckler, The human auditory pathways: A quantitative study: The human lateral lemniscus and its nuclei, *Brain Language 4*, 277–294 (1977).

98. J. A. Ferraro and J. Minckler, The human auditory pathways: A quantitative study: The brachium of the inferior colliculus, *Brain Language 4*, 156–164 (1977).

99. J. A. Winer, The human medial geniculate body, *Hearing Res. 15,* 225–247 (1984).

100. N. L. Strominger, L. R. Nelson, and W. J. Dougherty, Second order auditory pathways in the chimpanzee, *J. Comp. Neurol. 172,* 349–366 (1977).

101. M. D. Carpenter, *Human Neuroanatomy,* 7th Ed., Williams and Wilkins, Baltimore, 1976.

102. D. N. Pandya, M. Hallett, and S. Mukherjee, Intra- and inter-hemispheric connections of neocortical auditory system in the rhesus monkey, *Brain Res. 14,* 49–65 (1969).

103. E. A. Karol and D. N. Pandya, The distribution of the corpus callosum in the rhesus monkey, *Brain 94,* 471–486 (1971).

104. G. D. Luk, D. K. Morest, and N. M. McKenna, Origins of the crossed olivocochlear bundle shown by an acid phophatase method in the cat, *Ann. Otol. 83,* 382–392 (1974).

105. W. B. Warr, The olivocochlear bundle: Its origins and terminations in the cat, in *Evoked Electrical Activity in the Auditory Nervous System* (R. F. Naunton and C. Fernandez, eds.), Academic Press, New York, 1978, pp. 43–65.

106. W. B. Warr and J. J. Guinan, Efferent innervation of the organ of Corti: Two separate systems, *Brain Res. 173,* 152–155 (1979).

107. J. Strutz and W. Spatz, Superior olivary and extraolivary origin of centrifugal innervation of the cochlea in guinea pig: A horseradish perioxadase study, *Neurosci. Lett. 17,* 227 (1980).

108. J. J. Guinan, W. B. Warr, and B. E. Norris, Diffrential olivocochlear projections from lateral vs medial zones of the superior olivary complex, *J. Comp. Neurol. 221,* 358–370 (1983).

109. J. J. Guinan, W. B. Warr, and B. E. Norris, Topographic organization of the olivocochlear projections from the lateral and medial zones of the superior olivary complex, *J. Comp. Neurol. 226,*21–27 (1984).

110. J. S. White and B. B. Warr, The dual origins of the olivocochlear bundle in the albino rat, *J. Comp. Neurol. 219,* 203–214 (1983).

111. D. Robertson, Brainstem localization of efferent neurons projecting to the guinea pig cochlea, *Hearing Res. 20, 79–84* (1985).

112. R. A. Altschuler and J. Fex, Efferent transmitters, in *Neurobiology of Hearing: The Cochlea* (R. A. Altschuler, R. P. Bobbin, and D. W. Hoffman, eds.), Raven Press, New York, 1986, pp. 383–396.

113. M. C. Liberman and M. C. Brown, Physiology and anatomy of single olivocochlear neurons in the cat, *Hearing Res. 24,* 17–36 (1986).

114. G. L. Rasmussen, The olivary peduncle and other fiber projections of the superior olivary complex, *J. Comp. Neurol. 84,* 141–219 (1946).

115. G. L. Rasmussen, Efferent fibers of the cochlear nerve and cochlear nucleus, in *Neural Mechanisms of the Auditory and Vestibular Systems* (G. L. Rasmussen and W. F. Windle, eds.), Thomas, Springfield, Illinois, 1960.

116. G. L. Rasmussen, Anatomical relationships of the ascending and descending auditory systems, in *Neurological Aspects of Auditory and Vestibular Disorders* (W. S. Field and B. R. Alford eds.), Thomas, Springfield, Illinois, 1964.

117. G. L. Rasmussen, Efferent connections of the cochlear nucleus, in *Sensorineural Hearing Processes and Disorders* (A. B. Graham, ed.), Little, Brown, Boston, 1967.

118. J. M. Harrison and M. E. Howe, Anatomy of the descending auditory system (mammalian), in *Handbook of Sensory Physiology V5/1* (W. D. Keidel and W. D. Neff, eds.), Springer, Berlin, 1974, pp. 363–388.

119. A. J. Rockel and E. G. Jones, The neuronal organization of the inferior colliculus of the adult cat: I. The central nucleus, *J. Comp. Neurol. 147*, 11–60 (1973a).

120. A. J. Rockel, and E. G. Jones, The neuronal organization of the inferior colliculus of the adult cat: II. The precentral nucleus, *J. Comp. Neurol. 147*, 301–334 (1973b).

121. I. T. Diamond, E. G. Jones, and T. P. S. Powell, The projection of the auditory cortex upon the diencephalon and the brain stem of the cat, *Brain Res. 15*, 305 (1969).

122. D. K. Morest, Synaptic relationship of Golgi type II cells in the medial geniculate body of the cat, *J. Comp. Neurol. 162*, 157–194 (1975).

123. J. A. Winer, I. T. Diamond, and D. Raczkowsky, Subdivisions of auditory cortex of the cat, the retrograde transport of horseradish peroxidase to medial geniculate body, and posterior thalamic nuclei, *J. Comp. Neurol. 176*, 387–418 (1977).

3

Conductive Mechanism

This chapter deals with the routes over which sound is conducted to the inner ear. The first section is concerned with the usual air conduction path through the outer and middle ear. The second section briefly discusses the bone conduction route. In the last section, we shall go into some detail about the acoustic reflex, which is a topic of growing scientific and clinical interest.

AIR CONDUCTION ROUTE

Outer Ear

Pinna

The pinna has traditionally been credited with funneling sounds into the ear canal and enhancing localization. It has been demonstrated, however, that hearing sensitivity is not affected when the pinna is excluded from sound conduction by bypassing it with tubes to the canal and by filling its depressions [1]. Thus, the sound collecting/funneling function is not significant for the human pinna.

The pinna's greatest contribution to hearing is probably in sound source localization. The obvious example occurs when a pet turns its ears toward a ringing doorbell. This action is impossible for man, whose extrinsic ear muscles are vestigial. However, head turning in both humans and animals orients the ears relative to the stimulus, which, along with differences in the intensity and time of arrival of a sound at the two ears, permits accurate localization. The pinna itself contributes to localization in man, particularly when listening with only one ear (monaurally) and when the sound source is in the median plane of the head rather than off to one side. Pinna effects are important in these two situations because monaural hearing precludes the use of the interaural differences available during binaural hearing, and because these interaural differences are minimized in the median plane, where the sound source is equidistant from both ears.

The depressions and ridges of the pinna contribute to median-plane localization [2–5], as is shown by increases in the number of localization errors made when the various depressions are filled. The contribution of the pinna to localization is due to variations in the stimulus spectrum caused by the structure of the pinna. Blauert [6] suggested that the pinna acts as a filter that attenuates or passes frequencies depending on their direction. Batteau [7] showed that sounds reflected from the structures of the pinna cause time delays between the reflected and direct sounds on the order of under 300 μsec. Since these very small delays are detectable [4], they may be used in median-plane and monaural localization. Pinna effects also contribute to correct horizontal plane localization of the front versus rear quadrants (see Chap. 13). The frequencies over 4000 Hz are particularly important in the effects associated with the pinnae.

Ear Canal

The eardrum is located at the end of the ear canal rather than flush with the skull surface. Sounds reaching the drum are thus affected by the acoustic characteristics of the canal, as well as by those of the pinna. Sounds at the eardrum are also affected by the azimuth—the angle at which the ear is oriented toward the sound source (Fig. 3.1). This effect is due to the reflection and diffraction of sounds from the head and other body parts, and also to the acoustic shadow cast by the head.

A head shadow occurs when the head is between the sound source and the ear being investigated, and may be thought of as analogous to an eclipse. The signal coming from the left speaker (at 225° azimuth) in Fig. 3.1 will be attenuated at the right ear because the head is, so to speak, blocking the path. This head shadow is significant for frequencies over 1500–2000 Hz because their wavelengths are small compared to the size of the head.

The ear canal may be conceived of as a tube open at one end and closed at the other. Such a tube resonates at the frequency with a wavelength four times the length of the tube. Since the human ear canal is about 2.3 cm long, its resonance should occur at the frequency of wavelength 9.2 cm, i.e., at about 3800 Hz. One could test his hypothesis by

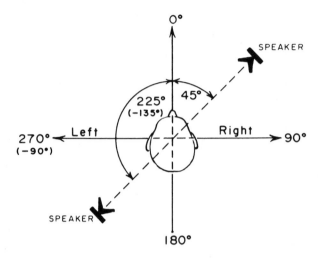

Figure 3.1   Azimuth angles around the head. The loudspeaker toward the right is at an azimuth of 45°; the one at the left has an azimuth of 225° (or −135°).

directing a known sound into a sound field, and then monitoring the sound pressure at the eardrum of a subject sitting in that sound field. This test has been done in various ways in many studies. Figure 3.2 shows the results of three studies [8–10] in the form of transfer functions. (Transfer functions show the relationship between the input to a system and its output. See Dallos [11] for a complete discussion.) The figure shows how sounds presented from a speaker in front of the subject are affected by the ear canal. The common finding of these studies is a wide resonance peak in the vicinity of 4000 Hz. The peak is relatively smooth and extends from below 2000 Hz to above 5000 Hz. It does not resemble the sharp resonance of a rigid tube. However, the ear canal is an irregular rather than a simple tube, and the drum and canal walls are absorptive rather than rigid. These factors introduce damping. Also, group (averaged) data are shown in the figure. Since resonant frequency depends on canal length, variations in ear canal length among subjects will widen and smooth the averaged function. The important point, however, is that the resonance characteristics of the canal serve to boost the level of sounds in the mid-high frequencies by as much as ∼15 dB at the eardrum compared to the sound field.

Stinton and Lawton [12] have recently reported extremely accurate geometric specifications of the human ear canal based upon impression taken in cadavers. They found that there is considerable variability from

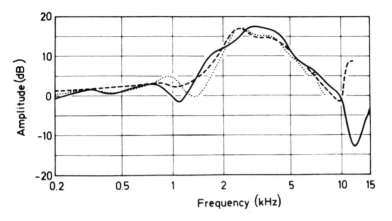

Figure 3.2 Ear-canal transfer functions at 0° azimuth (Wiener and Ross [8], dotted; Shaw [9], dashed; Mehrgardt and Mellert [10], solid). (From Mehrgardt and Mellert [10], with permission of *J. Acoust. Soc. Amer.*)

canal to canal, resulting in differences greater than 20 dB for the higher frequencies (particularly over 10 KHz.).

The sound field to eardrum transfer function varies with azimuth. Figure 3.3 shows data by Shaw [9] at 45° azimuth increments. Positive azimuth angles denote sounds coming from the same side as the test ear, whereas negative azimuths indidate that the sound source is on the opposite side of the head. In particular, one should note that there is a steady increase in sound pressure going from −45° to +45°. Physical factors of this type provide the basis for sound localization in space. In light of the wide range of applications for these curves, Shaw and Vaillancourt [13] have recently published this information in a very useful tabular form.

The interested reader should be aware that a number of extensive theoretical papers on ear canal and eardrum acoustics have appeared in recent years [14–17], although these are beyond the current scope.

Middle Ear

Sound reaches the ear by way of the air, a gas. On the other hand, the organ of Corti is contained within the cochlear fluids, which are physically comparable to seawater. This difference between these media is of considerable import to hearing, as the following example will show. Suppose you and a friend are standing in water at the beach. He is speaking, and in the middle of his sentence you dunk your head under the water. However

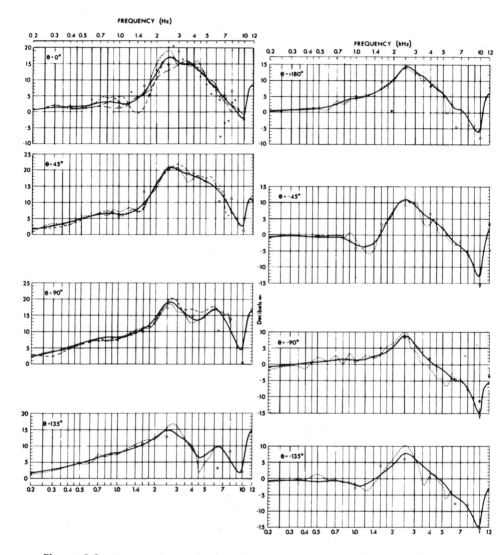

Figure 3.3 Ear canal transfer functions at various azimuths. (From Shaw [9], with Permission of *J. Acoust. Soc. Amer.*)

loud and clear your friend's voice was a moment ago, it will be barely, if at all, audible while your head is submerged. Why?

   The answer to this question is really quite straightforward. Air offers less opposition to the flow of sound energy, or impedance, than does sea water. Since the water's impedance is greater than that of the air, there is an impedance mismatch at the boundary between them. Airborne sound thus meets a substantial increase in the opposition to its flow at the water's surface, and much of the energy is reflected back rather than being transmitted through the water. The impedance mismatch between the air and cochlear fluids has the same effect. The middle ear system serves as an impedance-matching transformer that makes it possible for the sound energy to be efficiently transmitted from the air to the cochlea.

As in any other system, the impedance of the middle ear is due to its stiffness, mass, and resistance. Figure 3.4 is a block diagram of the middle ear with respect to its impedance [18], revised from Zwislocki's earlier model [19]. One may think of the upper row of boxes as the line of energy flow from the eardrum to the cochlea, and of the boxes coming down from them as the ways energy is shunted from the system. The first box represents the middle ear cavities, which contribute significantly to the stiffness of the system. The next two boxes, "eardrum/malleus" and "eardrum (decoupled)," should be thought of together. The former represents the proportion of sound energy transmitted from the drum to the malleus. It includes the inertia of the malleus; the elasticity of the drum, tensor tympani muscle, and mallear ligaments; and the friction caused by the strain on these structures. "Eardrum (decoupled)"is the proportion of energy diverted from the system when the drum vibrates independently (decoupled from) the malleus, which occurs particularly at high frequencies. The box labeled "incus" is the effective mass of the incus and the stiffness of its supporting ligaments. The energy lost at the two ossicular joints is represented by "incudomalleal joint" and "incustapedial joint," which shunt energy off the main line of the diagram. The last box shows the effects of the stapes, cochlea, and round window in series. The attachments of the stapes as well as the round window membrane contribute to

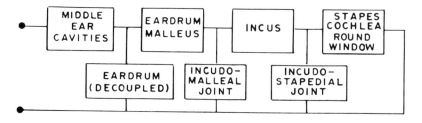

Figure 3.4 Block diagram of the middle ear. [From Zwislocki [18], in *Acoustic Impedance and Admittance—The Measurement of Middle Ear Function* (A.S. Feldman and L. A. Wilber, eds.), © 1976 by Williams and Wilkins.]

the stiffness component. Most of the ear's resistance to due to the cochlea. Zwislocki [20] has pointed out that a major effect of this resistance is to smooth out the response of the middle ear by damping the free oscillations of the ossicular chain.

Middle Ear Transformer Mechanism

The ratio between the impedances of the cochlear fluids and the air is approximately 4000:1. To find out how much energy would be transmitted from the air to the cochlea without the middle ear, we apply the simple formula $T = 4r/(r + 1)^2$, where T is transmission and r is the ratio of the impedances. The result is approximately 0.001. In other words, only about 0.1% of the airborne energy would be transmitted to the cochlea, while about 99.9% would be reflected back. This corresponds to a 30 dB drop going from the air to the cochlea.

The middle ear thus "steps up" the level of airborne sound to overcome the impedance mismatch between the air and cochlear fluids. As we shall see in the next chapter, early place theory [21] held that the middle ear transformer was the source of various nonlinearities in hearing, such as combinations tones. These distortion products of the middle ear's hypothetical nonlinear response were ostensibly transmitted to the cochlea, where the nonlinearities were analyzed according to the place principle as though they were present in the original signal. However, Wever and Lawrence [22] have demonstrated that the middle ear performs its function with elegant linearity, and we must accordingly regard it as a linear transformer, and look elsewhere (to the cochlea) for the sources of nonlinear distortions.

Several factors, discussed below, contribute to the transformer function of the middle ear. They include the areal ratio of the eardrum to the oval window, the curved-membrane mechanism of the drum, and the level action of the ossicular chain.

Areal Ratio

We know that pressure (p) is equal to force (F) per unit area (A); or p = F/A. If we therefore exert the same pressure over two areas, one of which is five times large than the other, then the pressure on the smaller surface will be five times greater. Examples of this fundamental principle are shown in Fig. 3.5a.

The area of the human eardrum is roughly 64.3 mm^2, while that of the oval window is about 3.2 mm^2 [22]. Thus the drum:oval window ratio is about 20.1 to 1, as shown in Fig. 3.5b. If we assume that the ossicles act as a simple rigid connection between the two membranes, then there would be a pressure amplification by a factor of 20.1 going from the eardrum to the oval window.

Eardrum Mechanism

Helmholtz [21] suggested that the eardrum contributes to the effectiveness of the middle ear transformer by lever action according to the curved membrane principle (Fig. 3.6). The drum's rim is firmly attached to the annulus, and curves down to the attachment of the malleus, which is mobile, as in the figure. A given force increment ΔF thus displaces the membrane with greater amplitude than it displaces the manubrium. Since the products of force and distance (amplitude of dis-

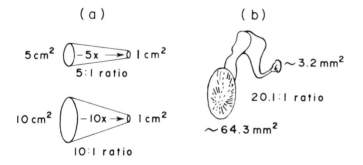

Figure 3.5 The areal ratio. General principal (a), and areal ratio of the middle ear ossicles (b).

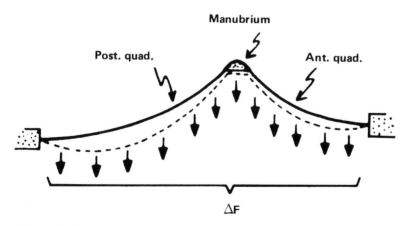

Figure 3.6 Curved membrane principle. (From Tonndorf and Khanna [23], with permission of *Ann. Otol.*)

placement) on both legs of the lever are equal (F1D1 = F2D2), the smaller distance traveled by the manubrium is accompanied by a much greater force. In this way, Helmholtz proposed that lever action of the eardrum would result in an amplification of force to the ossicles.

Subsequent experiments led to the abandonment of this principle, since studies of drum movement were inconsistent with it, and since Helmholtz's results were not replicated [22]. Bekesy [24] uses a capacitive probe to measure human eardrum displacement at various frequencies. The capacitive probe used a very fine wire as one plate of a capacitor and the drum surface as the other plate. Sound causes the drum to vibrate, which in turn varies its distance from the wire. If a current is passed through this capacitor, the movement of the drum will affect current flow. Monitoring the current flow at different spots on the drum enabled Bekesy to determine its displacement with considerable accuracy.

Figure 3.7a shows Bekesy's results for a 2000 Hz tone in the form of equal displacement contours. For frequencies up to approximately 2000 Hz, the eardrum moved as a stiff plate or piston, hinged superiorly at

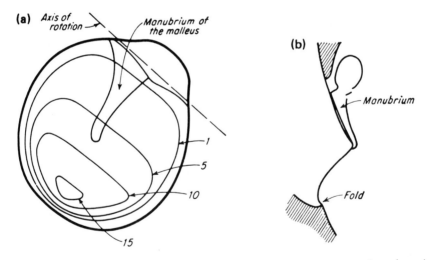

Figure 3.7 (a) Equal relative eardrum displacement contours (numbers indicate the relative amplitudes) for a 2000 Hz stimulus. (b) Cross-section of the eardrum showing a loose-fitting inferior edge. (From G. Bekesy, *Experiments in Hearing*, © 1960 by McGraw-Hill. Used with permission of McGraw-Hill Book Company.)

the axis of the ossicles. The greatest displacement occurred inferiorly. Bekesy attributed the drum's ability to move in this manner, without significant deformation, to a highly elastic or loose-fitting fold at its inferior edge (Fig. 3.7b). Above about 2400 Hz the membrane's stiffness broke down, and movement of the manubrium lagged behind that of the membrane rather than being synchronized with it. The stiffly moving portion of the drum had an area of 55 mm^2 out of a total area of 85 mm^2. This area seemed to constitute an "effective area" for the drum of about 70% of its total area. Applying the drum's effective area to the overall areal ratio (20.1 × 0.7) would result in an effective areal ratio of 14.1:1.

The eardrum's role was reevaluated by Tonndorf and Khanna [23], who used time-averaged holography to study drum movement in the cat. Holography is an optical method that reveals equal-amplitude contours as alternating bright and dark lines on the vibrating membrane. Figure 3.8 shows the isoamplitude contours for a 600 Hz tone. These contours show that the drum actually does not have an effective area that moves like a stiff plate. Instead, there are two areas of peak displace-

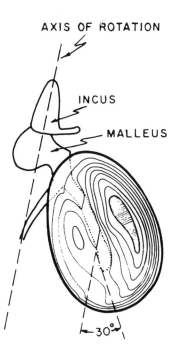

AXIS OF ROTATION

INCUS

MALLEUS

30°

Figure 3.8 Vibration patterns of the cat's eardrum in response to a 600 Hz tone. (From Tonndorf and Khanna [23], with permission of *Annal. Otol.*)

ment, consistent with Helmholtz's curved-membrane concept. This mode of vibration is seen up to about 1500 Hz. The pattern becomes more restricted at higher frequencies, and increasingly complex subpatterns occur in the vibrations as frequency rises above approximately 3000 Hz. Thus, the entire drum area contributes to the areal ratio, as opposed to just an effective portion of it. In addition, the curved membrane principle contributes to the transformer ratio (by a factor of 2.0 in the cat). If we accept an areal ratio of 39.8:1.4 = 34.6 for the cat [22], then the middle ear transfer ratio as of this point becomes 34.6 × 2.0 = 69:2:1. This value must be multiplied by the lever ratio of the ossicles to arrive at the final transformer ratio of the middle ear.

Ossicular Lever

Helmholtz [21] proposed that nonlinear distortions are introduced by the ossicular chain, and are largely due to what he conceived of as a cog-wheel articulation between the malleus and incus. This situation would allow for relative movement in one direction at the malleoincudal joint. The resulting distortions would simulate the cochlea at places corresponding to the receptors for those frequencies, as though they were present in the original signal. Barany [25] demonstrated, however, that except during intense stimulation these two bones are rigidly fixed at the malleoincudal joint and move as a unit in response to sound stimulation.

Bekesy [24] has reported that the stapes moves differently in response to moderate and intense stimulation in human cadavers (Fig. 3.9). At moderate intensities, the stapes footplate rocks with a piston-

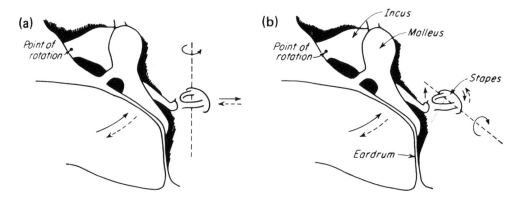

Figure 3.9 Stapes movement at (a) moderate and (b) intense levels in cadavers. (From G. Bekesy, *Experiments in Hearing*, © 1960 by McGraw-Hill. Used with permission of McGraw-Hill Book Company.)

like motion in the oval window, with greater amplitude anteriorly (Figs. 3.9 a). Intense stimulation results in rotation of the footplate around its longitudinal axis (Fig. 3.9 b). Rocking of the stapes around the longitudinal axis substantially reduces the energy transmitted to the cochlea, which most likely serves as a protective device. However, the cat stapes has been observed to maintain essentially piston-like movements even at very high intensities, at least for low frequencies [26].

The ossicular chain rotates around in axis, illustrated in Fig. 3.10, corresponding to a line through the long process of the malleus and the short process of the incus [25]. The ossicular chain is delicately balanced around its center of gravity so that the inertia of the system is minimal [25]. The ossicles act as a lever about their axis. The lever ratio is on the order of 1.3 in humans and 2.2 in cats. However, the actual lever ratio is smaller, because of the interaction of the curviture of the drum and the length of the ossicular chain lever [23].

Recall that the drum curves more toward the umbo, and may be regarded as a curved string. The transformer ratio of a curved string decreases as the curviture becomes stronger (1/curviture). On the other hand, the transformer ratio of the ossicular level increases with length. Note in Fig. 3.11 that the ossicular lever is long (with respect to the point of attachment of the malleus on the drum) where the curviture is strong, and that it is short where the curviture is small. This interaction results in an essentially constant lever ratio, with a value of about 1.4 for the cat ossicular chain.

We may now apply the ossicular level ratio to the intermediate solution of 69.2 obtained above for the middle ear transfer ratio. The final value is 69.2 × 1.4 = 96.9:1. Therefore, the total transformer ratio, found

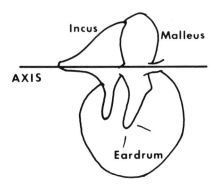

Figure 3.10   Axis of the ossicular chain. (After Barany [25].)

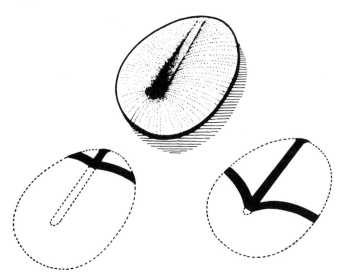

Figure 3.11 Interaction between the length of the ossicular chain and the inverse of drum curvature according to the relation (1/small curvature) (short lever) ~ const. ~ (1/strong curvature) (long lever). (From Tonndorf and Khanna [23], with permission of *Ann. Otol.*)

using the areal ratio, the curved membrane mechanism, and the ossicular lever, is 96.9:1, which corresponds to 39.7 dB. This closely approximates the 40 dB loss that results when the cat's middle ear is entirely obliterated [27].

Middle Ear Response

The middle ear transfer function is to a large extent responsible for the shape of minimal audibility curves (see Chap. 9). These curves show the amount of sound energy needed to reach the threshold of hearing as a function of frequency.

Bekesy [24] reported that the resonant frequency of the middle ear is in the 800 1500 Hz region. Recall that resonance occurs when mass and stiffness reactance are equal, cancelling out. Impedence is then entirely composed of resistance, and accordingly the opposition to energy flow is minimal at the resonant frequencies. Møller [28] found the major resonance peak of the middle ear to be about 1200 Hz, with a smaller resonance peak around 800 Hz. Normal ear reactance and resistance values obtained by Zwislocki [20] are shown in Fig. 3.12. Note that the ear's impedance results primarily from negative reactance up to about 800 Hz.

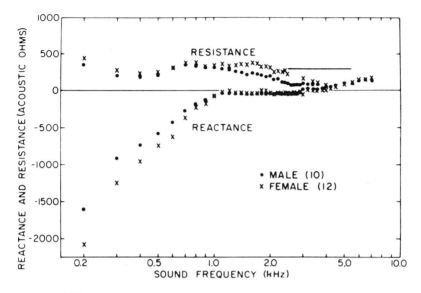

Figure 3.12   Acoustic resistance and reactance at the eardrum as a function of frequency. [From Zwislocki [20], in *The Nervous System, Vol. 3: Human Communication and Its Disorders* (D. B. Tower and E. L. Eagles, eds.), © 1975 by Raven Press.]

This effect is due to the middle ear mechanism itself, which is stiffness-controlled below the resonant frequency. There is virtually no reactance between 800 and 6000 Hz, indicating that energy transmission from the drum to cochlea is maximal in this range. Positive reactance takes over at higher frequencies as a result of the effective mass of the drum and ossicles. We thus expect sound transmission through the middle ear to be frequency-dependent with emphasis on the mid-frequencies; and the minimal audibility curves of the ear should reflect this relation.

The open circles in Fig. 3.13 show the middle ear transfer function based on data from anesthesized cats [11,26]. The filled circles are the behavioral thresholds of waking cats in a sound field [29]. The binaural threshold and transfer function are generally similar, but the threshold curve is steeper at low frequencies and flatter at high. This may reflect several factors [11,30–32]: First, since the thresholds show mean group data, the curve is probably somewhat flattened by the averaging among subjects; the transfer function is from a single representative animal. In addition there is a peak at around 4000 Hz in the middle ear response of anesthesized animals, which is much smaller when they are awake due to damping of the system by the tonus of the stapedius muscle. A second factor has to do with the effects of head diffraction, the pinna, and

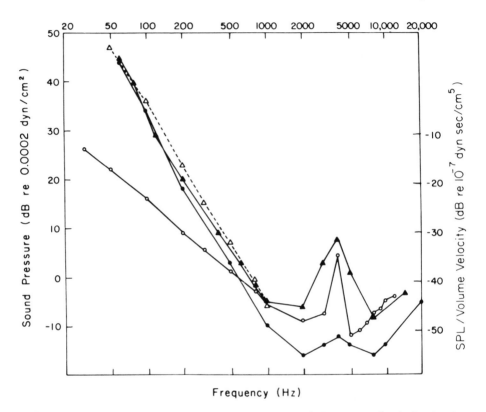

Figure 3.13   Middle ear transfer function (open circles) compared to behavioral thresholds (closed circles) and SPL at the drum (closed triangles). Open triangles show the transfer function corrected for cochlear input impedance. (From Dallos [11], *The Auditory Periphery,* © 1973 by Academic Press.)

the ear canal, as discussed in the section on the outer ear in this chapter. These effects are accounted for by viewing the behavioral thresholds in terms of the SPL near the eardrum at threshold, as is shown by the filled triangles in Fig. 3.13. The relationship of the threshold curve to the transfer function is closer when considered in these terms. The disparity between the transfer function and thresholds below about 1000 Hz is reconciled by correcting the transfer function for the input impedance of the cochlea (open triangles).

These factors show a remarkable degree of correspondence between the middle ear transfer function and the threshold curve, at least for the cat. Reasonable agreement between the transfer function based upon a model of the middle ear and the threshold curve has also been shown for humans [20]. Thus, we find that the impedance matching job of the middle ear is accomplished quite well for the mid-frequencies, although the frequency-dependent nature of the middle ear reduces its efficiency at higher and lower frequencies.

BONE CONDUCTION ROUTE

Until now we have dealt with the usual route from the air to the cochlea. The discussion would be incomplete, however, without at least a brief consideration of bone conduction—the transmission of sound to the cochlea by the bones of the skull. For this to occur, a sound must be strong enough to cause the bones to vibrate, or else the stimulus must be delivered by way of a vibrator applied to the skull. The impedance mismatch between air and bone is even greater than between air and cochlear fluid: An airborne sound must exceed the air conduction threshold by at least 50–60 dB before the bone conduction threshold is reached [33]. Direct stimulation with a vibrator is routinely employed in audiological evaluations to separate hearing losses attributable to the outer and/or middle ear from those due to impairments of the sensorineural mechanisms.

Two experiments prove that both air conduction and bone conduction initiate the same traveling waves in the cochlea (see Chap. 4). Bekesy [34] showed that air- and bone-conduction signals cancel one another when their phases and amplitudes are appropriately adjusted. Lowy [35] demonstrated that this cancellation occurs in the cochlea, since repetition of the Bekesy experiment on guinea pigs resulted in cancellation of the cochlear microphonic. (The cochlear microphonic is an electrical potential that reflects the activity of the basilar membrane; see Chap 4.) The implications of these experiments are monumental, since they demonstrate that the final activity in the cochlea is the same regardless of the mode of entry of the sound. Furthermore, this result gives support to the use of bone conduction as an audiological tool the results of which can validly be compared with those of air conduction in determining the locus of a lesion (assuming appropriate calibration of both signals).

Bekesy [34] found that below 200 Hz the human skull vibrates as a unit (Fig. 3.14 a). At about 800 Hz the mode of vibration changes (Fig. 3.14 b), and the front and back of the head vibrate in opposite phase to one another, with a nodal line of compression between them. About 1600 Hz the head begins to vibrate in four segments (Fig. 3.14c).

Tonndorf [36,37] demonstrated that the mechanism of bone conduction includes contributions from the outer, middle, and inner ear. For clarity, let us look at these components beginning with the inner ear.

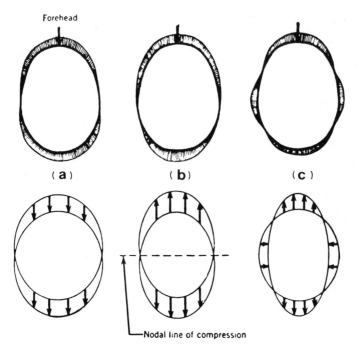

Figure 3.14 Patterns of skull vibration at (a) 200 Hz, (b) 800 Hz, and (c) 1600 Hz, with bone conduction stimulus applied for forehead. (After Bekesy [34].)

Compressional bone conduction is illustrated in Fig. 3.15. Vibration of the temporal bone results in alternate compression and expansion of the cochlear capsule. Since the cochlear fluids are incompressible, there should be bulging at compliant points. Bulging would occur at the oval and round windows without displacement of the cochlear partition if both windows were equally compliant (Fig. 3.15a). However, since the round window is much more compliant than the oval window, compression of the cochlear capsule pushes the fluid in the scala vestibuli downward, displacing the basilar membrane (Fig. 3.15b). This effect is reinforced since the sum of the surface area V of the vestibule and the surface area of the scala vestibuli is greater than that of the scala tympani (Fig. 3.15c). The possibility of a "third window" for the release of this pressure is provided by the cochlear aqueduct.

Tonndorf [38], however, found that the primary mechanism of bone conduction in the inner ear involves distortional vibrations of the cochlear capsule which are synchronous with the signal (Fig. 3.16). Since the volume of the scala vestibuli is greater than that of the scala tympani, these

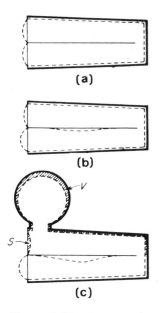

Figure 3.15 Compressional bone conduction (see text). (After Bekesy [34].)

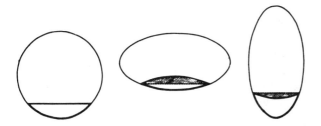

Figure 3.16 Effect of distortional vibrations on displacement of the cochlear partition. (From Tonndorf [38]; with permission of *J. Accoust. Soc. Amer.*)

distortions result in compensatory displacements of the cochlear partition even in the absence of compliant windows. The above-mentioned "window effects" modify the distortional component.

The contribution of the middle ear to bone conduction was demonstrated by Barany [25]. Recall that the ossicles move side-to-side rather than front-to-back. Barany found that for low frequencies bone conduction was maximal when a vibrator was applied to the side of the head and was minimal when it was applied to the forehead. This occurs because the lateral placement vibrates the skull in the direction of

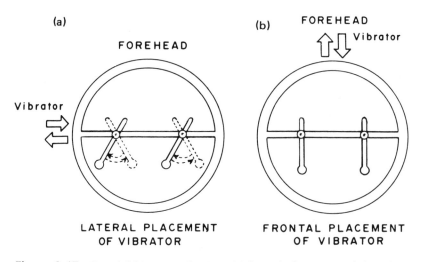

Figure 3.17 Inertial bone conduction: (a) lateral placement of the vibrator; (b) forehead placement. (Abstracted from Barany [25].)

ossicular movement (Fig. 3.17a) whereas frontal placement vibrates the skull perpendicular to their movement (Fig. 3.17b). In other words, the signal was transmitted best when it was applied in the direction of rotation of the ossicular chain about its axis. The mechanism is as follows: Since the ossicles are suspended analogously to pendulums, as shown in Fig. 3.17, their inertia cuases them to move relative to the skull when the latter is vibrated. *Inertial* bone conduction, then, stimulates the cochlea by the relative movement of the skull and ossicles, the effect of which is a rocking motion of the stapes at the oval window.

The middle ear component of bone conduction is of particular interest in otosclerosis, a disorder in which hearing loss results from fixation of the stapes in the oval window. A hearing loss results because the fixated stapedial footplate cannot effectively transmit energy to the cochlea. Although one might expect bone conduction to be impaired at low frequencies, impairment occurs instead at about 2000 Hz. This phenomenon is called "Carhart's notch" [39]. Bone conduction is impaired at 2000 Hz because this is the resonant frequency of the ossicular chain in man (the resonant frequency of the ossicular chain is species-specific [36]).

The contribution of the outer ear to bone conduction is most readily observed during occlusion of the cartilaginous part of the ear canal. Vibration of the skull under these conditions leads to the radiation of sound energy into the enclosed canal from its walls. These radiations then stimulate the eardrum and finally the cochlea along the familiar air conduction route [36]. This enhancement of the low frequencies for bone conduction is not seen when the ear is unoccluded, because the open ear canal acts as a high-pass (low-cut) filter. The occlusion effect occurs because the lows are not lost when the outer ear canal is closed off, so that sensitivity for these frequencies is enhanced.

In summary, the bone conduction mechanism appears to be primarily due to distortion of the inner ear capsule, to the relative movements of the skull and ossicles due to the inertial lag of the latter, and to the sound radiated into the ear canal from its walls. Tonndorf et al. [36] found in cats that the outer and middle ear components are dominant below about 1000 Hz, but that all three mechanisms are about equally important in the 1000–6000 Hz range.

ACOUSTIC REFLEX

Early experiments on dogs revealed bilateral tensor tympani contractions when either ear was stimulated by intense sound [40,41]. It was later demonstrated that the stapedius muscle also responds to intense sound stimulation in cats and rabbits [42]. However, whether the acoustic reflex *in man* is due to contractions of one or of both intratympanic muscles has been the subject of some controversy.

Direct observation through perforated eardrums revealed stapedius muscle contractions in man as a consequence of intense sound stimulation [43–45]. Terkildsen [46,47] indirectly examined middle ear muscle activity by monitoring changes in air pressure in the ear canal in response to sound stimulation. Stapedius contraction would result in an outward movement of the drum, while tensor concentration would pull the drum inward (see Chap. 2). The drum movement in turn, results in changes in ear canal pressure. Terkildsen could thus infer the nature of muscle activity by monitoring the air pressure in the ear canal during sound stimulation. Most of his subjects manifested on outward deflection of the drum, suggesting that the stapedius muscle was active. There were, however, some cases showing tensor activity as well (inward drum displacement). Similar findings were reported by Mendelson [48,49].

Perhaps the greatest contribution to what is known about the acoustic reflex (AR) comes from measurements of acoustic impedance at the plane of the eardrum using an impedance bridge. The mechanical acoustic impedance bridge was first applied to the study of the AR by Metz [50] and was improved and made clinically efficient by Zwislocki [51]. An electroacoustic impedance bridge was introduced by Terkildsen and

Nielsen [52]. Almost all AR research since the introduction of the electroacoustic bridge has used this method or variations of it. The principle is straightforward: Since contractions of the intratympanic muscles stiffen the middle ear system (including the drum), the impedance is increased. (The reflex primarily affects the compliance component of impedance rather than resistance because the system is stiffened.) It is this change in acoustic impedance that is measured by the device.

Let us now consider how the ear's impedance can be used to infer information about the activities of one intratympanic muscle vs. the other. (Recall that the AR is bilateral, so we can stimulate one ear and monitor the impedance change in the other.) In the normal ear we really cannot tell whether the AR is due to contractions of the stapedius and/or of the tensor. However, if the reflex is present when the stapedius muscle is intact but not when the muscle (or its reflex arc or attachment) is impaired, then we may conclude that the stapedius muscle contributes to the AR in man. The same argument applies to the tensor tympani. (Remember at this point that the stapedius is innervated by the seventh cranial nerve and the tensor by the fifth; and that the former inserts via its tendon on the more medial stapes while the latter connects to the more lateral malleus.)

Several studies have demonstrated that the acoustic reflex is absent when there is pathology affecting the stapedius muscle [53–55]. However, the AR was still obtained in two cases of tensor tympani pathology [53]. It might be added at this point that a measurable tensor reflex does occur as part of a startle reaction to very intense sound [56], or in response to a jet of air directed to the eye [54]. Based on these observations, one is drawn to conclude that in man the AR to sound stimulation is at least primarily a stapedius reflex.

Reflex Parameters

Several parameters of the AR should be discussed before describing its effect upon energy transmission through the ear, or its suggested roles within the auditory system. The possible relationship between the AR and loudness will also be covered.

We have been referring to the AR as occurring in response to "intense" sound stimulation. Let us now examine just how intense a sound is needed. With a reasonable amount of variation among studies, the AR thresholds in response to pure tone signals from 250 to 4000 Hz range from about 85 to 100 dB SPL [57–64]. The reflex threshold is approximately 20 dB lower (better) when the eliciting stimulus is wide-band noise [61,63–66]. In general, the AR is obtained at a lower intensity when it is monitored in the ear being stimulated instead of in the opposite ear [67,68]. For an extensive discussion of the acoustic reflex threshold and its parameters, see the review by Gelfand [64].

The lower reflex threshold for noise than for tones suggests that the AR is related to the bandwidth of the stimulus. Flottrop et al. [69] studied this relationship by measuring AR thresholds elicited by successively wider bands of noise and complex tones. They found that the increasing bandwidth did not cause the threshold to differ from its value for a pure tone activator *until* a certain bandwidth was exceeded. At this point there was a clear-cut break, after which increasing the bandwidth resulted in successively lower reflex thresholds. This study was replicated at 1000 Hz with similar results [70]. These findings suggest that there is a *critical band* for the AR, above which widening the bandwidth results in lower thresholds. Confirmation was obtained by Djupesland and Zwislocki [71], who found that increasing the separation in frequency between the two tones in a two-tone complex caused a lowering of the reflex threshold once a particular bandwidth was exceeded.

Although the existence of a critical bandwidth was a constant finding in the noise and two-tone studies, the thresholds were lower for noise. Popelka et al. [72] replicated this work using tone complexes made up of many components which were equally spaced (on a log scale) in frequency. Their findings, which are shown in Fig. 3.18, confirm the critical band phenomenon. The width of the critical band (shown by the break from the horizontal on each function in Fig. 3.18) increases with center frequency. It is important to note that the critical bandwidth for the AR is substantially wider than the psychoacoustic critical bands discussed in chapters that follow. However, Hellman and Scharf [73] have recently pointed out that the differences between acoustic reflex and psychoacoustic critical bands may not be as substantial as has been supposed.

The AR does not occur instantaneously upon presentation of the activating signal. Instead, a measurable impedance change is observed only after a latency, the length of which depends on both the intensity and frequency of the stimulus. Metz [74] found that this latency decreased from about 150 msec at 80 dB above the threshold of hearing [80 dB sensation level (SL)] to 40 msec at 100 dB SL in response to a 1000 Hz activating signal. Møller [75] reported latencies of 25–130 msec for 500 and 1500 Hz pure tones. As a rule, latencies were shorter for 1500 Hz than for 500 Hz tones. Dallos [76] found a similar inverse relationship between activator intensity and reflex latency for white noise. These findings were confirmed and expanded upon by Hung and Dallos [77], who found that AR latencies were shorter for noise signals than for pure

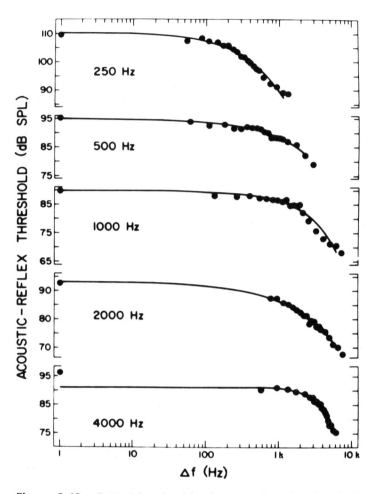

Figure 3.18 Critical bandwidths for acoustic reflex thresholds at center frequencies of 250–4000 Hz. Dots to the left of functions show corresponding pure tone reflex thresholds. (From Popelka et al. [72], with permission of *J. Acoust. Soc. Amer.*)

tones, with the longest latencies for tones below 300 Hz. The shortest latencies, on the order of 20 msec, were in response to noise activators.

These measurements were based upon changes in acoustic impedance. However, the latency of the impedance change is a measure of the latency of the *mechanical* response of the middle ear rather than of the neural transport time for the reflex arc alone [78]. Zakrisson et al. [79]

found that the electromyographic (EMG) response of the stapedius muscle in man has a latency as short as 12 msec. They also reported that the EMG "threshold" is about 6 dB lower than that for the impedance change measured as the lower stimulus level needed to yield 10% of the maximum response. Since we are concerned with the effect of the AR on the transmission of energy through the middle ear, we are most interested in the mechanical-response latency. However, one should be aware that changes in muscle potentials occur in the stapedius prior to the measured impedance change.

Hung and Dallos [77] reported that some of their subjects demonstrated a "latency relaxation" at the onset of the AR response. That is, there was an actual *decrease* in impedance prior to the impedance increase. This decrease was routinely observed by Silman, Popelka, and Gelfand [63]. It appears that it reflects a partial relaxation of the stapedius muscle before contraction. The interested reader should refer to Bosatra, Russolo, and Silverman [80] for an in-depth discussion on the latency of the acoustic reflex.

We have already seen that AR latency shortens with increasing stimulus intensity. Similarly, increasing stimulus level also causes an increase in reflex magnitude (i.e., in the amount of impedance change associated with the reflex) [63,74,75,81–83], and a faster rise time of the reflex response [76,77]. We shall call the relationship between stimulus intensity and reflex magnitude the growth function of the reflex.

The acoustic reflex growth function has been studied in response to pure tone and wide-band and narrow-band noise activating signals [58,62,63,76,77,81–83]. An extensive and insightful analysis of this topic is available in the review by Silman [83]. The reflex growth functions of four subjects studied by Hung and Dallos [76] are presented in Fig. 3.19. It illustrates that the growth of AR magnitude is essentially linear for pure tones as high as about 120 dB SPL. The functions for wide-band noise are essentially linear up to approximately 110 dB SPL. These data are substantially supported by the other studies cited. Thus, AR magnitude tends to increase linearly with a stimulus intensity of 85–120 dB SPL for tones and roughly 70–110 dB SPL for wide-band noise. Saturation occurs at higher levels.

Møller [58,67] reported steeper reflex growth functions with increasing frequency in the 300–1500 Hz range. Flottrop et al. [69] found greater impedance changes at 250 Hz than at 4000 Hz. They also reported that although signals at 1000 and 2000 Hz elicited the same maximum reflex magnitude as at 250 Hz, about 10 dB more (re: reflex threshold) was needed for the two higher frequencies. Furthermore, while some studies have suggested that a 2000 Hz tone elicits the greatest impedance

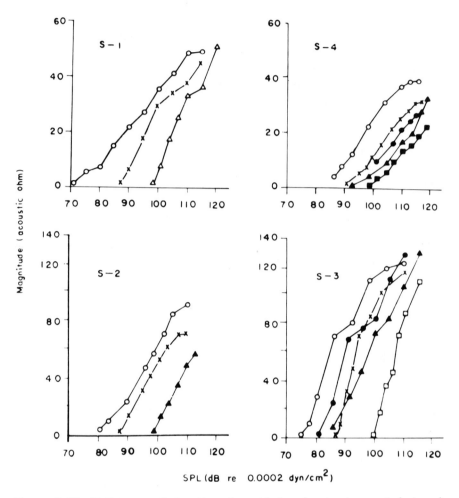

Figure 3.19 Reflex growth functions for wide-band noise (open circles) and pure tones (250 Hz, open squares; 300 Hz, filled squares; 500 Hz, filled triangles; 600 Hz, open triangles; 1000 Hz, crosses; 1500 Hz, filled circles). (From Hung and Dallos [77], with permission of *J. Acoust. Soc. Amer.*)

change [84,85], others suggest that 1000 HZ and wide-band stimuli produce maximal responses [62,86]. On the other hand, Borg and Møller [87] found no significant differences in the slopes of the AR growth functions in the 500–3000 Hz range for laboratory animals. It thus appears that any clear-cut relationship between activator frequency and reflex magnitude is still undetermined.

Two temporal parameters of the AR are particularly interesting. One deals with stimulus durations below about one second and the other has to do with long stimulus durations. The former is temporal summation and the latter is adaptation.

Temporal summation deals with the relationship between stimulus duration and intensity when the time frame is less than about 1 sec (see Chap. 9). It is most easily understood by example. Suppose a subject's threshold for a tone that lasts 200 msec happens to be 18 dB. Will the threshold remain at 18 dB when the same tone is presented for only 20 msec? It is found that when the 20 msec tone is used the threshold changes to 28 dB. (A similar trade-off is needed to maintain the stimulus at a constant loudness.) This illustrates the general psychoacoustic observation that when a signal is shortened by a factor of 10 (e.g., from 200 to 20 msec), the signal level must be increased by as much as 10 dB to offset the decade decrease in duration. This is understandably called a time-intensity trade.

Temporal summation also occurs for the acoustic reflex [81,88–91]. However, it appears that the amount of intensity change needed to counteract a given decrease in stimulus duration is greater for the AR than for psychoacoustic phenomena. Figure 3.20 summarizes the gen-

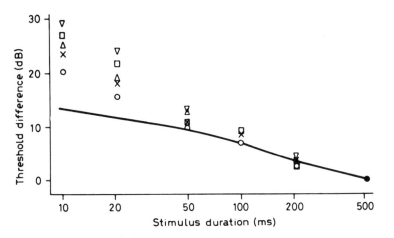

Figure 3.20   Temporal summation for the acoustic reflex threshold. This figure shows the trade off between activator duration and level at 500 Hz (crosses), 1000 Hz (circles), 2000 Hz (triangles), 3000 Hz (squares), and 4000 Hz (upside down triangles). A typical psychoacoustic temporal summation function is represented by the solid line for comparison. (From Woodford, Henderson, Hamernick, and Feldman [89].)

eral nature of temporal summation for the acoustic reflex [89]. Unfortunately, there are rather large differences between the results of various studies reporting the intensity needed to offset a given duration change. For example, decreasing the duration of a 2000 Hz tone from 100 to 10 msec was offset by an increase in stimulus level by about 25 dB in one study [88] as opposed to roughly 15 dB in another [89]. In the 500–4000 Hz range, Djupesland et al. [90] studied the time-intensity trade-off relation for the AR with one-octave wide-noise bands. They used as their comparison point the stimulus level/duration needed to maintain the reflex magnitude at half the maximum impedance change. Djupesland et al. found that a 10-fold decrease in duration was offset by a 20–25 dB increase in signal level. In contrast, Gnewikow (in 1974, cited by Jerger, Mauldin and Lewis [91]) has found that a 12–23 dB intensity increase was needed to offset decade reductions in duration for 500 and 4000 Hz pure tones. Jerger et al. [91] found less temporal summation than the other studies, as shown in Fig. 3.21 for 500–4000 Hz. Notice that the amount of temporal integration increases with frequency, which is a common finding among the studies.

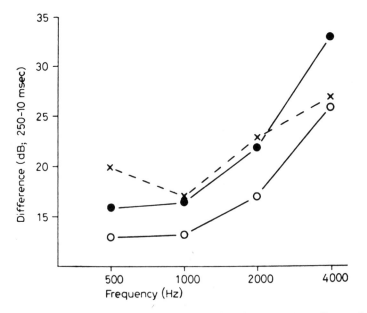

Figure 3.21 Temporal summation for the acoustic reflex at four frequencies obtained by Jerger et al.[91] (open circles); Gnewikow (1974) (filled circles); and Woodford et al.[89] (crosses). [From Jerger, Mauldin, and Lewis, Temporal summation of the acoustic reflex, *Audiology 16,* 177–200 (1977).]

These discrepancies have yet to be resolved. However, Jerger et al. [91] suggested that at least some of the differences are to problems associated with the visual detection threshold (in which the experimenter looks for the smallest noticeable impedance change on a meter or oscilloscope) and with constant percentage of maximum impedance change [90] methods of obtaining the data.

Let us now examine stimulus durations of several seconds and longer. Early studies on laboratory animals showed that the degree of muscle contraction due to the AR decreases as stimulation is prolonged [42,92]. This decrease is referred to as reflex decay or adaptation; it has been demonstrated as a decrease in reflex magnitude in man by numerous investigators [76,85,93–98]. An extensive review of this topic is provided by Wilson, Shanks, and Lilly [98]. In spite of wide differences among subjects, the common finding is that reflex adaptation increases as the frequency of the pure tone stimulus is raised.

Particular attention should be given to the findings of Kaplan et al. [85], who studied reflex adaptation to pure tones of 500–4000 Hz at 6, 12, and 18 dB above the reflex threshold. Figure 3.22 summarizes their median data at the three SLs re: reflex threshold, with frequency as the parameter. There is greater reflex adaptation as frequency increases. Also, adaptation tends to begin sooner after stimulus onset for higher frequencies. These data are normalized in Fig. 3.23, in which the point of greatest impedance change is given a value of 100% and the other points are shown as percentages of the maximum impedance change. In this plot the data are shown separately at each frequency with the suprathreshold level as the parameter. In addition to clearly showing the frequency effect, Fig. 3.23 demonstrates that the course of the adaptation function is similar at various levels above reflex threshold, at least up to +18 dB.

Tietze [94,95] proposed that the course of AR adaptation could be described by the time constants of reflex rise time and adaptation. These time constants refer respectively to how long it takes for reflex magnitude to attain 63% of the maximum value (rise) and then to decrease to 63% of it (adaptation); both are measured from the moment of AR onset. The time constants are functions of frequency. Tietze's [95] model describes reflex adaptation by the formula

$$Zn = \frac{1}{1 - \tau_{an}/\tau_{ab}} \left[\exp(-t/\tau_{ab}) - \exp(-t/\tau_{an}) \right]$$

where Zn is the normalized maximum impedance change; τ_{an} and τ_{ab} are the time constants of reflex rise and adaptation, respectively; and t is the time (sec) of reflex rise from onset. Kaplan et al. [85] applied this formula

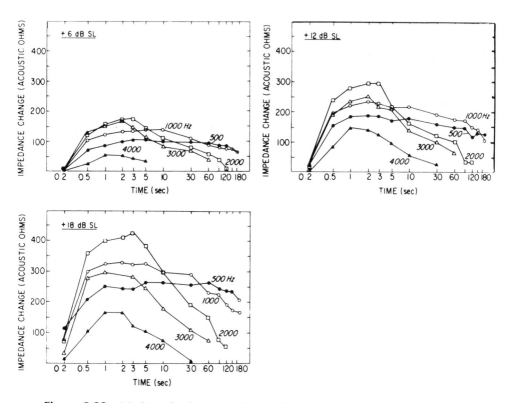

Figure 3.22   Median absolute impedance change (acoustic ohms) as a function of time for three suprareflex threshold levels. (From Kaplan et al. [85], with permission of *Ann. Otol.*)

to their data, using the ratio τ_{an}/τ_{ab} to generate the dotted lines in Fig. 3.23. (Note that, expect at high frequencies where rapid adaptation reduces the maximum impedance change, τ_{an} is generally quite small relative to τ_{ab}.) As Fig. 3.23 shows, Kaplan's data support the exponential adaptation predicted by Tietze's model.

Loudness is the perceptual correlate of the intensity of the acoustic stimulus (see Chap. 11); other things being equal, loudness increases as stimulus level as increased. An abberation of the intensity-loudness relationship is found in patients with cochlear disorders. Once the signal is increased above the impaired threshold of such an ear, the loudness grows at a faster rate than normal in response to increasing stimulus level. This is called loudness recruitment. What has the AR to do with loudness and recruitment? Since both loudness and the AR are related to

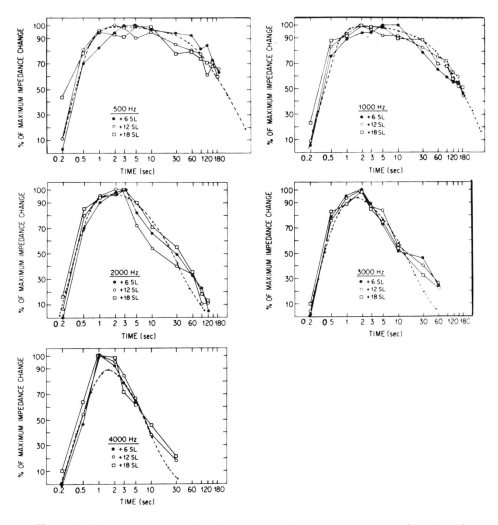

Figure 3.23 Median normalized impedance change (percent) as a function of time for each frequency. (From Kaplan et al. [85], with permission of *Ann. Otol.*)

stimulus intensity, at least some association between them is understandable. The question is whether the AR is a function of loudness.

Metz [57] obtained AR thresholds at lower SLs from patients with presumably cochlear sensorineural hearing loss than from normal subjects. In other words, the spread between the threshold of hearing and the AR threshold was smaller for those with the hearing losses. Since the impaired subjects also had loudness recruitment, Metz proposed that the lower SL of the reflex reflected recruitment. In other words, it was argued that the AR was elicited by the loudness of the signal. Jepsen [59] reported that, while the auditory thresholds of his subjects increased with age, the reflex thresholds tended to decrease, especially at 1000 Hz and above. He attributed this to presbycusis (hearing loss associated with aging), and assumed that it was due to recruitment.

The relationship between loudness and the AR, however, is not nearly as clear-cut as these early findings suggest. Ross [99] compared the equal-loudness and equal-reflex contours of four subjects. The contours were similar for two, while the others had systematic differences between the loudness and AR contours (the loudness curves were flatter). Ross suggested that the latter two equal-loudness contours might have been aberrant, but in fact they were quite similar to those reported by Fletcher and Munson [100], among others.

Margolis and Popelka [61] compared the loudness of a variety of stimuli set to the AR threshold level. There was a range of about 17 dB in the loudness levels, suggesting that the AR is not a manifestation of a critical loudness level. Block and Wightman [101] suggested that the loudness-reflex relationship is supported by their finding of similarly shaped equal-loudness and equal-reflex contours. However, they often found that the same reflex magnitude was elicited by stimulus levels as much as 10 dB apart. Such a spread corresponds to a doubling of loudness [102]; in this light their findings appear to support rather than refute those of Margolis and Popelka. The substantially wider critical bands for the AR than for loudness discussed previously provide a further basis for questioning to concept that the AR is loudness-based.

Returning to patient data, Beedle and Harford [103] found steeper AR growth functions for normal ears than for ears with cochlear dysfunction. This result is, of course, inconsistent with a loudness basis for the reflex. The impact of their data, however, was impaired by the fact that their normal subjects averaged 24 years old, compared to 47 years old for the pathological group. The reflex growth functions of age-matched normal and hearing-impaired subjects were studied by Silman et al. [63]. Examples of their findings are shown in Fig. 3.24. If the reflex were loudness determined, then the function for the impaired groups, although displaced along the intensity axis, would be expected to approach the normal curves at higher stimulus levels. This expectation is based on the notion that loudness recruitment should result in equal loudness for both groups at equal suprathreshold levels. Equal loudness would in turn elicit equal reflex magnitudes at those levels. As the figure shows, this is not the case. Yet, in spite of this point and the previous

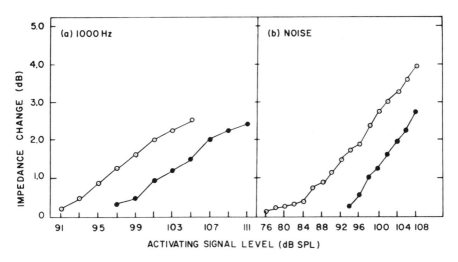

Figure 3.24 Reflex growth as a function of SPL for 1000 Hz (a) and a broad-band noise (b). Open symbols, Normal ears; closed symbols, impaired ears. (Adapted from Silman, Popelka, and Gelfand [63].)

ones, the acoustic reflex-loudness problem remains unresolved and subject to further investigation.

Hellman and Scharf [73] have provided the most extensive and insightful review of this issue to date. They have shown that the arguments (such as those above) against a loudness-reflex relationship are not as convincing as they might seem. Just two examples will be briefly mentioned. Consider first the material in Fig. 3.24, just discussed. These data could be explained by the fact that both loudness and reflex magnitude increase as power functions of the stimulus level at the SPLs where these functions are obtained. Second, they demonstrated that for given subjects, equally loud sounds elicited equal reflex magnitudes when the criteria were defined precisely. Given that both loudness and the acoustic reflex reflect the neural coding of the stimulus level at the periphery, it is thus understandable that the two phenomena should be related. The controversial and unresolved issue is whether one is dependent upon the other. It is apparent that the AR is largely stimulus dependent. Furthermore, it should not be surprising that the parameters of the reflex response reflect the sensory (and neural) processing of relatively intense stimulation. It is equally apparent that the AR is a feedback or control mechanism—although its exact purpose(s) remains unclear. Given these points, what effect does the AR have on energy transmission through the conductive mechanism?

Recall that the AR stiffens the conductive mechanism so that sound is reflected at the eardrum [76]. Since the effect of stiffness is inversely related to frequency, we would expect the AR to affect middle ear transmission most strongly at low frequencies.

Smith [104] and Reger [105] compared the pure-tone thresholds of human subjects to the thresholds during voluntary contractions of the middle ear muscles. Thresholds were shifted by about 20–40 dB at 125–500 Hz, and by 15 dB at 1000 Hz, and there was little or no change at higher frequencies. While the expected frequency relation is maintained, voluntary contractions may not yield the same transmission loss as the AR [105]. Perhaps the most impressive data on how the AR affects middle ear transmission come from animal studies.

The cochlear microphonic (CM) is an electrical potential of the cochlea which is proportional to the intensity of the stimulus over a wide dynamic range. This is discussed in Chap. 4. Changes in the magnitude of the CM will thus reflect remarkably well the transmission loss resulting from the AR. Simmons [106] found that, while the AR in cats shifted the CM response in a manner that decreased with frequency up to 7000 Hz, the effect of the reflex was greatest below 2000 Hz and was only slight at higher frequencies. Figure 3.25 shows the change in the CM due to stapedius muscle contraction in the cat [107]. Møller [107] found that impedance change data and CM findings in response to the AR were within 5 dB over a substantial portion of the frequency range. The figure shows that the AR affects primarily the frequencies below about 2000

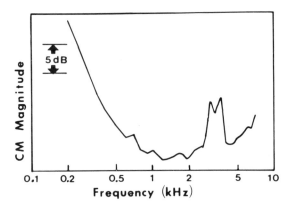

Figure 3.25   Effect of the acoustic reflex on transmission in the cat's middle ear. (Adapted from Møller [107].)

Hz. Similar low-frequency changes have been reported in response to electrically elicited contractions of the tensor tympani [108].

Several recent studies [109–112] have dealt with the effects of middle ear muscle contractions on absolute thresholds and loudness in humans. Rabinowitz [109] has reported a 10 dB change in the low-frequency transmission characteristics of the middle ear due to the AR. However, Morgan and Dirks [111] found that reflex-eliciting stimulus levels up to 100 dB SPL did not result in a change in the loudness of a test tone presented to the opposite ear. Stimuli greater than 100 dB SPL caused a decrease in loudness for low-frequency tones but not the 1500 Hz. Furthermore, Morgan et al. [112] demonstrated that the absolute thresholds are not affected by the AR. These findings do not fully support earlier observations. It may be that there is no clear relationship between the amount of impedance change and the amount of threshold shift caused by the reflex [112]. This lack of correspondence between the animal and human data might also reflect species differences.

Reflex Theories

There are many theories and speculations about the purpose of the acoustic reflex. Space and scope preclude more than a cursory review here; and the reader is urged to consult Simmons [30], Jepsen [59], and Borg, Counter, and Rosler [113].

Since the reflex is elicited by relatively high stimulus levels, and its magnitude grows with increasing stimulus level, one would expect that a primary purpose of the AR would be protection of the cochlea from damaging stimulation. This "protection theory" is weakened by the facts that the latency and adaptation of the reflex cause it to respond too slowly to sudden sounds, and make it inefficient against prolonged sounds. Also, sounds intense enough to elicit the AR are virtually nonexistent in nature. Nevertheless, the protection offered by the AR is a beneficial side effect if not the main purpose.

The "accommodation theory" states that the action of the two middle ear muscles modifies the conductive mechanism so as to optimize the absorption of sound energy. According to the "fixation theory," the intratympanic muscles help keep the ossicles in proper position and appropriately rigid, particularly at high frequencies when acceleration is great. Other theories have asserted that these muscles contribute to changes in labyrinthine pressure and to the formation of aural overtones.

Simmons [30] found a sharp antiresonance peak around 4000 Hz in the middle ear transmission function of cats whose intratympanic muscles were removed, as well as in normal cats under anesthesia. Normal, waking cats whose intratympanic muscles have normal tonus showed greatly reduced dips in this region. Simmons reasoned that tonus of the middle ear muscles smooths the frequency response of the conductive system. He suggested that modulation of muscle tonus would have the effect of enhancing attention by changing the intensity and frequency characteristics of environmental sounds. This modulation would be analogous to the constant motion of the extraocular muscles in vision. Also, several skeletal movements as well as unexpected and novel environmental sounds elicit the AR. Since the reflex mainly attenuates low frequencies, and since most of an organism's own physiologic noises are low in frequency, such a reflex response would have the effect of reducing the animal's internal noise. A better signal-to-noise ratio would result, which is of obvious importance to the survival of any species, whether predator or prey. This idea agrees with Borg's [78] position that the qualitative purpose of the AR is to attenuate low-frequency sounds, thereby improving the auditory system's dynamic range.

REFERENCES

1. G. Bekesy and W. A. Rosenblith, The mechanical properties of the ear, in *Handbook of Experimental Psychology* (S. S. Stevens, ed.), Wiley, New York, 1958, pp. 1075–1115.
2. M. Gardner, Some monaural and binaural facets of median plane localization, *J. Acoust. Soc. Amer. 54*, 1489–1495 (1973).
3. M. Gardner and R. Gardner, Problem of localization in the median plane: Effect of pinnae cavity occlusion, *J. Acoust. Soc. Amer. 53*, 400–408 (1973).
4. D. Wright, J. Hebrank, and B. Wilson, Pinna reflections as cues for localization, *J. Acoust. Soc. Amer. 56*, 957–962 (1974).
5. J. Hebrank and D. Wright, Spectral cues used in the localization of sound sources in the median plane, *J. Acoust. Soc. Amer. 56*, 1829–1834 (1974).
6. J. Blauert, Sound localization in the median plane, *Acoustica 22*, 205–213 (1969).
7. D. W. Batteau, The role of the pinna in human localization, *Proc. Roy. Soc (London) B168*, 158–180 (1967).
8. F. M. Wiener and D. A. Ross. The pressure distribution in the auditory canal in a progressive sound field, *J. Acoust. Soc. Amer. 18*, 401–408 (1946).
9. E. A. G. Shaw, Transformation of sound pressure level from the free field to the eardrum in the horizontal plane. *J. Acoust. Soc. Amer. 56*, 1848–1861 (1974).
10. S. Mehrgardt and V. Mellert, Transformation characteristics of the external human ear, *J. Acoust. Soc. Amer. 61*, 1567–1576 (1977).
11. P. Dallos, *The Auditory Periphery*, Academic Press, New York, 1973.

12. M. R. Stinton and D. W. Lawton, Specification of the geometry of the human ear canal for the prediction of sound-pressure level distribution, *J. Accoust. Soc. Am. 85*, 2492–2530 (1989).

13. E. A. G. Shaw and M. M. Vaillancourt, Transformation of sound-pressure level from the free field to the eardrum presented in numerical form, *J. Acoust. Soc. Am. 78*, 1120–1123 (1985).

14. S. M. Khanna and M. R. Stinton, Specification of the acoustical input to the ear at high frequencies, *J. Acoust. Soc. Am. 77*, 577–589 (1985).

15. R. D. Rabbitt and M. H. Holmes, A fibrous dynamic continuum model of the tympanic membrane, *J. Accoust. Soc. Am. 80*, 1716–1728 (1986).

16. G. R. J. Funnell, W. F. Decraemer, and S. M. Khanna, On the damped frequency response of a finite-element model of the cat eardrum, *J. Acoust. Soc. Am. 81*, 1851–1859 (1987).

17. M. R. Stinton, and S. M. Khanna, Sound propagation in the ear canal and coupling to the eardrum, with measurements on model systems, *J. Acoust. Soc. Am. 85*, 2481–2491 (1989).

18. J. Zwislocki, The acoustic middle ear function, in *Acoustic Impedance and Admittance—The Measurement of Middle Ear Function* (A. S. Feldman and L. A. Wilber, eds.), Williams & Wilkins, Baltimore, 1976, pp. 66–77.

19. J. Zwislocki, Analysis of the middle-ear function. Part I: Input impedance, *J. Acoust. Soc. Amer. 34*, 1514–1523 (1962).

20. J. Zwislocki, The role of the external and middle ear in sound transmission, in *The Nervous System* (D. B. Tower and E. L. Eagles, eds.), Vol. 3: *Human Communication and Its Disorders*, Raven Press, New York, 1975, pp. 45–55.

21. H. Helmholtz, Die Mechanik der Gehorknöchelchen und des Trommelfells, *Pflüg. Arch. Ges. Physiol. I*, 1–60 (1868).

22. E. G. Wever and M. Lawrence, *Physiological Acoustics*, Princeton Univ. Press, Princeton, New Jersey, 1954.

23. J. Tonndorf and S. M. Khanna, The role of the tympanic membrane in middle ear transmission, *Ann Otol. 79*, 743–753 (1970).

24. G. Bekesy, *Experiments in Hearing*, McGraw-Hill, New York, 1960.

25. E. Barany, A contribution to the physiology of bone conduction, *Acta Otol.*, Suppl 26 (1938).

26. J. Guinan and W. T. Peake, Middle ear characteristics of anesthesized cats, *J. Acoust. Soc. Amer. 41*, 1237–1261 (1967).

27. J. Tonndorf, S. M. Khanna, and B. J. Fingerhood, The input impedance of the inner ear in cats, *Ann, Otol. 75*, 752–763 (1966).

28. A. R. Møller, improved technique for detailed measurements of the middle-ear impedance, *J. Acoust. Soc. Amer. 32*, 250–257 (1960).

29. J. D. Miller, C. S. Watson, and W. P. Covell, Deafening effects of noise on the cat, *Acta Otol.*, Suppl, 176 (1963).

30. F. B. Simmons, Perceptual theories of middle ear function, *Ann. Otol. 73*, 724–740 (1964).

31. F. N. Wiener, R. R. Pfeiffer, and A. S. N. Backus, On the pressure transfor-

mation by the head and auditory meatus of the cat, *Acta Otol.* 61, 255–269 (1966).

32. P. Dallos, Low-frequency auditory characteristics: Species dependencies, *J. Acoust. Soc. Amer. 48,* 489–499 (1970).

33. G. Bekesy, Vibrations of the head in a sound field and its role in hearing by bone conduction, *J. Acoust. Soc. Amer. 20,* 749–760 (1948).

34. G. Bekesy, Zur Theories des Hörens bei der Schallaufnahme durch Knochenleitung, *Poggendorff's Annln Phys. Chem. 13,* Ser. 5. 111–136 (1932).

35. K. Lowy, Cancellation of the electrical cochlear response with air- and bone-conduction. *J. Acoust. Soc. Amer. 14,* 156–158 (1942).

36. J. Tonndorf et al., Bone conduction: Studies in experimental animals; A collection of papers, *Acta Otol., Suppl 213* (1966).

37. J. Tonndorf, A new concepts of bone conduction, *Arch Otol. 87,* 49–54 (1968).

38. J. Tonndorf, Compressional bone conduction in cochlear models, *J. Acoust. Soc. Amer. 34,* 1127–1132 (1962).

39. R. Carhart, Clinical application of bone conduction audiometry, *Arch. Otol. 51,* 798–808 (1950).

40. V. Hensen, Beobachtungen über die Thätigkeit des Trommellspanners bei Hund und Katze, *Arch, Anat, Physiol. II,* 312–319 (1878).

41. J. Pollack, Über die Function des Musculus tensor tympani, *Med. Jahrbuch 82,* 555–582 (1886).

42. T. Kato, Zur Physiologie der Binnenmuskeln des Ohres, *Pflüg. Arch. ges. Physiol. 150,* 569–625 (1913).

43. E. Lüscher, Die Function des Musculus stapedius beim Menschen, *Zeitsch. Hals-Nasen-und-Ohrenheilkunde 23,* 105–132 (1929).

44. J. R. Lindsay, H. Kobrack, and H. B. Perlman, Relation of the stapedius reflex to hearing sensitivity in man, *Arch, Otol. 23,* 671–678 (1936).

45. A. B. Potter, Function of the stapedius muscle, *Ann. Otol. 45,* 639–643 (1936).

46. K. Terkildsen, Movements of the eardrum following inter-aural muscle reflexes, *Arch, Otol. 66,* 484–488 (1957).

47. K. Terkildsen, Acoustic reflexes of the human musculus tensor tympani, *Acta Otol., Suppl. 158* (1960).

48. E. S. Mendelson, A sensitive method for registration of human intratympanic muscle reflexes, *J. Appl. Physiol. 11,* 499–502 (1957).

49. E. S. Mendelson, Improved method for studying tympanic reflexes in man, *J. Acoust. Soc. Amer. 33,* 146–152 (1961).

50. O. Metz, The acoustic impedance measured on normal and pathological ears, *Acta Otol., Suppl. 63* (1946).

51. J. Zwislocki, An acoustic method for clinical examination of the ear, *J. Speech Hearing Res. 6,* 303–314 (1963).

52. K. Terkildsen and S. S. Nielsen, An electroacoustic measuring bridge for clinical use, *Arch. Otol. 72,* 339–346 (1960).

53. O. Jepsen, Studies on the acoustic stapedius reflex in man: Measurements

of the acoustic impedance of the tympanic membrane in normal individuals and in patients with peripheral facial palsy, Thesis, Universitetsforlaget, Aarhus, Denmark, 1955.

54. I. Klockhoff, Middle-ear muscle reflexes in man, *Acta Otol.*, Suppl. 164 (1961).

55. A. Feldman, A report of further impedance studies of the acoustic reflex, *J. Speech Hearing Res. 10*, 616–622 (1967).

56. G. Djupesland, Middle ear muscle reflexes elicited by acoustic and non-acoustic stimulation, *Acta Otol.*, Suppl 188 (1964).

57. O. Metz, Threshold of reflex contractions of muscles of the middle ear and recruitment of loudness, *Arch. Otol. 55*, 536–593 (1952).

58. A. Møller, The sensitivity of contraction of tympanic muscle in man, *Ann. Otol. 71*, 86–95 (1962).

59. O. Jepsen, The middle ear muscle reflexes in man, in *Modern Developments in Audiology* (J. Jerger, E.), Academic Press, New York, 1963, pp. 194–239.

60. J. Jerger, Clinical experience with impedance audiometry, *Arch. Otol. 92*, 311–321 (1970).

61. R. Margolis and G. Popelka, Loudness and the acoustic reflex, *J. Acoust Soc. Amer. 58*, 1330–1332 (1975).

62. R. H. Wilson and L. M. McBride, Threshold and growth of the acoustic reflex, *J. Acoust. Soc. Amer. 63*, 147–154 (1978).

63. S. Silman, G. Popelka, and S. A. Gelfand, Effect of sensorineural hearing loss on acoustic stapedius reflex growth functions, *J. Acoust. Soc. Amer. 64*, 1406–1411 (1978).

64. S. A. Gelfand, The contralateral acoustic-reflex threshold, in *The Acoustic Reflex: Basic Principles and Clinical Applications* (S. Silman, E.), Academic Press, New York, 1984, pp. 137–186.

65. L. Dutsch, The threshold of the stapedius reflex for pure tone and noise stimuli, *Acta Otol. 74*, 248–251 (1972).

66. J. L. Peterson and G. Liden, Some static characteristics of the stapedial muscle reflex, *Audiology 11*, 97–114 (1972).

67. A. Møller, Bilateral contraction of the tympanic muscles in man examined by measuring acoustic impedance-change, *Ann. Otol. 70*, 735–753 (1961).

68. K. W. Green, and R. H. Margolis, The ipsilateral acoustic reflex, in *The Acoustic Reflex: Basic Principles and Clinical Applications* (S. Silman, ed.), Academic Press, New York, 1984, pp. 275–299.

69. G. Flottrop, G. Djupesland, and F. Winther, The acoustic stapedius reflex in relation to critical bandwidth, *J. Acoust. Soc. Amer. 49*, 457–461 (1971).

70. G. Popelka, R. Karlovich, and T. Wiley, Acoustic reflex and critical bandwidth, *J. Acoust. Soc. Amer. 55*, 883–885 (1974).

71. G. Djupesland and J. Zwislocki, On the critical band in the acoustic stapedius reflex, *J. Acoust. Soc. Amer. 54*, 1157–1159 (1973).

72. G. Popelka, R. Margolis, and T. Wiley, Effects of activating signal bandwidth on acoustic-reflex thresholds. *J. Acoust. Soc. Amer. 59*, 153–159 (1976).

73. R. Hellman, and B. Scharf, Acoustic reflex and loudness, in *The Acoustic*

Reflex: Basic Principles and Clinical Applications (S. Silman, ed.), Academic Press, New York, 1984, pp. 469–516.

74. O. Metz, Studies on the contraction of the tympanic muscles as indicated by changes in impedance of the ear, *Acta Otol. 39*, 397–405 (1951).

75. A. Møller, Intra-aural muscle contraction in man examined by measuring acoustic impedance of the ear, *Laryngoscope 68*, 48–62 (1958).

76. P. Dallos, Dynamics of the acoustic reflex: Phenomenological aspects, *J. Acoust. Soc. Amer. 36*, 2175–2183 (1964).

77. I. Hung and P. Dallos, Study of the acoustic reflex in human beings: I. Dynamic characteristics, *J. Acoust. Soc. Amer. 52*, 1168–1180 (1972).

78. E. Borg, Dynamic characteristics of the intra-aural muscle reflex, in *Acoustic Impedance and Admittance—The Measurement of Middle Ear Function* (A. S. Feldman and L. A. Wilber, eds.), Williams & Wilkins, Baltimore, 1976, pp. 236–299.

79. J. E. Zakrisson, E. Borg, and S. Blom, The acoustic impedance change as a measure of stapedius muscle activity in man: A methodological study with electromyography, *Acta Otol. 78*, 357–364 (1974).

80. A. Bosatra, M. Russolo and C. A. Silverman, Acoustic-reflex latency: State of the art, in *The Acoustic Reflex: Basic Principles and Clinical Applications* (S. Silman, ed.), Academic Press, New York, 1984, pp. 301–328.

81. S. A. Gelfand, S. Silman, and C. A. Silverman, Temporal summation in acoustic reflex growth functions, *Acta Otol. 91*, 177–182 (1981).

82. S. Silman and S. A. Gelfand, Effect of sensorineural hearing loss on the stapedius reflex growth function in the elderly, *J. Acoust. Soc. Am. 69*, 1099–1106 (1981).

83. S. Silman, Magnitude and growth of the acoustic reflex, in *The Acoustic Reflex: Basic Principles and Clinical Applications* (S. Silman, ed.), Academic Press, New York, 1984, pp. 225–274.

84. S. Silman, Growth function of the stapedius reflex in normal heating subjects and in subjects with sensorineural hearing loss due to cochlear dysfunction, Ph.D. Dissertation, New York University, New York, 1976.

85. H. Kaplan, S. Gilman, and D. Dirks, Properties of acoustic reflex adaptation, *Ann. Otol. 86*, 348–356 (1977).

86. D. Cunningham, Admittance values associated with acoustic reflex decay, *J. Amer. Aud. Soc. I*, 197–205 (1976).

87. E. Borg and A. Møller, The acoustic middle ear reflex in man and in anesthesized rabbits, *Acta Otol. 65*, 575–585 (1968).

88. G. Djupesland and J. Zwislocki, Effect on temporal summation on the human stapedius reflex, *Acta Otol. 71*, 262–265 (1971).

89. C. Woodford, D. Henderson, R. Hamernick, and A. Feldman, Threshold-duration function of the acoustic reflex in man, *Audiology 14*, 53–62 (1975).

90. G. Djupesland, A. Sundby, and G. Flottrop, Temporal summation in the acoustic stapedius reflex mechanism, *Acta Otol. 76*, 305–312 (1973).

91. J. Jerger, L. Mauldin, and N. Lewis, Temporal summation of the acoustic reflex, *Audiology 16*, 177–200 (1977).

92. R. Lorente de Nó, The function of the central acoustic nuclei examined by means of the acoustic reflexes, *Laryngoscope 45*, 573–595 (1935).

93. E. Borg, A quantitative study of the effects of the acoustic stapedius reflex on sound transmission through the middle ear, *Acta Otol. 66*, 461–472 (1968).

94. G. Tietze, Zum zeitverhalten des akustischen reflexes bei reizung mit dauertonen, *Arch. Klin. Exp. Ohren. Nasen. Kehlkpfheilkd 193*, 43–52 (1969).

95. G. Tietze, Einge eigenschaften des akustischen reflexes bei reizung mit tonimpulsen, *Arch. Klin. Exp. Ohren. Nasen. Kehlkopfheilkd 193*, 53–69 (1969).

96. T. L. Wiley and T. S. Karlovich, Acoustic reflex response to sustained signals, *J. Speech Hearing Res. 18*, 148–157 (1975).

97. R. H. Wilson, J. K. McCollough, and D. J. Lilly, Acoustic reflex adaptation: Morphology and half-life data for subjects with normal hearing, *J. Speech Hear. Res. 27*, 586–595 (1984).

98. R. H. Wilson, J. E. Shanks, and D. J. Lilly, Acoustic-reflex adaptation, in *The Acoustic Reflex: Basic Principles and Clinical Applications* (S. Silman, ed.), Academic Press, New York, 1984, pp. 329–386.

99. S. Ross, On the relation between the acoustic reflex and loudness, *J. Acoust. Soc. Amer. 43*, 768–779 (1968).

100. H. Fletcher and W. A. Munson, Loudness: Its definition, measurement and calculation, *J. Acoust. Soc. Amer. 5*, 82–108 (1933).

101. M. G. Block and F. L. Wightman, A statistically based measure of the acoustic reflex and its relation to stimulus loudness, *J. Acoust. Soc. Amer. 61*, 120–125 (1977).

102. S. S. Stevens, The direct estimation of sensory magnitude—loudness, *Amer. J. Psychol. 69*, 1–25 (1956).

103. R. K. Beedle and E. R. Harford, A comparison of acoustic reflex growth in normal and pathological ears, *J. Speech Hearing Res. 16*, 271–280 (1973).

104. H. D. Smith, Audiometric effects of voluntary contraction of the tensor tympani muscle, *Arch. Otol. 38*, 369–372 (1943).

105. S. N. Reger, Effect of middle ear muscle action on certain psycho-physical measurements, *Ann. Otol. 69*, 1179–1198 (1960).

106. F. B. Simmons, Middle ear muscle activity at moderate sound levels, *Ann. Otol. 68*, 1126–1143 (1959).

107. A. R. Møller, An experimental study of the acoustic impedance and its transmission properties, *Acta. Otol. 60*, 129–149 (1965).

108. A. Starr, Regulatory mechanisms of the auditory pathway, in *Modern Neurology* (S. Locke, ed.), Little, Brown & Co., Boston, 1969.

109. W. M. Rabinowitz, Acoustic-reflex effects on the input admittance and transfer characteristics of the human middle-ear, unpublished Ph.D. dissertation, MIT, Cambridge, Massachusetts, 1976.

110. M. Loeb and A. J. Riopelle, Influence of loud contralateral stimulation on the threshold and perceived loudness of low-frequency tones, *J. Acoust. Soc. Amer. 32*, 602–610 (1960).

111. D. E. Morgan and D. D. Dirks, Influence of middle ear muscle contraction on pure tone suprathreshold loudness judgments, *J. Acoust. Soc. Amer. 57,* 411–420 (1975).

112. D. E. Morgan, D. D. Dirks, and C. Kamm, The influence of middle-ear contraction on auditory threshold for selected pure tones, *J. Acoust. Soc. Amer. 63,* 1896–1903 (1978).

113. E. Borg, S. A. Counter, and G. Rosler, Theories of middle-ear muscle function, in *The Acoustic Reflex: Basic Principles and Clinical Applications* (S. Silman, ed.), Academic Press, New York, 1984, pp. 63–99.

4

Cochlear Mechanisms and Processes

We have already discussed the manner in which the conductive mechanism influences the signal and transmits it to the inner ear. In this chapter we will concentrate upon the sensory mechanism. The cochlea may be conceived of as a transducer that converts the vibratory stimulus into a form usable by the nervous system. However, this is far from the whole picture. We shall see that the cochlea performs a considerable amount of analysis, that it is the major source of aural distortion, and that it is involved in processes that are active as well passive.

Before proceding to examine the processes of the cochlea, it is desirable to briefly review the traditional theories of hearing as well as some principles of sensory receptor action. These two topics provide a useful general framework as well as an important historical perspective within which the student can consider the material that follows.

THEORIES OF HEARING

The study of the auditory system is practically and historically intertwined with the traditional theories of hearing. Broadly speaking, these theories fall into two general categories—place (resonance) theories and frequency (temporal, periodicity) theories—as well as the combined place-frequency theory. A detailed review of these theories goes beyond the current scope or intent; the student is referred to Wever's [1] classic work, *Theory of Hearing,* for an excellent critical review of these theories.

Place Theories

Although place (or resonance) theories existed since the beginning of the 1600s, modern versions began with the resonance theory of Helmholtz [2] in the late 1800s. Helmholtz relied to a large extent upon Ohm's auditory "law" and Müller's doctrine of specific nerve energies. Ohm's auditory law states that the ear performs a Fourier analysis upon complex periodic sounds; i.e., that it breaks the complex wave down into its components regardless of their phase relationships. A major problem with Ohm's auditory law is that it precludes temporal analysis. We shall see, however, that the auditory system is sensitive to temporal as well as frequency parameters. Müller's doctrine refers to the specificity of the different senses. It states that the neural signal coming from the ear is interpreted as sound whether the actual stimulus was a tone or a blow to the head; the eye elicits a visual image whether the stimulus is light or pressure on the eyeball, etc. This doctrine appears to hold on the periphery although there are dramatic commonalities among the various senses in terms of their fundamental principles of operation (see Action of Sensory Receptors, below) and central mechanisms.

The mechanism of the place theory proposed by Helmholtz is relatively simple and straightforward. It assumes that the basilar membrane is composed of a series of segments, each of which resonates in response to a particular frequency. Thus, an incoming stimulus results in the vibration of those parts of the basilar membrane whose natural frequencies correspond to the components of the stimulus. Since these resonators are arranged by place along the cochlear partition, the precise place of the vibrating segment would signal the existence of a component at the natural frequency of that location. Nonlinear distortions introduced by the ear (such as combination tones due to the interaction of two stimulus tones, or harmonics of the stimulus tone) are viewed as being generated by a nonlinear response of the middle ear mechanism. These distortion products are then transmitted to the cochlea, where they cause vibrations at the places whose resonant frequencies correspond to the frequency of the combination tone (or harmonic). The distortion product is thus perceived as though it were present in the original signal.

Such a strict place theory is faced with several serious problems. To begin with, in order to account for the sharp frequency tuning of the inner ear, the theory demands that the basilar membrane contain segments which are under differing amounts of tension in a manner analogous to the tension on variously tuned piano strings. However, Bekesy [3] demonstrated that the basilar membrane is under no tension at all.

A second problem is that strict place theory cannot account for the perception of the "missing fundamental" (Chap. 12), the phenomenon in which the presence of harmonics of a tone (e.g. 1100, 1200, and 1300 Hz) results in the perception of the fundamental frequency (100 Hz) even though the latter is not physically present.

Place theory is also plagued by the relationship between the sharpness of a system's tuning and the persistence of its response. In order for the ear to achieve the required fine frequency discriminations, the various segments of the basilar membrane must be sharply tuned. In other words, they could each respond only to a very narrow range of frequencies. A segment could not respond to higher or lower frequencies, or else the necessary discriminations would be impossible. The problem is that such a narrowly tuned system must have very low damping—its response will take a relatively long time to die away after the stimulus stops. In other words, if there were sharp tuning of the resonators along the basilar membrane, then their responses would persist long after the stimulus has ceased. This situation would cause an interminable echo in our ears, precluding any functional hearing. On the other hand, if the resonators were less sharply tuned, they would not have the persistence problem, but they would be unable to support the necessary fine frequency discriminations.

Place theory ascribed aural distortions to the middle ear. However, as we saw in the last chapter, it is now known that the middle ear operates in a manner that is astoundingly linear. Moreover, we shall see later in this chapter that the inner ear is the site of active processes, and that most nonlinear distortions are attributable to the cochlea. These notions are obviously inconsistent with strict place theory.

A variety of other place theories followed that of Helmholtz [2]. Of particular interest is the traveling wave theory of Nobel laureate Georg von Bekesy [3]. Bekesy's traveling wave theory has been confirmed by many investigators using a multiplicity of approaches, and is discussed in detail later in this chapter.

Frequency Theories

Frequency (or temporal) theory proposes that the peripheral hearing mechanism does not perform a frequency analysis, but rather that it transmits the signal to the central auditory nervous system for processing. Such theories have been referred to as "telephone theories" by analogy with the manner in which a telephone signal is transmitted in toto. Though there are several such theories, Rutherford's [4] telephone theory, proposed not long after Helmholtz's theory, has been the best known. This theory states that the cochlea is not frequency-sensitive along its length, but rather that all parts respond to all frequencies. The job of the hair cells is simply to transmit all parameters of the stimulus waveform to the auditory nerve, and analysis is performed at higher levels.

Since a neuron can only respond in an all-or-none manner, the only way in which it can of itself transmit frequency information is to discharge the same number of times per second as there are cycles in the stimulus (e.g., it must fire 720 times per second to transmit a 720 Hz tone). Frequency theory thus presumes that auditory nerve fibers can fire fast enough to represent this information. There is no problem at low frequencies; however, an upper limit on the number of discharges per second is imposed by the absolute refractory period of the neuron. The absolute refractory period is the time required after discharging for the cell to reestablish the polarization it needs to fire again; it lasts about 1 msec. The fiber cannot fire during the absolute refractory period, no matter how intensely stimulated. This period is followed by a relative refractory period during which the neuron will respond provided the stimulus is strong enough. The 1 msec absolute refractory period corresponds to a maximum firing rate of 1000 times per second. Thus, simple frequency theory is hard pressed to explain how sounds higher in frequency than about 1000 Hz can be transmitted by the auditory nerve and perceived by the listener.

A second problem of the telephone theories is that damage to the apical parts of the cochlea result in high-frequency hearing loss. This is contradictory to frequency theory, which states that the different parts of the cochlea are not differentially sensitive to frequency. Furthermore, we shall see that there is actually a remarkable degree of frequency selectivity along the cochlear partition.

Rutherford's telephone theory was by no means the only frequency theory of hearing, but it serves to demonstrate the fundamental approach and associated problems. The most important modification of frequency theory was the volley principle advanced by Wever [1]. Instead of suggesting that any one neuron must carry all of the information burden, the volley principle states that groups of fibers cooperate to represent the stimulus frequency in the auditory nerve. This is shown in Fig. 4.1. The sinusoid (sound wave) at the top of the figure has a frequency too high to be represented by a series of spike discharges from a single auditory nerve fiber. Instead, fibers work in groups so that in the total response of the group there is a spike corresponding to each cycle of the stimulus. This cooperation is accomplished by having each individual neuron respond to cycles separated

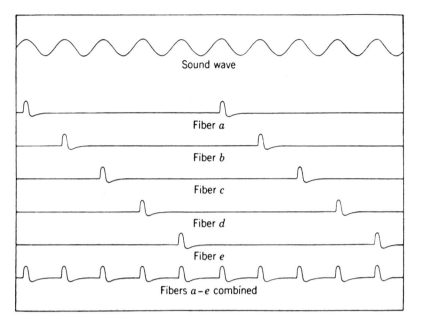

Figure 4.1 Diagrammatic representation of the volley principle (see text). (From Wever [1], *Theory of Hearing,* Dover, 1949.)

by some interval. In Fig. 4.1 this interval is every 5 cycles. Thus, fiber a discharges in response to cycles 1, 6, and 11; fiber b to cycles 2, 7, and 12; fiber c to 3, 8, and 13; etc. The result is that each cycle is represented by a spike in the combined response of the fiber group (bottom line in the figure). We shall see in Chap. 5 that the discharges of auditory nerve fibers do appear to follow the periodicity of the stimulus for frequencies as high as about 4000–5000 Hz. However, these responses are probabilistic rather than one-to-one.

Place-Volley Theory

Even at this early point it should be apparent that neither the place nor frequency theory alone can explain the selectivity of the ear. Both are operative. A frequency or periodicity mechanism is most important for low frequencies, while a place mechanism is paramount for high-frequency representation [1,5]. The question is not one of where the "cutoff points" are, since these do not exist. As we shall see in the following chapters, place coding below approximately 300–400 Hz is too broad to reasonably account for frequency discrimination, and periodicity coding is not supported for frequencies above roughly 4000–5000 Hz. Frequency coding in the wide range between these two extremes appears to occur by the interaction of both mechanisms.

ACTION OF SENSORY RECEPTORS

The auditory system is one of several specialized sensory systems. Although there is specificity of the senses at the periphery, there are nevertheless remarkable similarities among them. The following is a brief overview of sensory receptor action [6,7,8] with particular reference to the ear.

Davis [6] proposed a general plan of sensory receptor action, which is outlined schematically in Fig. 4.2. This model describes how external stimulus energy is transmitted and coded into a form which is usable by the central nervous system. The sensory neuron is common to all sen-

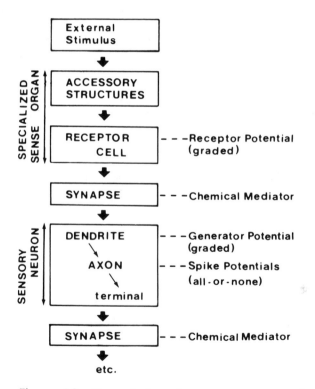

Figure 4.2 General plan of sensory receptor action (efferent feedback not shown). (Adapted from Davis [6].)

sory systems, although specialized receptor cells (sense organ) and accessory structures may or may not be present, and are different for the various senses. In the ear, the conductive mechanisms and the parts of the cochlea other than the hair cells constitute the accessory structures. The hair cells are the specialized receptors for hearing.

The accessory structures assist in the action of the sense organ, but do not actually enter directly into the sensory transduction process, per se. In other words, the conductive and cochlear structures have the hair cell to do its job, but are not themselves receptors. In the ear, the accessory structures carry out a large variety of vital functions. They receive, amplify, and analyze the stimulus, and convert it into a form usable by the hair cells. They also perform feedback and inhibitory functions (under the control of efferent neurons), and protect the sensory receptors from external damage.

The receptor cell transduces the stimulus and transmit it to the afferent neuron, an electrochemical event. Electrical potentials associated with this process can be detected within the hair cells and outside of them as receptor potentials. These receptor potentials are graded, meaning that their magnitudes depend upon the intensity of the stimulus. The potential reflects the activity of the sensory cell, but does not directly transmit information to the neuron. The receptor cell also emits a chemical mediator which is transmitted across the synapse between the hair cell and the afferent neuron. It is this chemical mediator which excites the neuron.

Exactly what substance constitutes the neurotransmitter from the hair cells to the afferent auditory neurons is still not firmly established. However, the amino acid glutamate is the most likely candidate. Acetylcholine is accepted as the efferent mediator in the cochlea. A detailed discussion of neurotransmitters in the cochlea is provided in a recent review by Klink [9].

The neuron's dendrite receives an amount of chemical mediator from the hair cell, which elicits a graded postsynaptic potential. The postsynaptic potential is called a generator potential because it provides the electrical stimulus which triggers the all-or-none spike discharges from the axon. When the magnitude of the generator potential is great enough, it activates the initial segment of the axon, which in turn produces the spike potential (nerve impulse). The material in Chap. 5 on the activity of the auditory nerve is based upon these action potentials. The spikes travel down the axon to its terminus, where the presynaptic endings emit a chemical mediator. This chemical mediator crosses the synaptic junction to excite the dendrites of the next neuron, and the process is repeated.

TRAVELING WAVES

Classic resonance theory envisioned the basilar membrane to be under varying degrees of tension along its length to account for frequency tuning by place. However, Bekesy [3]* demonstrated that the basilar membrane is not under tension at all. Instead, its elasticity per unit area is essentially uniform, while there is a widening of the membrane with distance along the cochlea from base to apex (see Fig. 2.13). This widening of the membrane results in a gradation of stiffness along the cochlear partition such that the membrane is about 100 times stiffer near the stapes that at the helicotrema. Because of this stiffness gradient, stimulation of the cochlea results in the formation of a pressure wave that travels from the base toward the apex. In fact, the traveling wave proceeds toward the helicotrema regardless of where the stimulus is applied.

Before examining the details of the traveling wave, let us explore why it occurs. To begin with, the wavelengths of all audible sounds are much larger than the length of the outstretched cochlea. The result is that the pressure exerted on the cochlear partition is uniform over its length. The stiffness gradient of the basilar membrane causes it to act as a series of low-pass filters. Thus, no matter where applied, successively higher frequencies can only initiate vibrations of the cochlear duct closer and closer to the base (where they fall within the passband) [10]. Since the partition's impedance is composed of both stiffness and resistive components[†] toward the base, and virtually only of resistance toward the apex, the traveling wave is propagated up the partition from places of greater impedance to places of lesser impedance. The speed of the traveling wave decreases with distance from the stapes as it proceeds up the cochlear duct [3].

The pendulum analogy suggested by Bekesy [3] should make the nature of the traveling wave clear. Suppose there is a rod to which a series of progressively longer pendulums are attached (Fig. 4.3). Each pendulum has its own natural frequency; the shorter the string the higher the resonant frequency. We may think of each pedulum as representing a place along the basilar membrane, with the length of the pendulum string corresponding to the stiffness gradient. A driving force is supplied by swinging the heavy pendulum rigidly attached to the rod. If the rod is rotated back and forth at a particular frequency, the resulting stimulus is applied over the entire rod just as the pressure from a sound

---

*Much of Bekesy's work is reproduced in his book *Experiments in Hearing* [3]. For simplicity, this reference will be cited whenever possible.

[†]Refer to Chap. 1 for an overview of the components of impedance.

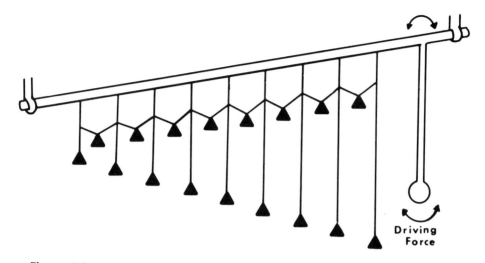

Figure 4.3 Pendulum analogy of traveling wave motion. (Adapted from various drawings by Bekesy [3].)

stimulus is exerted over the entire cochlear duct. The motion of the rod will cause the pendulum to swing at the stimulus frequency. Of course, the closer the natural frequency of a particular pendulum is to the frequency being applied to the rod, the larger will be its amplitude of swing. There will thus be a particular pendulum that swings with maximum amplitude for each frequency applied to the rod; and changing the frequency at which the rod rocks will move the location of maximum swing to the pendulum whose resonant frequency corresponds to the new stimulus frequency. Note at this point that each pendulum is connected to its neighbor, so that the vibrations of the pendulums interact. The different string lengths cause phase differences between the pendulums, which produces waves. The result is that a sinusoidal motion applied to the rod causes a wave which travels from shorter (higher frequency) to longer (lower frequency) pendulums, with the maximum of the wave occurring at the pendulum which resonates at the frequency of the stimulus.

Let us now proceed to the vibration pattern of the basilar membrane in response to sinusoidal stimulation. The abscissa in Fig. 4.4 is distance (in mm) from the stapes along the basilar membrane, and the ordinate is amplitude of membrane displacement. Two types of information are shown in this figure. The outer dashed lines represent the envelope of the traveling wave as a whole. This envelope outlines the displacement

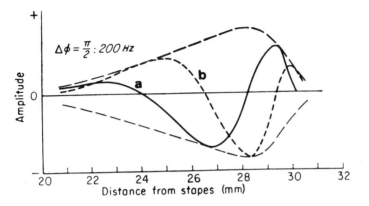

Figure 4.4 Traveling wave pattern for a 200 Hz tone. (From G. Bekesy [3], *Experiments in Hearing,* © 1960 by McGraw-Hill. Used with permission of McGraw-Hill Book Company.)

of the cochlear partition during an entire cycle of the wave. Note that the displacement pattern builds gradually with distance from the stapes, reaches a maximum in the vicinity of 28–29 mm, and then decays rapidly beyond the point of maximal displacement. The peak of the traveling wave envelope occurs at the place along the basilar membrane where vibration is greatest in response to the stimulus frequency (200 Hz in this case). The traveling wave envelopes for several low frequencies are shown in Fig. 4.5. Observe that these low frequencies results in a displacement pattern covering most of the basilar membrane, although the places of maximum vibration move toward the base with increasing frequency. Standing waves do not arise because there are virtually no reflections from the apical end of the cochlear duct. For very low frequencies (50 Hz) the entire membrane vibrates in phase, so that no traveling wave arises. For higher frequencies, however, notice that there is an increasing phase lag with distance from the stapes; this lag reflects the increasing propagation time and shortening wavelength as the wave proceeds toward the apex.

Figure 4.4 also shows the peak-to-peak amplitudes of membrane displacement are two discrete phases of the wave cycle. For simplicity, assume that the solid line *a* occurs at 0° (time zero) and that the dashed line *b* occurs at 90° (¼ cycle later). The difference between the two instantaneous displacements depends on what phase of the cycle the wave is in. A full cycle would include a complete set of instantaneous displace-

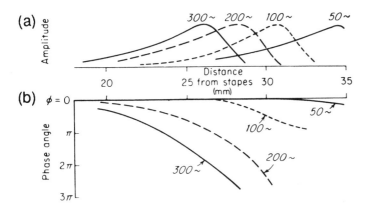

Figure 4.5 Traveling wave envelopes (a) and phase curves (b) for several low frequencies. (From Bekesy [3], *Experiments in Hearing* © 1960 by McGraw-Hill. Used with permission of McGraw-Hill Book Company.)

ment patterns back and forth within the traveling wave envelope, which would begin and end at the solid curve *a* we have designated as our reference for 0° phase. If one imagines this series of instantaneous displacement curves in rapid succession (as in a motion picture with a successive phase in each frame) then the resulting image would be a traveling wave with a maximum at the palce shown by the peak of the envelope.

How does the cochlear partition respond to an impulsive stimulus, such as a click? Think again of the pendulum analogy. Since an impulsive stimulus, at least ideally, contains energy at all frequencies, it will cause each pendulum to vibrate at its own resonant frequency. Recall that the stiffness of the basilar membrane decreases with distance from the stapes (which is analogous to the increasing lengths of the pendulum strings), and that wave movement is in the direction of decreasing stiffness. Therefore, the vibratory pattern over time is a traveling wave which migrates from the equivalents of shorter (higher frequency) to the longer (lower frequency) pendulums. As expected, the traveling wave envelope is not nearly as peaked as when there is a sinusoidal stimulus. Figure 4.6 shows the envelope and several instantaneous displacements of such a traveling wave in a cochlear model [11]. Such models of the cochlea as the one in which these data were generated maintain the known properties of the cochlear duct, and greatly facilitate experimental manipulations and measurements.

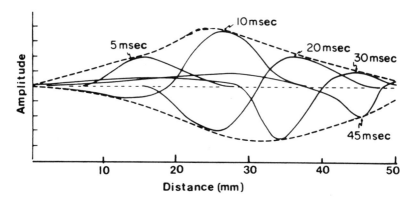

Figure 4.6 Traveling wave in a cochlear model (impulsive stimulus). (From Tonndorf [11], with permission of *J. Acoust. Soc. Amer.*)

HAIR CELL ACTIVATION

A primary task is to determine exactly what it is that stimulates the sensory cells of the organ of Corti. It is clearly established that sensory hair cells transduce mechanical into electrochemical activity when their stereocilia are bent [12–15]. Specifically, sensory hair cells like those in the cochlea are activated when their stereocilia are bent in a particular direction and that inhibition occurs when they are bent in the opposite direction [16,17]. This concept is shown in Fig. 4.7. Here we see that bending of the stereocilia toward the longer kinocilium results in excitation (measured by the activity of the associated neuron), while bending in the opposite direction (away from the kinocilium) is inhibitory. Cochlear HCs do not have this kinocilium. However, the analogous structure is a basal body (centriole or rudimentary kinocilium) found at the base of the "W"-shaped arrangement of stereocilia on the OHC's. Recall that the base of the W faced toward the outside of the cochlear duct (away from the modiolus). Therefore, the process of cochlear HC activation involves the bending of the stereocilia away from the modiolus.

Having established that the mechanical stimulus to the sensory cells is to bend their stereocilia away from the modiolus, we are left with two key questions. First, how does the mechanical activity along the cochlear partition get translated into such bending forces upon the sensory hairs. Second, what is it about the bending of these cilia which causes the hair cells to become activated?

Bending of the HC stereocilia to away from the modiolus involves a motion that is *across* the cochlear duct (radially). Yet, the traveling wave

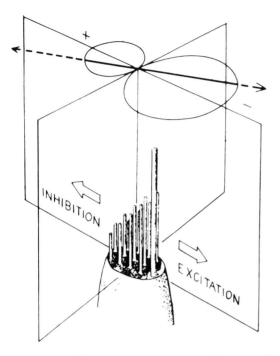

Figure 4.7 Directional sensitivity of sensory hair cells. (From Flock [16], with permission of Springer-Verlag, Inc.)

runs longitudinally in the direction of the cochlea. Classical findings by Bekesy [3] demonstrated that such radial motion is actually achieved in the vicinity of the traveling wave peak. Specifically, he observed that the nature of the shearing forces changes at different locations long the traveling wave envelope. As shown in Fig. 4.8, the shearing vibrations basal to the point of maximal displacement (toward the stapes) were found to be in the radial direction, as required to eventuate the properly oriented stimulation of the stereocilia. The shearing forces apical to the peak of the traveling wave (toward the helicotrema) were in the longitudinal direction; i.e., in the direction followed by the cochlear duct.

Tonndorf [18] explained how this change from longitudinal to radial shearing can come about. Figure 4.9a shows how the basilar membrane might move if it were like a freely vibrating ribbon. Note how the pattern is all in the longitudinal direction. However, this is not the case. Instead, the membrane is actually constrained on both sides by its attachments to the walls of the cochlea. The result is a vibration pattern more like the one depicted in Fig. 4.9b, which is based upon observations of the instan-

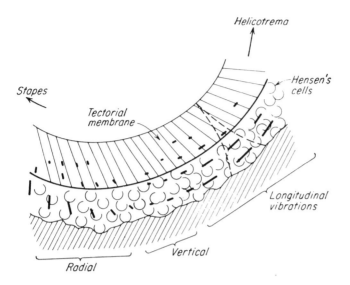

Figure 4.8 Schematic diagram showing radial and longitudinal shearing observed by Bekesy in the vicinity of the traveling wave peak. (From Bekesy [3], *Experiments in Hearing*, © 1960 by McGraw-Hill. Used with permission of McGraw-Hill Book Company.)

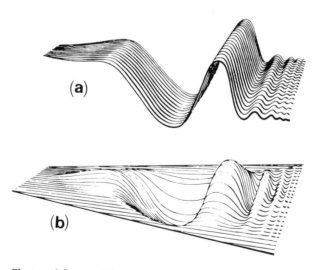

Figure 4.9 (a) Vibration patterns of the basilar membrane that would be expected if it vibrated like a ribbon; and (b) when it is constrained by its lateral attachments. (From Tonndorf [18], with permission of *J. Acoust. Soc. Am.*)

taneous pattern in a cochlear model. Notice that the vibrations under these lateral constraints induce radially directed forces on the stapedial (high frequency) side of the traveling wave peak. In the cochlea, these forces which would be across the direction of the duct.

Having established a mechanism to generate radial forces, we may focus upon how these forces are caused to act upon the HCs. It has long been established that the bending of the HC stereocilia in the proper direction (away from the modiolus) occurs when the cilia are sheared between the tectorial membrane above and the reticular lamina below. Recall here that the hair cells (HCs) are seated on the basilar membrane with the reticular lamina on top, and with their cilia associated in various ways with the tectorial membrane (Chap. 2). The shearing effect takes place because the tectorial and basilar membranes are hinged at different points. Specifically, whereas the basilar membrane extends from the bottom of the osseous spiral lamina, the tectorial membrane is hinged at the upper lip of the limbus. As a result, the axes of rotation are different for these two membranes, so that their displacement causes them to move relative to one another. The result is a shearing force upon the cilia between them.

The essence of the notion just described appears to have been introduced by Kuile [19,20]. The most widely accepted mechanism for this concept was proposed by Davis [21], and is shown schematically in Fig. 4.10. Frame (a) in the figure shows the relative positions of the basilar membrane and tectorial membrane at rest; and frame (b) shows their relative positions when the scala media is deflected upward toward the scala vestibuli. Notice that the membranes are viewed as operating as stiff boards that pivot around the hinge-points. The resulting motions shear the cilia so that they bend outward (away from the modiolus) when the membranes are deflected upward (toward scala vestibuli), resulting in depolarization of the hair cell.

The idea that shearing of the stereocilia away from the modiolus results from basilar membrane displacements upward toward the scala vestibuli has enjoyed almost universal acceptance. However, recent findings and theoretical arguments have uncovered several problems with this conceptualization. First, recall from Chap. 2 that the underlying assumption that the tectorial membrane moves about its pivot point as a stiff board is not supported by data on its physical characteristics. Second, auditory nerve excitation has been shown to be associated with downward displacement of the basilar membrane [23–26]. Third, different periods of the basilar membrane's motion may be associated with HC stimulation at different places along the cochlear duct [27]. Several of these discrepancies may be resolved by Zwislocki's [28–30] modifica-

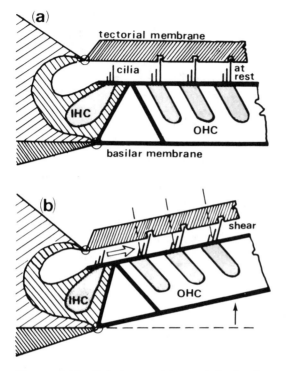

Figure 4.10 Relative positions of the basilar membrane and tectorial membrane at rest (a) and during elevation toward the scala vestibuli (b). Davis' [21] model calls for upward deflection to result in outward bending of the stereocilia, as shown in (b). (Adapted from Ryan and Dallos [22], Courtesy of Little, Brown and Company, © 1976.)

tion of the model, in which the tectorial membrane is conceived as bending over the internal sulcus in a manner that is consistent with its physical attributes. Clearly, these issues go far beyond the intended scope of this text. The interested reader should refer to discussions by Steel [27] and Zwislocki [29,30] for detailed coverages of this controversial area. However, two conclusions do seem clear. First, the mechanical process by which the HC cilia are stimulated is a shearing action directed away from the modiolus. Second, the nature and direction(s) of the membrane motions which precipitate the outward shearing of the HC cilia is at the very least far more complex than what was previously almost universally accepted.

The stereocilia of the outer hair cells (OHCs) are in intimate contact with the overlying tectorial membrane (except for the shorter ones);

whereas the preponderance of information suggests that the inner hair cell (IHC) cilia do not make such contact. These differences imply alternative means of communicating the movements of the membranes to the stereocilia of the two types of HCs. To study this, Dallos and associates [31] compared the cochlear microphonics (see the section on Cochlear Electrical Potentials, below) generated by the IHCs and OHCs on the guinea pig. It is possible to differentiate the responses of the two cell groups, since the normal cochlear microphonic is derived chiefly from the OHCs, and ototoxic drugs tend to obliterate these same cells. Thus, the cochlear microphonic responses of the two cell groups were separated by measuring the responses before and after the animals were injected with an ototoxic drug (kanamycin). The output of the OHCs was found to be proportional to the basilar membrane *displacement*. In contrast, the response of the IHCs was proportional to the *velocity* of basilar membrane displacement. Subsequent studies have confirmed that the IHCs are activated by the velocity of basilar membrane movement [32–35]. In other words, the OHCs respond to the amount of displacement and the IHCs respond to the rate at which the displacement changes.

The reason for this difference in the mode of activation is consistent with the different relationships of the inner and outer HC cilia to the tectorial membrane. Since the OHC cilia attach to the tectorial membrane, an effective stimulus is provided by the relative movement of the reticular and tectorial membranes, which depend upon basilar membrane displacement. The IHC, on the other hand, stand free of the tectorial membrane. Their stimulus is thus provided by the *drag* imposed by the surrounding viscous fluid as the basilar membrane is displaced; the greater the velocity of basilar membrane displacement, the greater the drag exerted upon the cilia.

Suppose that all the necessary events have brought the signal to the relevant location along the organ of Corti, and that whatever relative appropriate movements of the reticular and tectorial membranes have operated in order to impart outward shearing forces upon the hair cells. We already know that the HCs are activated by the ensuing deflections of their stereocilia away from the modiolus. How does this occur? In other words, what is the process by which the bending of the sterocilia translates into sensory transduction?

A theory that explains this transduction process has been· described by Pickles et al. [36] and Hudspeth [15]. Recall from Chap. 2 that the stereocilia bundles are composed of rows stiff cilia that are cross-linked by fine fibers (Fig. 4.11). One general class of cross-linking fibers connect the cilia laterally within and between rows. The other general category of fibers is made up of filaments that go from the tip of a shorter ste-

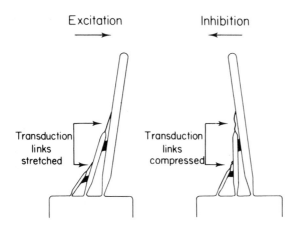

Figure 4.11   Cross-links among hair cell stereocilia (see text). (From Pickles et al. [36], with permission of *Hearing Research*.)

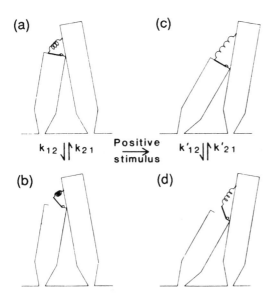

Figure 4.12   The opening and closing of the "trap door" allows ions to pass through mechanoelectric transduction channels. (From Hudspeth [15], The cellular basis of hearing, *Science*, 230, 745–752 (1985). Copyright 1985 by AAAS.)

reocilium to the side of the adjacent higher one in the next row. Bending of the stereocilia away from the modiolus (associated with excitation) stretches these tip-to-side fibers, whereas movement in the opposite direction (associated with inhibition) compresses them.

Stretching the fiber opens a pore on the tip of the cilium. In contrast, the pore would be closed when opposite bending of the stereocilia compresses the rows together. This notion is depicted in Fig. 4.12. By analogy, the bending of the stereocilia in one direction or the other in effect pulls or pushes upon the filament, which in turn opens or closes a "trap door" in the cilium. Opening the pore grants access to a transduction channel through which ions may flow.

The springs indicated on the filaments in Fig. 4.12 imply that the pore will alternate between being open and closed even when there is no stimulation. Stimulation deflects the stereocilia so that the filaments are stretched, thereby causing the pore to be open for a greater proportion of the time; which, in turn, causes the ion current flow to be greater and causes the HC to be activated. This mechanism constitutes the process of mechano-electrical transduction at the HC, at least in general terms. A detailed description of the process, including underlying experimental findings and the nature of the ion transfer, is outlined by Hudspeth [15].

COCHLEAR ELECTRICAL POTENTIALS

Several electrical potentials may be recorded from various parts of the cochlea and its environs. References have already been made to the cochlear microphonic, which is one of these, and to the general conceptualization of the action of sensory receptors. Resting potentials are the positive and negative direct current (dc) polarizations of the various tissues and their surrounding fluids. Receptor potentials are electrical responses from a receptor cell (e.g., a cochlear hair cell) that result when the cell is stimulated. These may these may involving alternating current (ac) or dc. Note that the presence of a receptor potential does not necessarily mean that the nervous system is aware of the stimulus: it just reflects the fact that the hair cell itself has responded. It is the transmission of a chemical mediator across the synapse and the resulting neural firing that indicates that the signal has now activated the nervous system.

We may conceive of these potentials in terms of whether they are derived from a single cell or from many cells. This is an important dichotomy because compound potentials, which include the contributions of many cells at various distances from the electrode, may include responses to different phases of the same stimulus (or to different stimuli) at different times and in different ways. Thus, the electrode "sees" a much different picture than it would if it were recording from a single cell.

The method of measurement chosen determines whether single-cell or compound (gross) potentials are recorded. The differences among methods boil down to a dichotomy between microelectrodes and gross electrodes. Basically, microelectrodes are electrodes small enough to impale an individual cell, so that its activity can be motioned in relative isolation from other cells. Microelectrodes often have diameters much smaller than 1 μm. Gross electrodes on the other hand, are not small enough to enter a cell. They include electrodes ranging in size from those which can be inserted into a nerve bundle (which are sometimes themselves called microelectrodes) to the large surface electrodes used in EEG and other clinical applications. Gross electrodes are used in two general ways. The first method uses a single active electrode to measure the electrical activity in an area (relative to a ground electrode). The other method, that of differential electrodes, uses two active electrodes the signals of which are added, subtracted, or averaged, depending upon the specific need.

Resting Potentials

The unusual chemical situation in the cochlear duct was discussed in Chap. 2. Recall that endolymph is among the very few extracellular fluids to be high in potassium; and that the proper ionic balance of the cochlear fluids has a profound effect upon the functioning of the organ of Corti.

Bekesy [3] measured the cochlear resting potentials in the guinea pig by inserting an electrode into the perilymph of the scala vestibuli (which he set as a 0 mV reference), and then advancing it down through the scala media and the organ of Corti, and into the scala tympani. He found a positive 50–80 mV resting potential within the scala media. As the electrode was advanced through the organ of Corti, the voltage dropped from about +50 mV to about −50 mV, and then returned to near zero as the electrode passed through the basilar membrane into the perilymph of the scala tympani. Experiments [37] revealed the scala media potential to be about +100 mV. This positive resting voltage is called the endocochlear potential (EP). The EP is greatest near the stria vascularis [38]; and this is the only area that keeps a positive potential when the endolymph is drained from the cochlear duct [39]. Furthermore, the EP is still present after damage to or removal of the HCs, and is found even in the waltzing guinea pig, whose HCs are congenitally absent [39,40]. The stria vascularis is thus the source of the EP.

The negative resting potential in the organ of Corti was confirmed by Tasaki et al. [38], who found its magnitude to be about -60 to -70 mV. Two strong arguments lead one to conclude that it is an intracellular potential [41]. First, this potential cannot be recorded for more than a few minutes, which suggests that it is due to an individual cell which stops functioning after a while because of the damage caused by the invading electrode. The potential would be recordable for longer durations if it were extracellular. Second, if cortilymph had a negative potential, there could be no polarization difference between the insides of the HCs and the auditory nerve fibers and their surrounding fluid, because the functioning of these cells depends upon the presence of a polarization difference across their membranes. The net result of the positive EP and negative intracellular potential is an electrical polarity difference of as much as 160 mV or more across the reticular membrane.

Modern measurement techniques have enabled recent studies to provide a more accurate picture of the resting potentials of the inner and outer HCs [34,42–45]. For example, Dallos and colleagues measured the electrical potentials in the upper turns of the guinea pig cochlea using a precisely controlled microelectrode which was advanced across the organ of Corti below and parallel to the reticular lamina [43–45]. This approach enabled them to accurately establish the membrane potentials of both inner and outer HCs, as well as to describe the details of both ac and dc intracellular receptor potentials, addressed below. Although there is variability in the data, it now appears that representative membrane potential values are approximately -40 mV for the IHCs and -70 mV for the OHCs [44,45].

Receptor Potentials

The measurement of electrical potentials that depend on the stimulation of the ear have impacted upon virtually all aspects of our understanding of auditory physiology. In this section, we will explore several aspects of the cochlear receptor potentials. The parameters of these potentials to a large extent also describe many aspects of cochlear physiology. Consequently, such issues as the relative sensitivity of the inner versus outer hair cells and points which foreshadow the subsequent discussion of cochlear tuning will be explored in the context of this section.

Cochlear Microphonics

In 1930, Wever and Bray [46] reported that if the electrical activity picked up from the cat's auditory nerve is amplified and directed to a loudspeaker, then one can talk into the animal's ear and simultaneously hear himself over the speaker. This result demonstrated that the electrical potentials being monitored were a faithful representation of the stimulus waveform.

Wever and Bray originally thought that they were monitoring the auditory nerve alone. A major problem with this early interpretation is that no other nerve mimics the stimulus waveform, and why should the auditory nerve be the only exception? It was soon shown that the eighthnerve action potential was not the only signal being recorded. Instead, the Wever–Bray effect was actually due to an ac electrical potential being picked up by the electrodes placed near the nerve [47,48]. It was found, for example, that the response was stronger at the round window than at the nerve, and that the Wever–Bray effect could still be demonstrated even if the nerve was destroyed or anesthesized. Such findings demonstrated that the ac potential which reflects the stimulus with such remarkable fidelity is generated by the cochlea; and Adrian [47] coined the term cochlear microphonic (CM) to describe it.

The relationship between the HCs and the CM is firmly established [41,49]. Bekesy [3] demonstrated that CMs are elicited by basilar membrane deflections. An interesting experiment revealed that the CM is generated at the cilia-bearing ends of the HCs. This experiment was based on the fact that the polarity of an electrical potential is out of phase when measured from opposite sides of its generator. To locate the generator of the CM, the polarity of the potential was monitored in an electrode which was advanced through the cochlea from the scala tympani toward the scala vestibuli (Fig. 4.13). The polarity of the CM reversed when the electrode crossed the reticular lamina, suggesting that this is the location of the CM generator. The site of CM polarity reversal was localized to the cilia-bearing ends of the HCs (at the reticular lamina) because the dc resting potential changed dramatically to the positive EP at this point, indicating that the reticular membrane had been impaled.

Cochlear microphonics are produced by both the inner and outer HCs, although there is considerable evidence which indicates that they reflect a greater contribution by the OHCs [34,35,44,45,51]. The findings shown in Fig. 4.14 demonstrate one of the reasons for this conclusion. The figure shows the intracellular ac receptor potential relative to the ac potential as it exists outside of these cells in the fluid of the organ of Corti. The latter is, of course, the CM. A value of zero implies no difference between what is happening inside and outside of the cell, and any other value indicates the degree to which the intracellular activity differs from what is happening outside. These comparisons are made in terms of both the magnitudes and phases of these potentials and are made for

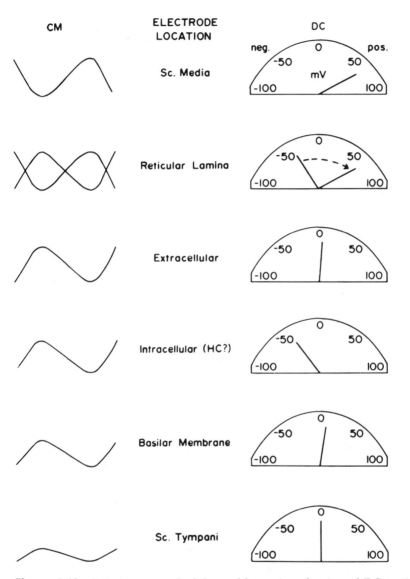

Figure 4.13 Polarity reversal of the cochlear microphonic and DC resting potentials recorded by an electrode being advanced through the cochlea. (Modified after Tasaki et al. [38].)

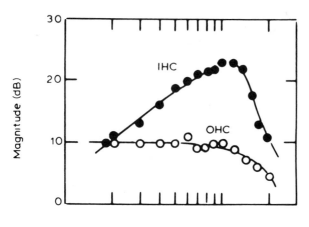

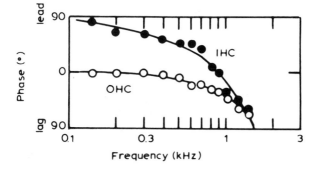

Figure 4.14   These figures compare the magnitudes (upper) and phases (lower) of intracellular ac receptor potentials to those in the organ of Corti outside of the hair cells (hence, HC re OC). Notice that for the IHC values change as a function of frequency relative to those in the organ of Corti, whereas those for the OHCs remain relatively constant. (From Dallos [35], with permission of *Hearing Research*.)

the frequency range involved in the experiment from which the data are derived. The IHC values change as a function of frequency relative to those in the organ of Corti. However, even though the potentials are about 10 dB greater inside the OHC than outside, there is little change in magnitude or phase as a function of frequency for the ac potentials inside the OHCs compared to the fluids of the organ of Corti. The readily apparent implication is that the OHCs must be making a principal contribution to the gross ac potential of the cochlea, namely the CM.

    How is the CM generated? There are several theories, but Davis' variable-resistance model has enjoyed the widest acceptance. Think of the sources of the cochlear resting potentials as biological batteries, generating a current flowing through the scala media, the basilar membrane, and the scala tympani. (One pole of the biological battery goes to the cochlear blood supply, completing the circuit.) A sound stimulus would then be represented electrically (the CM) if it caused the resistance to current flow to change in accordance with the stimulus waveform [3,52,53]. Davis [53] proposed that this variable resistance is provided by the movements of the HC cilia, which occur in response to basilar membrane displacement. In other words, the movements of the cilia modulate the resistance, which in turn sets up an alternating current. This ac potential is monitored as the CM. The amount of current (CM magnitude) depends on the forces exerted upon the hairs, which is ultimately determined by the intensity of the sound stimulus. Figure 4.15 shows a recent version of the model.

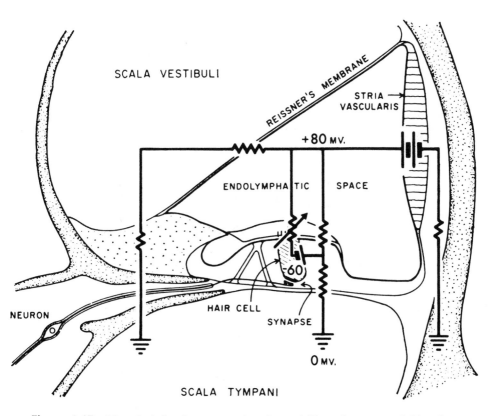

Figure 4.15   Electrical circuit representing the variable resistance model in relation to the major structures of the cochlea. (From Davis [53], with permission.)

Davis' variable resistance model is a widely accepted explanation of CM gneration. It is supported by the observation that changes in CM polarity and magnitude result from experimentally induced anoxia and electrical currents [54]. This evidence is supportive because, for example, one would expect an artificially induced current to enhance the one produced by the physiological battery, resulting in a larger CM. However, this model requires some modification in order to account for a number of findings dealing with electrical impedance changes at the base of the hair cells [55,56].

Two alternative models will be mentioned by way of examples. Wever [49] suggested that the CM is generated by the HC itself, rather than by the interaction of the HCs with other structures. Another mechanism was suggested by Katsuki [57]. He cited measurements by Tanaka et al. [58] which revealed that the CM within the guinea pig HC was small, whereas the CM was largest in the scala media. This result suggests that the origin of the CM might lie outside of the HC, and casts doubt on the generally accepted concept of CM phase reversal at the reticular lamina. Katsuki proposed that the CM may be generated by ion exchanges on the surface of the HCs or within the tectorial membrane.

The CM is a graded potential—its magnitude changes as the stimulus intensity is raised or lowered. This is shown by the CM input–output (I–O) function (Fig. 4.16). The magnitude of the CM increases linearly with stimulus level over a range of roughly 60 dB [59], as is shown by the straight line segment of the I–O function. This classic figure shows the linear response extending down to about 0.4 mV, but subsequent studies have recorded CM magnitudes as low as a few thousandths of a microvolt [49]. With adequate stimulation, the CM does not appear to have a threshold, per se; instead the smallest response seems to grow out of the noise floor, being limited by the recording method, equipment, and physiologic noise. Saturation occurs as the stimulus level is raised beyond the linear segment of the I–O function, as shown by the flattening of the curve. Increasing amounts of harmonic distortion occur in this region. Raising the intensity of the stimulus even further causes overloading, in which case the overall magnitude of the CM can actually decrease.

The graded nature of the CM is also observed in terms of the intracellular ac receptor potential which is its equivalent measured within the hair cells. In fact, because these potentials are recorded *within* a given cell, they enable one to compare the relative thresholds of the inner versus outer HCs. Using this approach, Dallos [44] clearly demonstrated that the *inner* HCs are on the order of 12 dB more sensitive than the outer HCs. This demonstration definitively negates the previously held notion that the OHCs are more sensitive than the IHCs; which was largely based

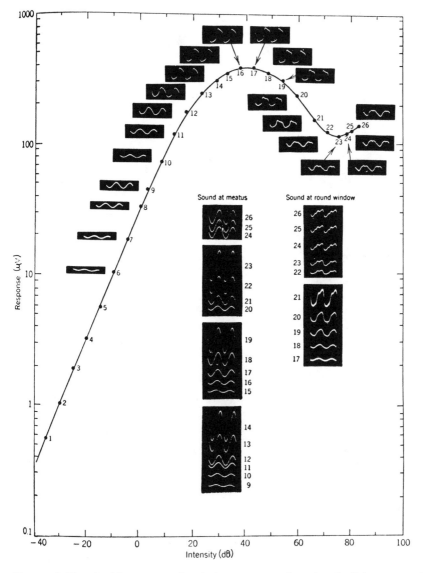

Figure 4.16 Cochlear microphonic input-output function (cat) for a pure tone stimulus. Inserts along the curve are CM responses at points on the function (the apparent decrease in size between points 9 and 10 is due to a change in oscilloscope sensitivity, not a drop in CM magnitude). Inserts below the function are sound levels at the ear canal and round window. (From Wever and Lawrence [59], *Physiological Acoustics,* © 1982 by Princeton University Press. Reprinted by permission of Princeton University Press.)

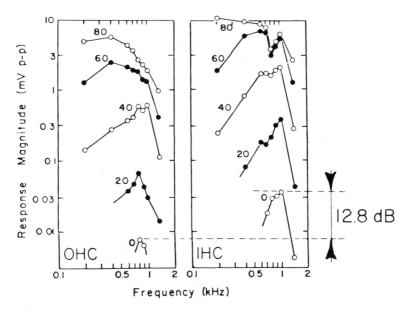

Figure 4.17   Effects of stimulus level on the magnitude of the intracellular ac receptor potential as a function of frequency for an IHC and an OHC (see text). (From Dallos [45], with permission of *Hearing Research*.)

upon studies that measured thresholds following the destruction of OHCs with ototoxic drugs [31,71]. (The more likely reason for the threshold drops found after OHC injury is discussed later in this chapter.)

Figure 4.17 shows how the intracellular ac receptor potential changes in magnitude as a function of frequency in response to stimuli that are increased in 20 dB steps. The IHC–OHC sensitivity difference is marked by the comparison of their response magnitudes at the best frequency for the lowest stimulus level (0 dB). (The best, or characteristic, frequency is the one for which the HC has the lowest thresholds or the greatest magnitude of response.) The graded nature of the response is revealed by the increasing magnitude of the potential as the stimulus level increases. The slowing down of response growth at higher levels is easily seen in the figure: Even though any two successive stimuli are 20 dB apart, the resulting curves become closer and closer for the higher stimulus levels.

Distribution of the CM

Recall that large CM responses are recorded from the round window [46]. This placement was used extensively by Wever and Lawrence [59].

Similar responses are recorded at the cochlear promontory [60]. It is thus important to know what contributes to the round-window response. To study this, Misrahy et al. [61] successively destroyed sections of the guinea pig's cochlea, beginning at the apex and working downward, while monitoring the CM in the basal turn. They found that the upper turns did not make significant contributions to the CM in the basal turn. It may thus be concluded that the CM recorded at the round window is for the most part derived from the activity of the basal turn.

Another approach to studying the distribution of the CM is to place electrodes along the cochlea to obtain CMs from more or less restricted locations. The space and time distribution of the CM along the cochlear spiral was first reported with this method by Tasaki et al. [62]. They inserted pairs of differential electrodes into the scalae tympani and vestibuili of the guinea pig. One electrode pair was placed in each of the four turns. This method allowed them to separate the CM, which is of opposite polarity in the two scalae, from the auditory nerve action potential (AP), which is always negative. (Addition of the two out-of-phase signals will cancel out the CM and enhance the AP, whereas subtraction will remove the AP and enhance the CM.) They found that the space–time distribution of the CM was consistent with the propagation pattern of the traveling wave. Low-frequency signals had large CMs at the apical turn and minimal responses at the base; while high frequencies had maximal CMs at the base and no response at the apex (Fig. 4.18). They also found that the velocity of the signal was very high in the first turn and smaller toward the apex.

Of particular interest are the findings of Honrubia and Ward [64]. They used microelectrodes in the scala media to measure the distribution of CM responses along the cochlear duct. The electrodes were precisely placed at intervals determined from place–frequency maps of the cochlear partition. Tones were then presented at fixed intensities, and CM magnitude was measured at various distances along the cochlear duct. For example, the CM was measured at each electrode site in response to a 1200 Hz tone at 78 dB, a 2500 Hz tone at 101 dB, etc. Figure 4.19 shows typical results, with stimulus level as the parameter. Consider first the distribution of CMs at the lowest stimulus levels (most sensitive curves). Consistently with the traveling wave envelope, the peaks of these curves occur closer to the apex as frequency decreases. However, the CM curves do not line up exactly with the basilar membrane displacement curve. This discrepancy is shown clearly in Fig. 4.20, in which the CM curve is wider and less peaked than the basilar membrane tuning curve. The difference is largely due to the fact that the electrode "sees" CMs generated by thousands of

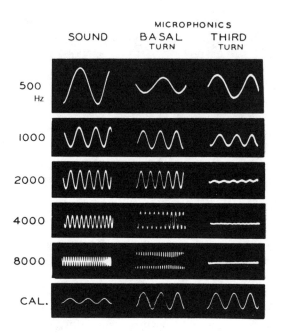

Figure 4.18 Cochlear microphonics recorded with differential electrodes in the first and third turns of the guinea pig cochlea. [From Davis [63], in *Neural Mechanisms of the Auditory and Bestibular Systems* (Rasmussen and Windle, eds.), © 1960 by Thomas Publishing.]

HCs in its general vicinity rather than by just those at its precise point of insertion [65]. In other words, the electrode really monitors a weighted average of many CMs, which has the effect of flattening the curve somewhat.

As shown in Fig. 4.19, we see that CM magnitude increases with stimulus level for each frequency. Also, the place of maximum CM magnitude shifts downward toward the base as intensity increases. This may at first seem inconsistent with the place principle. However, the basal shift of maximum CM response is probably due to the wider range over which the more basal generators respond linearly [41]. In other words, as stimulus intensity increases, the CMs from the most sensitive place along the basilar membrane become saturated sooner than do the responses from more basal regions. Thus, CMs generated toward the base continue to increase in magnitude when those from the most sensitive place have already become saturated. The place of maximal CM re-

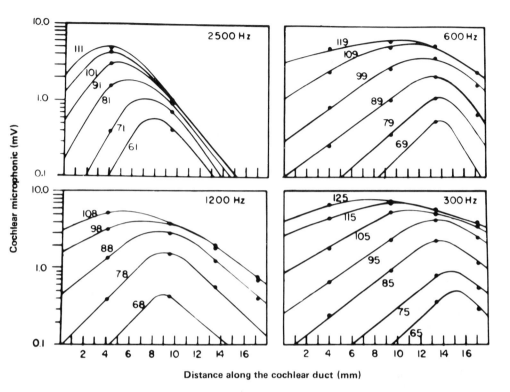

Figure 4.19 Cochlear microphonic magnitude as a function of distance along the basilar membrane for four frequencies presented at various intensities. (From Honrubia and Ward [64], with permission of *J. Acoust. Soc. Amer.*)

sponse therefore shifts downward along the cochlear partition (upward in frequency).

The the intracellular ac receptor potential also reveals a changing distribution with respect to frequency when the stimulus level increases, as shown in Fig. 4.17. Here, we see that the tuning of the ac potential is reasonably restricted around the best frequency when the stimulus level is low; and becomes wider, extending toward the low frequencies, when the stimulus level becomes greater. In other words, the intracellular ac receptor potential resembles a band-pass filter around the best frequency at low levels of stimulition and a low-pass filter at higher levels [44].

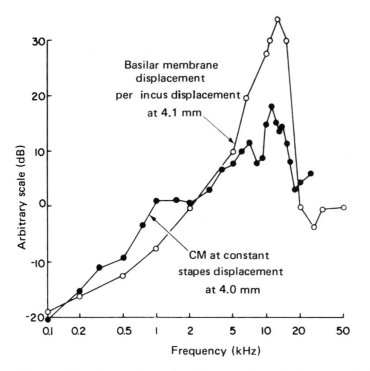

Figure 4.20 Comparison of basilar membrane tuning curves [95] and the CM curve at similar locations in the guinea pig cochlea. (From Dallos et al. [65], with permission of *J. Acoust. Soc. Amer.*)

Summating Potentials

The summating potential (SP) was first described by Davis, Fernandez and McAuliffe [66] and Bekesy [3]. Unlike the CM, which is an ac potential, the SP is a shift in the dc baseline in response to sound stimulation. In other words, the SP is a dc potential. Bekesy called this shift "dc fall." Subsequent research revealed that it may be a positive (SP+) or negative (SP−) baseline shift [18], and we will see that SP polarity depends is associated with the traveling wave envelope and the manner in which it is recorded. Like the CM, the SP is a graded potential, it increases in magnitude as stimulus level is raised [67]. Although the origin of the SP was one a matter of debate, it is now known that it is a receptor potential of the hair cells [34,42,44,45,51,68–70].

Davis et al. [71] produced relatively selective damage to the OHCs of guinea pigs with streptomycin and surgery. Although there was also damage of the IHCs and a few exceptional cases, they suggested that the

SP⁻ is produced by the IHCs while the SP⁺ is related to the OHCs. However, Dallos and Bredberg [41] found that both positive and negative SPs (measured as the potential difference between the scalae vestibuli and tympani, see below) are greatly affected by OHC destruction. Furthermore, Stopp and Whitfield [72] observed both SP⁺ and SP⁻ in pigeon cochleas, which do not have differentiated inner and outer HCs.

Honrubia and Ward [67] measured the SP and CM simultaneously in each turn of the guinea pig cochlea, using electrodes located in the scala media. We have already seen that the envelope (distribution of amplitude along the length of the cochlear duct) of the CM is a reasonable representation of the traveling wave envelope. Honrubia and Ward [75] found that the SP was positive on the basal side of the CM envelope and negative on the apical side. This result suggests that the SP is positive on the basal side of the traveling wave and becomes a negative apical to the traveling wave peak. Such a correspondance between the SP⁻ and the traveling wave peak supports the association, which has been suggested by several researchers [73,74], of the SP⁻ with auditory nerve excitation. Honrubia and Ward also proposed that the SP⁺ may inhibit neural excitation along the basal part of the traveling wave. This would restrict the part of the traveling wave envelope capable of causing neural excitation to the peak region, which would "sharpen" frequency selectivity.

Dallos and colleagues [41,75,76,77] used a somewhat different recording approach, which makes the important distinction between the average potential of both the scala vestibuli and the scala tympani on the one hand and the potential gradient (difference) across the cochlear partition on the other. This at first complicated distinction is clarified in Fig. 4.21. One electrode is in the scala vestibuli and the other is in the

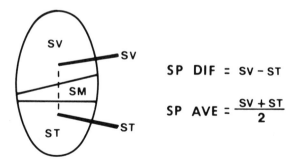

$$\text{SP DIF} = \text{SV} - \text{ST}$$

$$\text{SP AVE} = \frac{\text{SV} + \text{ST}}{2}$$

Figure 4.21 Recording DIF and AVE components of the summating potential from scala vestibuli (SV) and scala tympani (ST). (Modified from various drawings by Dallos.)

scala tympani. Each one registers the SP at the same cross-sectional plane along the cochlea, but from opposite sides of the scala media. Subtracting the SP in the scala tympani (ST) from the SP in the scala vestibuli (SV) (SV − ST) gives the potential difference of the SP across the coclear partition. This difference is called the DIF component. The average (AVE) component is obtained by simply averaging the SPs from both scalae [(SV + ST)/2]. The AVE component thus expresses the common properties (common mode) of the SP on both sides of scala media.

The spatial arrangements of the DIF SP and AVE SP are shown superimposed upon the traveling wave envelope in Fig. 4.22. Note that the DIF component becomes negative in the vicinity of the peak of the traveling wave envelope, a situation which resembles the spatial distribution of SP$^+$ and SP$^-$ discussed above. The polarity of the AVE component is essentially the reverse, being positive around the traveling wave peak and negative elsewhere. Figure 4.23 shows the relationships among the DIF and AVE components of the SP; the CM; and the traveling wave. These results were obtained from the third turn of one guinea pig cochlea, in which the electrodes were 14.5 mm from the base (the approximate location for 400 Hz). The traveling wave peaks at 400 Hz, with a rising slope of 6 dB per octave below the peak and a falling slope of −100 dB per octave above it. As in Fig. 4.22 the DIP SP is negative and the AVE SP is positive in the vicinity of the traveling wave peak. The figure also reveals that the SP curves are more localized than those for

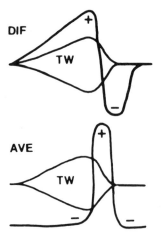

Figure 4.22   Spacial relationships of the AVE SP and the DIF SP to the traveling wave envelope (TW). (Modified from drawings by Dallos [75], with permission.)

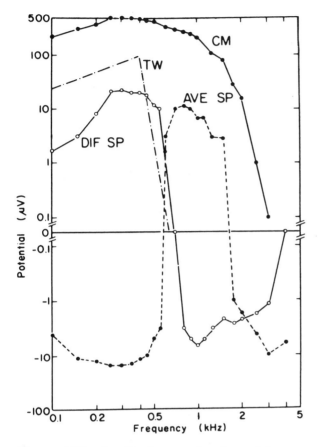

Figure 4.23 Amplitude as a function of frequency for the DIF and AVE summating potentials, cochlear microphonic (CM), and traveling wave (TW) for a 400 Hz stimulus (50 dB SPL). (From Dallos et al [77], with perission of *Acta Otol.*)

the CM. These two components (the AVE and DIF SP) ae probably produced by the same underlying processes [78].

As we have seen for the CM, intracellular recordings reveal that the SP is derived from the hair cells, with the principal contribution coming from the OHCs [34,45,46]. Figure 4.24 provides insight into this relationship. It shows tuning curves obtained at low levels of stimulation for the ac and dc intracellular receptor potentials (the intracellular versions of the CM and SP, respectively) of an IHC and an OHC having comparable best frequencies. The figure reveals that the polarity of the OHC's dc

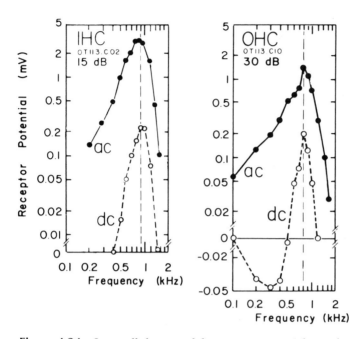

Figure 4.24   Intracellular ac and dc receptor potentials as a function of frequency at low levels of stimulation from an inner hair cell and an outer hair cell of comparable best frequency. (From Dallos [45], with permission of *Hearing Research*.)

receptor changes in both the positive and negative directions. In contrast, the dc receptor potential of the inner hair cell is positive only. Thus, the distribution of the SP is consisitent with that of the OHCs as opposed to the IHCs.

This negative–positive distribution of the intracellular dc receptor potential is in agreement with what we have just seen for the SP, which is gross extracellular potential representing the contribution of many cells. (The negative–positive shape of the dc receptor potential as a function of frequency at low stimulus levels becomes positive only at higher levels.)

The effects of increasing stimulus level upon the intracellular dc potential are largely similar to those observed above for the ac potential. Specifically, the magnitude of the potenial increases with stimulus level, compressing once moderate levels are achieved; and as a function of frequency, the response is sharply tuned and band-pass around the best frequency at low levels of stimulition, becoming wider and low-pass at higher levels.

Several other observations might be made from Fig. 4.24. The data were obtained using the lowest stimulus levels which allowed complete tuning curves to be generated. Note that this was 15 dB for the IHC and and 30 dB for the OHC. This difference should not be surprising if one recalls that the the IHCs are roughly 12 dB more sensitive than the OHCs. Second, notice that the tuning curves for the dc receptor potentials are sharper than those for the ac potentials. This observation is analogous to what we have seen for the CM and SP in Fig. 4.23. Finally, notice that these tuning curves, obtained at low levels of stimulation are very sharp; much sharper than what we have seen for the traveling wave envelope. The importance of this observation will become apparent when we address the issue of cochlear tuning later in this chapter.

DISTORTIONS IN THE COCHLEA

Pure place theory attributed aural distortions to the conductive mechanism. However, the middle ear system has been shown to be remarkably linear over a wide dynamic range [59,79]. Actually, no part of the ear is completely linear [41]; but the greatest proportion of nonlinear distortions are derived from the cochlea [2,41,59,80].

Bekesy [3] reported that eddy currents developed in opposite directions in the two scalae of a cochlear model (Fig. 4.25a). The locations of the eddies were related to the traveling wave maximum, being toward the base for high frequencies and toward the apex for low. As is shown by the lengths of the arrows in Fig. 4.25a, Tonndorf [81] found that the eddy currents accelerated in the narrower distal end and slowed in the wider proximal end. This effect occurs because, if the same amount of fluid per unit time is to flow through a narrow channel as through a wide one, then it must move faster in the narrow channel. The development of these eddy currents is analogous to the formation of undertow when seawater hits a beach (Fig. 4.25b). These eddies are inherently nonlinear; however, they are a reflection rather than the cause of the distortion process [82]. The distortion occurs because the inertia of the fluid and the restoring force of the basilar membrane are not exactly out of phase at high stimulus levels.

Tonndorf [10,80,83] suggested two merchanisms of distortion based on cochlear hydromechanics (mechanical properties of the cochlear fluids). Amplitude-dependent distortions occur at high stimulus levels, for which eddy currents appear. As stimulus level increases the elliptical eddies begin to flatten, which is a form of peak clipping. In addition, other eddies develop at places along the partition corresponding to the

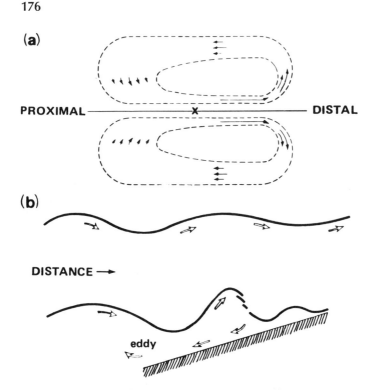

(a)

PROXIMAL ——————————— **X** ——————— DISTAL

(b)

DISTANCE ⟶

eddy

Figure 4.25 (a) Eddy currents in a cochlear model. The traveling wave peak is represented by the X. (From Tonndorf [81]. Permission *J. Acoust. Soc. Amer.*) (b) Surface waves in open water and in the production of eddies (undertow) when striking a surface. [From Tonndorf [80], Cochlear nonlinearities, in *Basic Mechanisms in Hearing* (Møller, ed.), © 1973 by Academic Press.]

harmonics of the original (primary) tone. This second mechanism is amplitude independent; i.e., it does not depend on stimulus level. Amplitude-independent distortion is schematically represented in Fig. 4.20. If two primary tones (500 and 510 Hz) are presented, a difference tone (or beat frequency) will be heard (510 − 500 = 10 Hz beat frequency). The beat frequency is caused by a distortion due to movements of individual fluid particles in elliptical orbits that are asymmetric (Fig. 4.26b) rather than symmetric (Fig. 4.26a). This asymmetry causes the particle orbits in the scalae vestibuli and tympani to be displaced relative to one another in a "push-pull" manner (Fig. 4.26c). The resultant energy at the difference (beat) frequency, which is lower in frequency than the primary tones, then proceeds up the cochlear partition (forming a new traveling wave if the beat frequency is high enough).

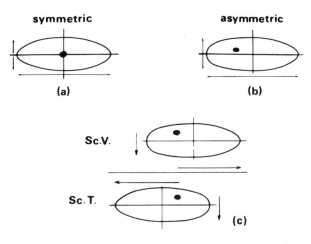

Figure 4.26 Fluid particle orbits in a cochlear model. (From Tonndorf [83], with Permission of *J. Acoust. Soc. Amer.*)

It is undisputed that distortions at high intensities are related to hydrodynamic nonlinearities which are amplitude dependent. However, CM data are inconsistent with the amplitude-independent mechanism at low and moderate levels. An alternate source of distortion is within the HC, and is most likely associated with the electrical generation of the CM [41,59]. This idea is supported by CM studies [41,79,84–87], and is likely because the variable-resistance model of CM production is inherently nonlinear [41].

Suppose that a distortion component were due to cochlear hydromechanics (mediated by a traveling wave). Such a traveling wave would result in basilar membrane displacement with a peak at the same place as would be produced by a real tone of the same frequency as the distortion product. Thus, a 300 Hz distortion product would produce the same traveling wave as a real 300 Hz tone; and the associated CM pattern would reach a maximum at the 300 Hz point (point a in Fig. 4.27). On the other hand, if the CMs associated with the distortion are not localized at point a, then it is unlikely that the distortion is the result of a traveling wave caused by a hydrodynamic nonlinearily. Several studies [41,79,85–87] demonstrated that the CMs corresponding to various kinds of distortion at low and moderate levels of stimulation were localized near the primary tones (point b) rather than at the place of a real tone of the same frequency (point a). This result suggests that distortions at low and moderate levels may be due to nonlinearities in the mechanoelectrical transducer; i.e., may be associated with the production of CMs at the HC level.

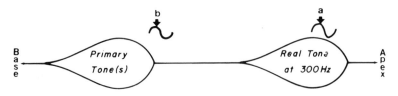

Figure 4.27 Highly schematic locations of maximum CM response for a 300 Hz distortion product mediated by a traveling wave (point a), and not mediated by a traveling wave (point b).

Two findings support this theory. Dallos [41] found that the magnitudes of CMs due to distortion products were greater than the magnitudes of CMs associated with actual tones of the same frequency. Dallos, et al. [84] found direct evidence that lower-level distortions are related to the electrical rather than the hydromechanical process. They polarized the cochlear partition with a dc current, which affects the electrical process that generates the CM. If the distortion products were due to traveling waves (hydrodynamic), then they would be affected by the dc current in the same way as the primary tones, because both were produced prior to the effects of the dc bias. However, if the distortion is due to the

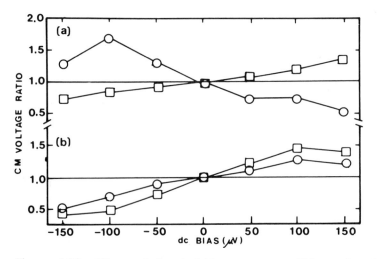

Figure 4.28 Effects of electrical bias current on CMs produced by primary tones (squares) and distortion components (circles) at low (a) and high (b) levels. (Redrawn from the data of Dallos et al. [84].)

electrical process at the HC, then it should be affected differently than the primaries because one is produced prior to the electrical process and the other is the result of it. Figure 4.28 shows an example of the results of this experiment. The CMs associated with the primary and the distortion product were affected (a) differently at low stimulus levels (67 dB SPL), but (b) similarly at high levels. The low-level distortion thus seems to result from electrical processes, whereas the high-level distortion is hydromechanical.

These studies suggest that distortions in the cochlea are due to a two-stage process, one mechanism operating at low, and the other at high, stimulus levels. The higher-level distortion products, which result from a chain of events similar to that for a directly presented sound (cochlear hydrodynamics), are the most certainly audible. Since the lower-level distortion products do not appear to occur by the same route, there is still some question as to their audibility [87].

COCHLEAR TUNING AND FREQUENCY SELECTIVITY

Basilar membrane displacement reaches a peak near the apex of the cochlea in response to low frequencies and near the base for higher frequencies. That is, the traveling wave causes a displacement pattern which is tuned as a function of distance along the basilar membrane. One may say that the cochlea is tuned to frequency as a function of distance along the cochlear partition. This relationship between the tuning of a location along the cochlear partition and the distance from the base to apex is depicted by Liberman's [88] cochlear frequency map shown in Fig. 4.29. This map was derived by determining the characteristic (best) frequencies of auditory neurons (see Chap. 5) which were labeled with horseradish peroxidase (HRP), and then tracing these neurons back to their respective hair cells along the cochlear duct. This method made it possible to precisely locate the places long the cochlea that correspond to particular frequencies. This cochlear map expresses distance along the cochlea in terms of percentage, thereby accounting for differences in cochlear length across specimens.

In the following chapters we shall see that fine frequency discriminations are made in psychoacoustic experiments, and that auditory nerve fibers are very sharply tuned. Can the mechanical displacement pattern in the cochlea account for this remarkable degree of frequency selectivity?

The key question is whether the sharpness of cochlear tuning approaches that of the auditory nerve. The upper curves in Fig. 4.30 show a set of response areas (tuning curves) for auditory nerve fibers in the guinea pig. Neural tuning curves will be discussed in Chap. 5. For now,

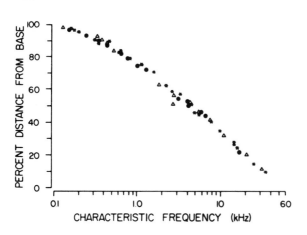

Figure 4.29 The cochlear map (cat) shows the relationship between frequency and distance (in percent) along the cochlear partition. (From Liberman [88], with permission of *J. Acoust. Soc. Am.*)

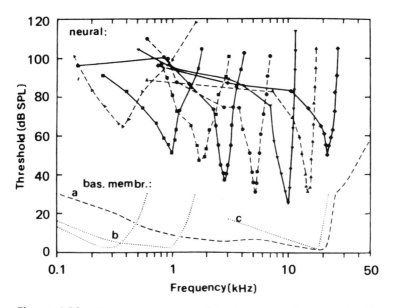

Figure 4.30 Upper curves: neural tuning curves (guinea pig). Lower curves: mechanical tuning (guinea pig) from (a) Wilson and Johnstone [95] at 20 kHz, (b) Bekesy [3] at 270 and 900 Hz, and (c) Johnstone et al. [96]. [From Evans [89], The sharpening of cochlear frequency selectivity, *Audiology 14*, 419–442 (1975).]

note their sharp peaks, which indicate that auditory nerve fibers re-spond best to a limited range of frequencies around a characteristic fre-quency. The low-frequency slopes of the neural tuning curves range from about 100 to 300 dB per octave, and the high-frequency slopes are approximately -100 to -600 dB octave in a variety of species [90–94].

The sharpness of tuning can also be described by a value Q, which is the ratio of the center (characteristic) frequency to the bandwidth. For a particular center frequency, the narrower the bandwidth is, the larger is the Q value (Fig. 4.31). Since it is difficult to determine the half-power points (which usually define the bandwidth) of physiologi-cal tuning curves, it has become standard practice to use the points on the curve 10 dB down from the peak ($Q_{10_{dB}}$). Auditory nerve fibers have $Q_{10_{dB}}$ values of about 2–10 for the mid-frequencies (Fig. 4.32). With this fact in mind, let us proceed to examine the nature of frequency selectiv-ity in the cochlea.

Bekesy [3] was the first to describe mechanical tuning in the cochlea. He used a binocular microscope to observe basilar membrane displace-

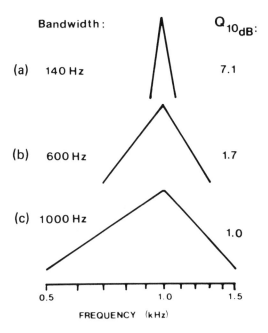

Figure 4.31 $Q_{10_{dB}}$ for three "tuning curves" centered at 1000 Hz. These curves were obtained as follows: (a) 1000/140 = 7.1; (b) 1000/600 = 1.7; (c) 1000/1000 = 1.0.

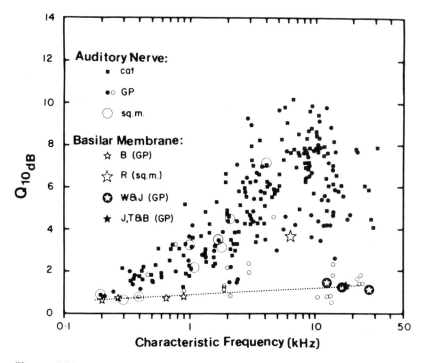

Figure 4.32 $Q_{10_{dB}}$ for auditory nerve and basilar membrane tuning curves. GP, guinea pig; sq. m., squirrel monkey. [From Evans and Wilson [92], Frequency selectivity in the cochlea, in *Basic Mechanisms in Hearing* (Møller, ed.), © 1973 by Academic Press.]

ment patterns in response to high-intensity stimuli. Figure 4.33 shows some of the basilar membrane tuning curves obtained by Bekesy. These curves are in terms of relative amplitude, so that the peak is assigned a value of 1.0 and the displacements at other points along the curves are in proportions of the peak amplitude. The tuning curves tend to become sharper with increasing frequency, but the low-frequency slopes of about 6 dB per octave are far from the sharpness of neural tuning. This fact is illustrated in Fig. 4.30, in which Bekesy's data curve (b) are compared with neural tuning curves having similar characteristic frequencies.

Although Bekesy's data were of monumental significance, several experimental limitations make it difficult to compare these early findings with neural tuning data: (1) Access to the cochlear partition was limited to the apical areas, so that Bekesy's observations were restricted to relatively low frequencies. (2) The observations were obtained visually. (3)

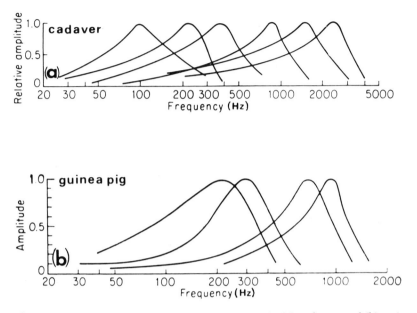

Figure 4.33   Basilar membrane tuning curves in (a) cadaver and (b) guinea pig. (From Bekesy [3], *Experiments in Hearing*, © 1960 by McGraw-Hill. Used with permission of McGraw-Hill Book Company.)

Absolute displacements were not specified. (Absolute values were re-ported in other contexts, however.) (4) Very high stimulus levels (roughly 120 dB SPL) were used, while neural data are available at much lower, including threshold, levels.

In 1967, Johnstone and Boyle [97] reported on the mechanical tuning of the guinea pig cochlea at a high frequency (about 18 kHz). Instead of visual observation, they used the Mössbauer technique. In this method, a radioactive source is placed on the basilar membrane and an absorber of the radiation is situated nearby. Vibration of the basilar membrane (on which the source is located) causes the amount of gamma rays absorbed to be modulated in a manner related to the vibration. Basilar membrane displacement is calculated based on these data. The Mössbauer method permits the use of stimulus levels as low as 60–70 dB SPL. Johnstone and Boyle found that the mechanical tuning of the basilar membrane is con-siderably sharper at 18 kHz than Bekesy's tuning curves at lower fre-quencies. Tuning in this area (about 1.2 mm from the stapes) had a 13 dB per octave slope on the low-frequency side of the peak and a slope of −70 dB per octave on the high-frequency side.

These results might at first seem to contradict Bekesy's findings at lower frequencies. Recall, however, that Bekesy's tuning curves became sharper as frequency increased (Fig. 4.33). Tonndorf and Khanna [98] calculated Q for both sets of data and found that the values fell along the same straight line. This result suggests that Bekesy's data are consistent with those of Johnstone and Boyle, which simply reflect sharper tuning along the basilar membrane as the base is approached.

Many studies investigated the tuning of the basilar membrane in the early 1970s using the Mössbauer [96,99–103] and other [95,104,105] techniques. Although data on specific aspects of the mechanical tuning curves vary, the important point is the considerable agreement among studies on the degree of mechanical tuning. This agreement is shown by the dotted line in Fig. 4.32, which joins the values of $Q_{10_{dB}}$ for several studies. Examples of mechanical tuning curves are shown in the lower part of Fig. 4.30 and in Fig. 4.34.

Wilson and Johnstone [95,105] measured basilar membrane tuning with a capacitance probe. This was a miniature version of the one used by Bekesy [3] (Chap. 3). Their findings are of particular interest because they confirmed the Mössbauer data with another technique, and also because the capacitance probe enabled them to measure basilar membrane vibrations for stimuli as low as 40 dB SPL. This level is in the range used in obtaining neural tuning curves, so that the problem of comparing mechanical tuning at high levels to neural tuning at low levels is overcome.

Such measurements of mechanical tuning have revealed high-frequency slopes as great as about -350 dB per octave, but the low-frequency slopes were not steeper than roughly 24 dB per octave. Clearly, these early results cannot account for the sharpness of the neural tuning data. The difference in terms of $Q_{10_{dB}}$ is dramatically evident in Fig. 4.32.

Moreover, Fig. 4.32 also shows a nonlinear response in the basilar membrane's vibration that was repeatedly reported by Rhode and colleagues in the squirrel monkey [101–103]. This nonlinearity appears as a lack of overlapping of the tuning curve peaks at different stimulus levels. The three curves in the figure would have overlapped exactly if the basilar membrane's vibration was linear because the amplitude (in dB) is derived from the ratio of basilar membrane-to-malleus displacement. In a linear system, this ratio would stay the same for different stimulus levels. This nonlinearity was the subject of some controversy because it was not observed in contemporary data obtained in the guinea pig. It will become evident in the following discussion that subsequent studies have shown that the *normal* basilar membrane is

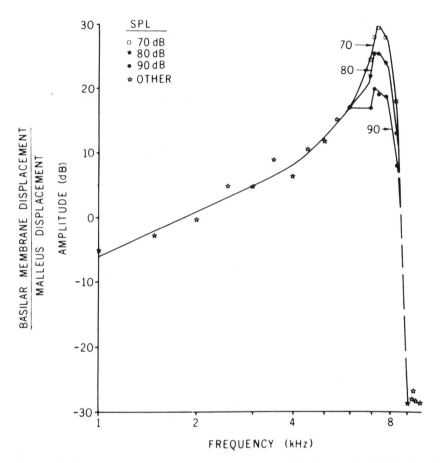

Figure 4.34 Basilar membrane tuning curves at 70, 80, and 90 dB SPL for the squirrel monkey. Lack of overlap around the peak indicates nonlinearity. (From Rhode [101]. with Permission of *J. Acoust. Soc. Amer.*)

nonlinear in the vicinity of the peak in other animals, as well. We shall see that the nonlinear mechanical response of the basilar membrane depends upon the integrity of the cochlea and is associated with the sharpness of cochlear tuning.

Since the perilymph was partially drained in some of the above-mentioned studies, Robertson [106] questioned the validity of some of the basilar membrane and neural tuning data. He found that perilymph drainage changed neural tuning curves, and suggested that the absence of perilymph from the cochlea might have resulted in widening of the basilar membrane tuning curves. In contrast to Robertson's findings, Evans and Wilson [107] observed that wide mechanical and sharp neural tuning were present in the same animals when there were various amounts of perilymph drainage. However, subsequent research by LePage and Johnstone [108] demonstrated that the perilymph drainage which is involved in capacitance probe measurements results in broad tuning and is associated with impaired threshold sensitivity. That is, the hearing sensitivity as measured by compound action potentials (see Chap. 5) became poorer by as much as about 70 dB due to perilymph drainage. Thus, it is apparent that perilymph drainage does result in widened mechanical tuning. As we shall see, a key issue seems to be the effect of the insult upon the integrity of the cochlea as a result of the experimental manipulations.

Evans and Wilson [91,92] hypothesized a "second filter" existing between the basilar membrane and neural responses, to account for the sharpness of neural tuning. As evidence for such a concept, they found that the sharpness of neural tuning curves is reduced when the metabolism of the cochlea is disturbed by interference with its oxygen supply or by chemical influences [89,92,93,109,110]. Under such circumstances, in fact, the resulting neural tuning curves resemble those of the basilar membrane. Further evidence suggesting a second filter comes from other observations: Auditory nerve fibers with the same most sensitive (characteristic) frequency vary in their degrees of tuning; neural frequency selectivity in guinea pigs appears to increase as thresholds decrease; and, in some guinea pigs a number of broadly tuned neurons are interspersed among sharply tuned units. These appeared to be inconsistent with sharp mechanical tuning, which would be expected to result in uniform tuning of the neural fibers. In summary, Evans and Wilson's hypothesized second filter has two distinctive characteristics: (1) the second filter is vulnerable to metabolic disturbances; (2) second filter units are "private" to single auditory neurons or groups of them, as opposed to being shared by a large number of neural fibers.

The appeal of the second filter concept to bridge the gap from broad mechanical to sharp neural tuning led to the proposal of several theories about its location and mechanism. A seemingly good candidate for the second filter mechanism is lateral inhibition, which involves the suppression of activity in weakly simulated neural units by more intense stimulation of adjoining units. An example from common experience is the sharply defined border that is seen between adjoining black and white bars (Mach bands). Lateral inhibition has been proposed as a sharpening mechanism in hearing [3,111–113]. Alternatively, there is evidence that lateral inhibition does not contribute to auditory frequency selectivity

[91,92,114–117]. Other proposed sharpening mechanisms have included IHC–OHC interactions [118–120]; radial shear displacements of the hair cells [121,122]; micromechanics associated with the tectorial membrane [29,123]; and hair cell membrane electrical resonances [124], among others. The interested reader should refer to Pickles [125] and Gelfand [126] for a more detailed review of second filter theories.

Subsequent findings have demonstrated that the mechanical properties of the cochlea can account for the sharpness of neural tuning. However, we shall also see that there appear to be active processes at work as well as the more traditionally conceived of passive ones, which together result in characteristics known to exist.

That sharp tuning already exists prior to the neural response was demonstrated by Russell and Sellick [42,68–70]. They measured the intracellular DC receptor potentials (SP) of guinea pig IHCs as a function of stimulus frequency and level. Typical findings are shown in Figure 4.35. Each curve shows the SPL needed to reach a certain magnitude of DC potential within the IHC as a function of frequency. These curves are called isoamplitude contours because each point on a given curve represents the SPL needed to achieve the same amplitude of SP. Russell and Sellick found that the smallest intracellular SP response that could result in a response from the auditory nerve was about 2.0 mV. At high stimulus levels (SPLs that result in larger SP amplitudes), the SP tuning is more or less like that of the mechanical data we have previously reviewed. Note, however, what occurs as the stimulus decreases toward the neural response thresholds: As the stimulus level decreases, the reduction in SP amplitude (A in mV) is accompanied by a clear increase in the frequency selectivity of IHC intracellular tuning curves. For example, when SP amplitude is 2.7 mV (within 10 dB of threshold), the value of $Q_{10_{dB}}$ is 9.2. This is as sharp as neural tuning. Similarly sharp tuning of intracellular potentials has been reported for OHCs as well [43]. One might note in this context that Cheatham and Dallos [78] showed that tuning curves for the SP are consistent with those of the basilar membrane and the auditory nerve action potential.

These findings demonstrate that frequency selectivity as sharp as what is found in the auditory neuron already exists within the HC and *before* it transmits to the nerve fiber. Clearly, the acuity of neural tuning does not require an intervening filter between the HC and the neuron.

What (and where), then, is the origin of the sharp tuning that is already seen in the hair cell? The answer comes from studies of the *in-vivo* mechanical responses of virtually undamaged cochleas at stimulus levels as low as those used to generate neural tuning curves.

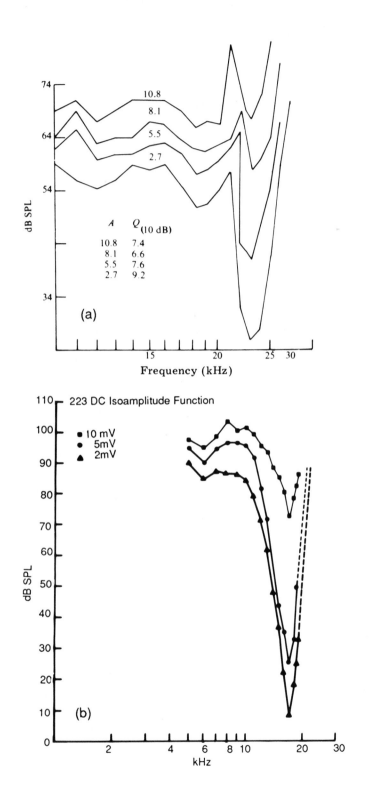

In 1982, Khanna and Leonard [127] demonstrated sharp basilar membrane tuning in the cat using laser inferometry. The interested reader should refer to a recent series of papers by Khanna and colleagues for a detailed discussion of this technique and its applications [128–131]. Also in 1982, Sellick, Patuzzi, and Johnstone [132] demonstrated similarly sharp mechanical tuning with the Mössbauer method in the guinea pig cochlea. The sharpness of the cochlea's mechanical tuning was subsequently corroborated by Robles, Ruggero and Rich [133].

Figure 4.36a shows the three cat basilar membrane tuning curves obtained by Khanna and Leonard. These curves show the SPL needed to yield a threshold amplitude (10–8 cm) of basilar membrane vibration as a function of frequency. The sharpest of these three curves is shown redrawn in Fig. 4.36b along with a neural tuning curve. The basilar membrane is strikingly similar to that of the neuron in the sharply tuned tip of the tuning curve, but deviates from the neural response at lower frequencies. These graphs reveal that the basilar membrane's response is as sharp as that of the neural tuning curve in the region of the most sensitive response (where $Q_{10_{dB}}$ is 5.9 for both curves in this example).   .

Similar findings for the guinea pig cochlea were obtained by Sellick, et al. Recall that the IHCs are activated by the velocity rather than the displacement of basilar membrane movement. As a consequence, they expressed the mechanical response of the basilar membrane in terms of the velocity of its motion. Figure 4.37a shows that the basilar membrane isovelocity curve (crosses) is remarkably similar to a representative neural tuning curve. The figure also shows the SPLs needed to yield an isoamplitude response of the basilar membrane. As in the previous figure, the isoamplitude response is similar to the neural response in the sharply tuned tip of the curve, but deviates at lower frequencies. Sellick, et al. also found that the basilar membrane response is nonlinear at and above the frequency of the sharply tuning peak, as shown in Fig. 4.37b. This nonlinear response is also seen in the sharply tuned intracellular tuning curves of the IHCs (Fig. 4.35). Dallos [44] has reported nonlinearities in the intracellular receptor potentials of both inner and outer HCs.

Sellick, et al. used the stimulus SPL needed to evoke an action potential from the auditory nerve (see Chap. 5) as a measure of the health of

---

Figure 4.35   Intracellular DC receptor potentials (SPs) from guinea pig IHCs as a function of frequency: (a) Receptor potential amplitude (A in mV) are shown with corresponding values of $Q_{10_{dB}}$. (From Russell and Sellick [68], courtesy of *Nature*. (b) Isoamplitude curves are shown for 2, 5, and 10 mV intracellular potentials. (From Russell and Sellick [69], The tuning properties of Cochlear hair cells, in *Psychophysics and Physiology of Hearing* (Evans and Wilson, eds.), © 1977 by Academic Press.)

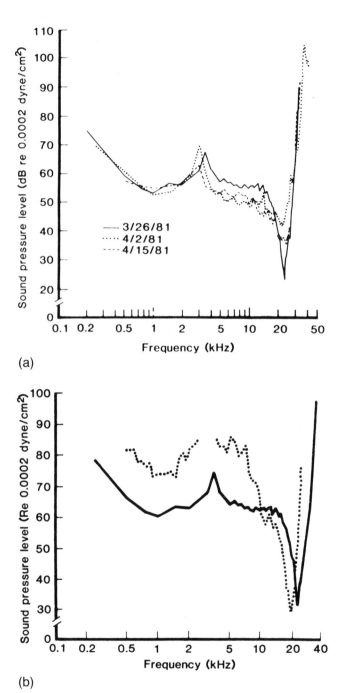

(a)

(b)

the cochlea over the course of their measurements. They found that these thresholds worsened as time passed, revealing that the experimental invasion of the inner ear itself caused progressive damage to the cochlea. Of particular importance is the fact that the sharpness of basilar membrane tuning deteriorated as the thresholds increased. This course of events is shown for two guinea pigs in Fig. 4.38, which also shows the post mortem tuning curves for these two animals. Moreover, basilar membrane's response, which showed nonlinearities while the cochlea was reasonably healthy early in the experiment, became linear as the experiment proceeded. In other words, as the state of the cochlea deteriorated, (a) thresholds became elevated, (b) mechanical tuning lost its sharpness, and (c) the nonlinear response of the basilar membrane became linear. Khanna and Leonard [127] also reported that trauma to the cochlea due to the experimental manipulations caused a loss of sharp mechanical tuning of the basilar membrane response. The vulnerability of the basilar membrane's nonlinear mechanical response has also been demonstrated by LePage and Johnstone [108].

Thus, it has been shown that the mechanical tuning of the cochlea can account for the sharpness of neural tuning and is nonlinear; and that this acute mechanical tuning and its nonlinearity are related and vulnerable to insult because they are lost when the state of the cochlea is compromised. It is now understood that the earlier studies failed to observe sharp mechanical tuning curves in the cochlea for one or more of several reasons: (a) the experimental manipulations themselves damaged or compromised the integrity of the cochlea, thereby obliterating the vulnerable sharp peaks and nonlinear response; (b) high SPLs were used, which involves broader responses and also may traumatize the cochlear structures; (c) post-mortem samples were used which no longer possessed the vulnerable aspects of the response.

It would appear that the mechanical tuning within the cochlea can account for the sharpness of neural tuning. A second filter, as such, is thus not needed. However, the important remaining question has to do with what is the nature of the mechanical tuning process. We must recall at this juncture that the real concern is with the sharpness of the mechanical stimulus actually transmitted to the hair cells. The traditional concept has been that this *mechanical* tuning of the cochlea is synony-

---

Figure 4.36 (a) The SPL necessary to achieve equal amplitudes of basilar membrane movements (10–8 cm) in three cats. (b) Comparison of the sharpest basilar membrane curve (3/26/81) with a neural tuning curve. (From Khanna and Leonard [127], Basilon membrane tuning in the cat cochlea, *Science*, 215, 305–306 (1982). Copyright 1982 by AAAS.)

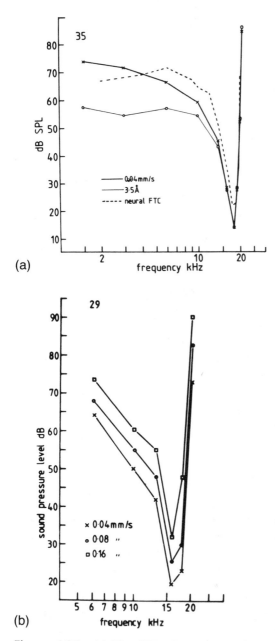

Figure 4.37 (a) The SPL necessary to achieve equal velocities (0.04 mm/s; crosses) amplitudes (3.5A; circles) of basilar membrane vibration, and a comparable neural tuning curve (dotted line) in the guinea pig. (b) The SPL needed to achieve three velocities of basilar membrane curve in the same guinea pig. (From Sellick, et al. [132], with permission of *J. Acoust. Soc. Am.*)

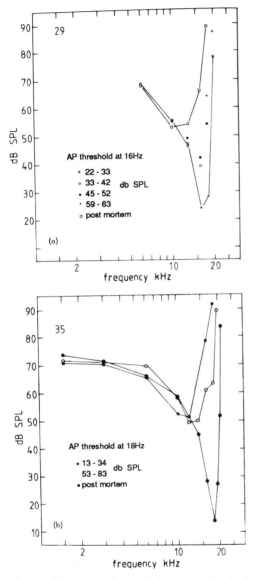

Figure 4.38 The loss of sharp mechanical tuning of the basilar membrane is observed as thresholds become elevated, revealing progressive damage to the cochlea over the course of the measurements, and post mortem, for two guinea pigs (a and b). (From Sellick, et al. [132], with permission of *J. Acoust. Soc. Am.*)

mous with that of the *basilar membrane*. However, convincing evidence is accumulating which suggests that the tuning of the cochlea is not just a passive response by the basilar membrane alone. Rather, there appears to be a contribution to tuning due associated with the hair cells and their connections to surrounding structures. Further, these effects appear to be active, affecting the micromechanics of the cochlear response, rather than just a passive response to an incoming signal.

Let us view the tuning curve somewhat differently in order to appreciate why the mechanical tuning of the cochlea must involve this second *component*, if not a second filter, per se. It has been demonstrated by Khanna and colleagues that the cochlea's mechanical response can be described as having two components [127,134–137]: One of these components has a broad, low-pass response. In the vicinity of the upper cut-off frequency of this broad response is a sharply tuned, band-pass filter. Together, the two components reveal the neural tuning curve's familiar sharp tip and broad tail. Injuries that affect the tip do not particularly affect the broad, low-pass component. In particular, injuries affecting the OHCs have been shown to affect the tip component but not the tail of the tuning curve, and the condition of the OHCs is correlated with the affect upon the tip of the tuning curve [131,137,138]. These changes in the tuning curve's tip are found in the absence of basilar membrane abnormalities [135,136]. The implication of these findings is that the tip component of the cochlea's mechanical tuning curve is associated with the OHCs in general and to the condition of their stereocilia in particular.

One might note in this context the classic observation that thresholds become 30–40 dB poorer when ototoxic drugs have destroyed the OHCs [31,71]. The long-held interpretation of this observation was that the IHCs, which survived the ototoxic assault, are not as sensitive as the OHCs. However, it is more likely that the drop in thresholds is due to the loss of the (probably) mechanical sensitizing effects of the OHCs [139]. Moreover, as previously noted and in contrast to previously held notions, intracellular recordings have established that the IHCs are on the order of 12 dB more sensitive than the OHCs [44].

The two-component nature of cochlear tuning has also been demonstrated by Liberman and colleagues, who determined how various cochlear manipulations affected the associated auditory neurons' responses [138,140–143]. Their findings are particularly intriguing because they identified individual auditory neurons with their associated hair cells. This association was made possible by marking the neurons with intracellularly injected horseradish peroxidase [144]. Labeling the neurons in this way avoids uncertainties about whether given neural tuning curve is actually associated with a particular location in the cochlea.

Figure 4.39 summarizes the findings obtained by Liberman and associates. In this figure, the upper frames show the location of damage or manipulation of the cochlea, and the lower frames show how the neural tuning curve is affected. In each case, the solid lines depict the normal tuning curve and the dotted lines show the curve that results from the indicated manipulation. In spite of the fact that the threshold of the sharply tuned tip is elevated in all cases, note that it is obliterated only for the case of the absent OHCs (b). Most certainly, both the IHCs and OHCs are needed to yield a normal neural tuning curve. However, it is clear that the presence of the sharply tuned component of the response depends upon the presence and condition of the OHCs.

A recent study by Smith et al. [145] provided behavioral support for the contribution of the OHCs to the sensitivity and fine-tuning of the cochlea. They obtained psychoacoustic tuning curves (PTCs), which are a behavioral measure of frequency selectivity akin to the auditory neuron tuning curve (see Chap. 6), from patas monkeys before and after producing OHC damage with the drug dihydrostreptomycin. The drug caused elevations of threshold sensitivity of 50 dB or more; and the loss the sharp tips of the PTCs to be obliterated, leaving only the broad, low-pass filter characteristic of the curves. Histological examination of the cochleas revealed that there was complete loss of OHCs but complete retention of the IHCs in the regions corresponding to the changes on the PTCs.

Another important observation links the mechanical response of the cochlea to the condition of the OHCs. Liberman [140] studied how cochlear damage due to acoustic trauma affected the threshold and characteristic frequency (CF) of the neural tuning curve. He found a downward shift in the CF as threshold sensitivity worsened, at least for neurons having an original CF above about 1000 Hz. Similarly, Leonard and Khanna [137] established that the mechanical tuning curve's CF became lower in frequency in cochleas having greater amounts of OHC damage.

It appears, then, that the sharpness of mechanical tuning in the cochlea depends upon micromechanical components related in some way to the OHCs. Several aspects of the OHCs and their associations have been identified as potential bases for the vulnerable and nonlinear fine-tuning of the cochlea's mechanical response. One factor concerns the stiffness of the OHC stereocilia, which we have seen is due to their internal structure. Moreover, we have seen that there is an organization of the physical characteristics of these cilia from the base to the apex of the cochlea. The capability to affect tuning is demonstrated by the existence of the expected inverse relationship between stereocilia stiffness and resonant frequency that occurs in many species [146–149], including

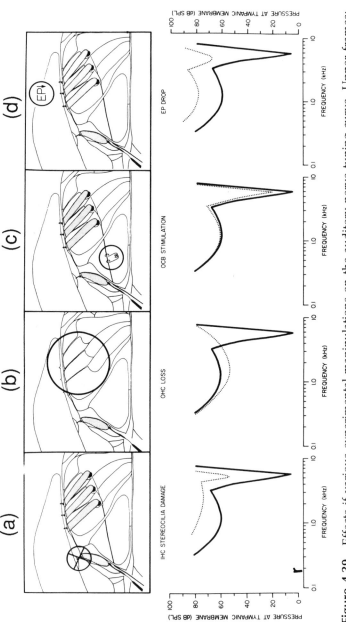 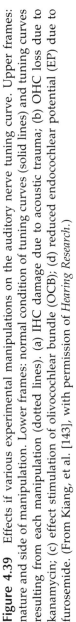

Figure 4.39 Effects if various experimental manipulations on the auditory nerve tuning curve. Upper frames: nature and side of manipulation. Lower frames: normal condition of tuning curves (solid lines) and tuning curves resulting from each manipulation (dotted lines). (a) IHC damage due to acoustic trauma; (b) OHC loss due to kanamycin; (c) effect stimulation of olivocochlear bundle (OCB); (d) reduced endocochlear potential (EP) due to furosemide. (From Kiang, et al. [143], with permission of *Hearing Research*.)

man [150]. Loss of the structural stiffness has been demonstrated as a consequence insults to the inner ear, and it appears that recovery from this "floppy" state is possible if the overall integrity of the HC is maintained [151]. These points all support an OHC basis for micromechanical tuning based. Moreover, as Khanna and Leonard [131] have pointed out, losing the stiffness of the OHC stereocilia should account for the downward shift of the characteristic frequency. This occurs because the effect of reducing the stiffness component of a filter is to lower its resonant frequency.

Otoacoustic Emissions

We have just seen that active processes play an interactive role in the transduction process transduction. Consistent with these concepts is a growing body of knowledge that began in 1978 when Kemp [152] demonstrated that the cochlea can issue sounds as well as receive them. He found that when a click is directed into the ear, it is followed by an echo that is emitted back from the cochlea, which can be detected roughly 5 msec or more after the click, typically peaking at latencies in the vicinity of approximately 5–15 msec. This phenomenon is called the stimulated or evoked (oto)acoustic emission, or the Kemp echo. Spontaneous acoustic emissions occur as well [153–156]. These are signals generated by the cochlea and measurable with a probe microphone in the ear canal. Figure 4.40 shows an example of a spontaneous otoacoustic emission. However, we will concentrate upon evoked emissions in man. Comprehensive reviews and discussions of the relationships among the various

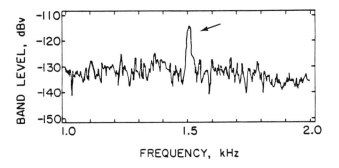

Figure 4.40 Example of a spontaneous otoacoustic emission at approximately 1500 Hz (arrow) detected above the noise floor in an occluded ear canal. Its level corresponds to about 11 dB SPL. (From Zurek [159] with permission of *J. Acoust. Soc. Am.*)

kinds of otoacoustic emissions may be found in recent articles McFadden and Wightman [157], Zwicker and Schloth [158], and Zurek [159].

It is worthwhile to review how the stimulated or evoked acoustic emission, or Kemp echo, is obtained. Suppose a probe device containing both a sound source (earphone) and a microphone (Fig. 4.41a) is inserted into someone's ear. A click is delivered to the ear, and the sound pressure is the occluded ear canal under the probe is measured over time. The resulting waveform will resemble the *middle* tracing in Fig. 4.41b. Here we see an initial damped oscillation lasting about 6 msec., followed by other oscillations several milliseconds later. The initial oscillations are the impulse response of the ear. A similar response would ensue if the click were directed into a metal-walled cavity designed to mimic the impedance characteristics of the human ear (Zwislocki coupler), as depicted in the *upper* tracing of Fig. 4.41b. The latter and much smaller oscillations, occurring after roughly 6–7 msec in this example, constitute the cochlear echo. The *lower* tracing of Fig. 4.41b shows just the Kemp echo after the response has been amplified and displaced by 5 msec. to remove the initial response.

The evoked acoustic emission has been described by numerous studies using clicks and/or tone bursts to elicit the response [152,153,158,160–168]. A number of findings have been derived from these and other studies [157–159]. To begin with, virtually all normal hearing humans appear to have a stimulated acoustic emission in response to clicks and/or tone bursts. A given ear's emission is extraordinary reproducible; however, the details of evoked emissions differ widely from ear to ear. Just as we have seen with respect to the sharpness and nonlinearity of the cochlea's mechanical tuning; the evoked acoustic emission is also vulnerable to such insults as ototoxicity and noise exposure and is obliterated by any substantive degree of sensorineural hearing loss.

The latency and magnitude of the echo depend on the level of the stimulus. Latency tends to decrease as the stimulus levels becomes greater. Although the magnitude of the evoked emission gets larger with increasing stimulus level, this relationship is linear only for low stimulus levels, above which the input-output curve becomes compressed, and saturates by the time the emission reaches about 20 dB SPL.

There are a number of interesting frequency relationships of the stimulated acoustic emission that are noteworthy. The latency of the emission decreases with increasing frequency. This association is important because it is consistent with the idea that the location within the cochlea from which the echo originates moves closer to the base with increasing frequency, as one would expect. A apparent problem with this point has been the observation that the actual latencies of the echo

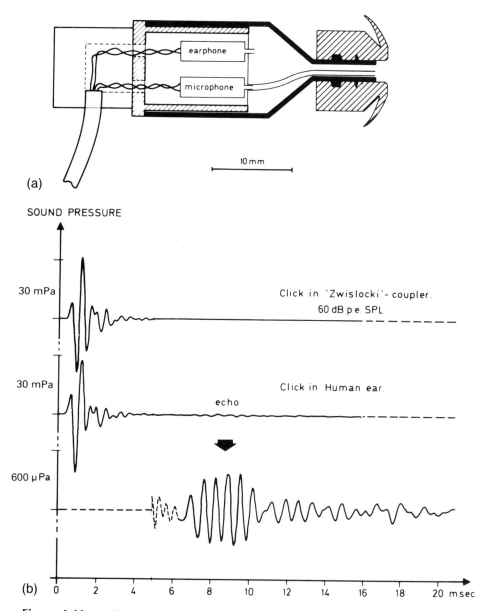

Figure 4.41 (a) Probe for eliciting and measuring otoacoustic emissions: It is inserted into the ear canal via the plastic ear tip at the right. The sound source is provided by the earphone and the microphone measures the sound pressure in the ear canal which is occluded by the ear tip. (b) Responses to a click: Upper: damped oscillations in a Zwislocki coupler. Middle: initial damped oscillations and the evoked emission (echo). Lower: amplified echo response displaced by 5 msec. (From Johnsen and Elberling [160], with permission of *Scandinavian Audiology*.)

199

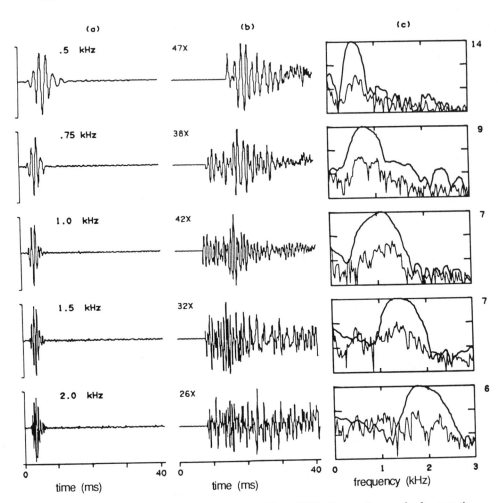

Figure 4.42 Effect of frequency from 500 to 2000 Hz on the evoked acoustic emission for one subject. Columns (a) and (b) show the evoked acoustic emission waveforms (before and after processing). Column (c) shows compares the spectra of the stimuli (smoother tracings) to those of the acoustic emissions. Note the orderly change in emission spectra with the changes in the stimulus spectra. (From Norton and Neeley [168], with permission of *J. Acoust. Soc. Am.*)

seem to be two or three times longer than the estimated time it would take the signal to reach and then return from a given place along the cochlear duct. However, it was recently pointed out that emission latencies correspond well with this expected round-trip travel time when the latter is based upon data obtained at low stimulus levels, similar to those employed in acoustic emissions work [168,169].

The spectral characteristics of click-evoked emissions do not exactly match those of the click used to elicit them. Instead, they tend to show an energy concentration in fairly narrow frequency ranges. Recent data using tone-bursts showed that the frequency concentrations in the spectra of acoustic emissions follow those of the stimuli, as exemplified in Fig. 4.42.

Acoustic emissions have been reported for the f2–f1 difference tone and the 2f1–f2 distortion product (the cubic difference tone) as long as the primary tones (f1 and f2) are close in frequency. An interesting example of distortion otoacoustic emissions is provided in Fig. 4.43 from an experiment by Burns et al. [170]. In the *lower* tracing, we see spontaneous otoacoustic emissions (SOAEs) at 1723 Hz and 2049 Hz. These act as primary tones (f1 and f2), yielding a cubic difference tone (2f1–f2) SOAE at 1397 Hz. In the *upper* tracing of the figure we see that the introduction of an external tone masks (see Chap. 10) the higher primary. As a result, this leaves only the lower primary SOAE, and the cubic difference tone which previously resulted from the interaction of f1 and f2 is now obliterated. These findings provide further evidence of active processes in the cochlea.

When continuous tones are presented to the ear, the acoustic emission has the same frequency as the stimulus but delayed by its latency.

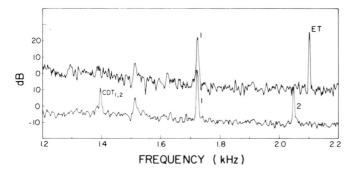

Figure 4.43 *Lower* tracing: primary (1, 2) spontaneous otoacoustic emissions (SOAEs) at 1723 Hz and 2049 Hz yield a cubic difference tone SOAE at 1397 Hz (CDT1,2). (The other (unlabeled) SOAE at 1520 Hz is not related to this effect.) *Upper* tracing: Adding an external tone (ET) masks f2, leaving only f1, thus obliterating the distortion product. (From Burns, Strickland, Tubis, and Jones [170].)

The interaction of the stimulus and emission will interact, resulting in peaks and valleys at frequencies with they are in and out of phase. This effect is seen at low levels of the stimulus, becoming less apparent and finally disappearing when the stimulus level exceeds 40 to 50 dB SPL. This level dependency is expected because of the emission's very low amplitude. That is, interference between the stimulus and emission can only occur when their levels are relatively similar; and due to the low level of the emission means that this condition can only be met at lower levels of the stimulus.

These phenomena are consistent with the concept that the evoked acoustic emissions monitored in the ear canal are cochlear in origin. It is apparent that active processes enable the cochlea to produce as well as receive acoustical signals. A detailed model for the production of acoustic emissions has yet to be generally accepted. Conceptually, it would probably employ active processes involving the motility of the OHCs, their connections with the tectorial membrane, and the efferent pathway. While the several models that have been proposed go well beyond the current scope, the interested reader may refer to discussions by Kemp [171], Kim [172], and Wilson [154].

Some Properties and Implications of Outer Hair Cells

The foregoing discussion revealed that the OHCs have a extensive impact upon the sharpness of cochlear tuning and the nonlinear response of the transduction process. This influence involves the role of the OHCs in the micromechanics of the cochlear response, which appears to involve an active contribution above and beyond passively responding to the stimulus. These special functions are founded upon by the various differences between the inner and outer HCs, which have been outlined in this chapter and also in Chap. 2. It is desirable to briefly recount some of the more salient IHC–OHC differences at this juncture. Moreover, such a recapitulation serves to point out the unique properties of the outer hair cells.

The inner and outer HCs both possess the essential elements of sensory receptor cells, yet they differ with respect to their architecture and location. The OHCs clearly make intimate contact with the tectorial membrane, whereas the IHCs either do not make such contact or have only a tenuous connection. The IHCs are now known to be roughly 12 dB more sensitive that the OHCs. About 95% of the afferent innervation (composed of Type I neurons) subserves the 3500 IHCs, and it is rather clear that the output of this system is the preponderant input to the auditory neural system. The 12,000 OHCs get only 5% of the afferent supply (which is made up of Type II units). In contrast to the afferent system, the efferent supply to the OHCs are the large neurons derived from the medial superior olive, which synapse directly to the hair cell. On the other hand, the IHCs' efferent supply is composed of the smaller fibers derived from the lateral superior olive, and which synapse on the afferent neurons instead of directly on the hair cell. Moreover, recall that several of the OHC's cellular structures bear a peculiar resemblance to muscle and that it contains a variety of contractile proteins.

The presence of contractile material leads one to ask whether the OHCs can actually contract in response to some sort of stimulation. In order to address this interesting question, scientists have removed OHCs from the cochlea and exposed them to a variety of stimuli under carefully controlled conditions. It should thus not be surprising that these isolated OHCs were found to contract when they were exposed to chemical agents known to effect contraction responses [173–178], electrical stimulation [175,179,180], and the efferent neurotransmitter, acetylcholine [175,178]. Moreover, recent findings by Slepecky et al. [178] have demonstrated that OHC elongation can occur as well as contraction in response to several of these agents.

An example of the contractile response of the OHC is shown in Fig. 4.44 for an isolated guinea pig OHC which was exposed to potassium gluconate [178]. Frame (a) shows the original length of the cell. The arrows in each frame show the original length of the cell. Notice that the cell shortened noticeably after being exposed to the potassium gluconate for one minute [frame (b)], and began to return to its original length after four minutes of exposure [frame (c)]. The HC became swollen and shorter when the chemical medium diluted with water [frame (d)]. This indicated that the cell membrane stayed intact during the experiment because it retained its normal osmotic characteristics.

The findings outlined in this and previous sections suggest that an active system which affects the micromechanics of the cochlea via the OHCs interacts with the traditionally envisioned system that passively transduces the signal and sends it off to the nervous system via the IHCs. Support for such a view comes from recent findings on how the olivocochlear bundle affects the afferent signals coming from the cochlea (see Chap. 2). The nature of these active mechanism goes well beyond the intended scope of this introductory text. Several interesting discussions address various aspects of these issues, several of which are listed in the references section [181–185].

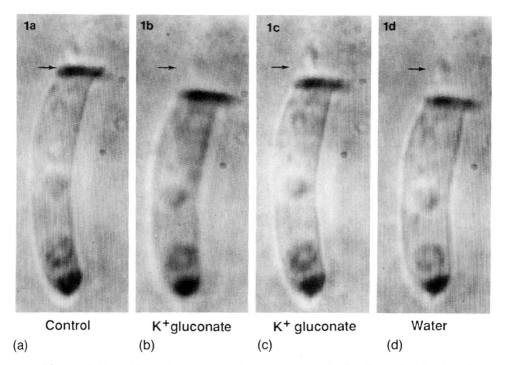

Control	K⁺gluconate	K⁺ gluconate	Water
(a)	(b)	(c)	(d)

Figure 4.44   Effect of potassium gluconate on an isolated OHC. (a) original length, (b) length after exposure to potassium gluconate for 1 minute, (c) length after 4 minutes of contact, (d) swelling and shortening when water was added to dilute the medium. Arrows show original length of the cell for comparison. (From Slepecky, Ulfendahl, and Flock [178], with permission of *Hearing Research*.)

REFERENCES

1. E. G. Wever, *Theory of Hearing*, Dover, New York, 1949, p. 167.
2. H. Helmholtz, *Die Lehre von den Tonempfindugen* (English translation: A. J. Ellis, *On the sensation of tones*, 1885).
3. G. Bekesy, *Experiments in Hearing*, McGraw-Hill, New York, 1960.
4. W. Rutherford, A new theory of hearing, *J. Anat. Physiol. 21*, 166–168 (1886).
5. E. G. Wever and M. Lawrence, *Physiological Acoustics*, Princeton Univ. Press, Princeton, New Jersey, 1954.
6. H. Davis, Some principles of sensory receptor action, *Physiol. Rev. 4*, 391–416 (1961).
7. H. Grundfest, The general electrophysiology of input membrane in electrogenic excitable cells, in *Handbook of Sensory Physiology* (W. R. Lowenstein,

ed.), Vol. 1: *Principles of Receptor Physiology*, Springer-Verlag, New York, 1971, pp. 136–165.

8. J. Tonndorf, Davis-1961 revisited: Signal transmission in the cochlear hair cell-nerve junction, *Arch. Otol. 101*, 528–535 (1975).

9. R. Klink, Neurotransmission in the inner ear, *Hearing Res. 22*, 235–243 (1986).

10. J. Tonndorf, Cochlear mechanics and hydro-mechanics, in *Foundations of Modern Auditory Theory* (J. Tobias, ed.), Vol. 1, Academic Press, New York, 1970, pp. 203–254.

11. J. Tonndorf, Response of cochlear models to aperiodic signals and to random noises, *J. Acoust. Soc. Amer. 32*, 1344–1355 (1960).

12. A. J. Hudspeth and D. P. Corey, Sensitivity, polarity, and conductance change in the response of vertibrate hair cells to controlled mechanical stimulation, *Proc. Nat. Acad. Sci. 74*, 2407–2411 (1977).

13. A. J. Hudspeth and R. Jacobs, Stereocilia mediate transduction in vertibrate cells, *Proc. National Acad. Sci. 76*, 1506–1509 (1979).

14. A. J. Hudspeth, Extracellular current flow and the site of transduction by vertibrate hair cells, *J. Neurosci. 2*, 1–10 (1982).

15. A. J. Hudspeth, The cellular basis of hearing; The biophysics of hair cells, *Science 230*, 745–752 (1985).

16. A. Flock, Sensory transduction in hair cells, in *Handbook of Sensory Physiology* (W. R. Lowenstein, ed.), Vol. 1: *Principles of Receptor Physiology*, Springer-Verlag, New York, 1971, pp. 396–441.

17. O. Lowenstein and J. Wersäll, A fundamental interpretation of the electron-microscopic structure of the sensory hairs in the cristae of the elasmobranch raja clavata in terms of directional sensitivity, *Nature 184*, 1807–1808 (1959).

18. J. Tonndorf, Shearing motion in scala media of cochlear models. *J. Acoust. Soc. Amer. 32*, 238–244 (1960).

19. E. ter Kuile, Die Ubertrungung der Energie von der Gundmembran auf die Haarzellan, *Pflug. Arch. ges Physiol. 79*, 146–157 (1900a).

20. E. ter Kuile, Die richtige Bewegungsform der Membrana basilaris, *Pflug. Arch. ges Physiol. 79*, 484–509 (1900b).

21. H. Davis, A mechano-electrical theory of cochlear action, *Annals Otol. 67*, 789–801 (1958).

22. A. Ryan and P. Dallos, Physiology of the inner ear, in *Hearing Disorders* (J. L. Northern, Ed.), Little, Brown, Boston, 1976, pp. 89–101.

23. T. Konishi and D. W. Nielsen, The temporal relationship between basilar membrane motion and nerve impulse inhibition in auditory nerve fibers of guinea pigs, *Japan J. Physiol. 28*, 291–307 (1973).

24. W. G. Sokolich, R. P. Hamernick, J. J. Zwislocki, and R. A. Schmiedt, Inferred response polarities of cochlear hair cells, *J. Accessed. Sac. Am. 59*, 963–974 (1976).

25. P. M. Sellick, R. Patuzzi, and B. M. Johnstone, Modulation of responses of spiral ganglion cells in the guinea pig by low frequency sound. *Hearing Res. 7*, 199–221 (1982).

26. M. A. Ruggero and N. C. Rich, Chinchilla auditory-nerve responses to low-frequency tones, *J. Accessed. Sac. Am. 73*, 2086–2108 (1983).

27. K. P. Steel, The tectorial membrane of mammals, *Hearing Res. 9*, 327–359 (1983).

28. J. Zwislocki, How OHC lesions can lead to neural cochlear hypersensitivity, *Acta Otol. 97*, 529–534 (1984).

29. J. Zwislocki, Cochlear function—An analysis, *Acta Otol. 100*, 201–209 (1985).

30. J. Zwislocki, Analysis of cochlear mechanics, *Hearing Res. 22*, 155–169 (1986).

31. P. Dallos, M. C. Billone, J. D. Durrant, C-Y. Wang, and S. Raynor, Cochlear inner and outer hair cells: Functional differences, *Science 177*, 356–358 (1972).

32. P. M. Sellick and I. J. Russell, The responses of inner hair cells to basilar membrane velocity during low frequency auditory stimulation in the guinea pig cochlea, *Hearing Res. 2*, 439–445 (1980).

33. A. L. Nuttall, M. C. Brown, R. I. Masta, and M. Lawrence, Inner hair-cell responses to velocity of basilar membrane motion in the guinea pig, *Brain Res. 211*, 171–174 (1981).

34. I. J. Russell and P. M. Sellick, Low frequency characteristics of intra-cellularly recorded potentials in guinea pig cochlear hair cells, *J. of Physiology 338*, 179–206 (1983).

35. P. Dallos, Some electrical circuit properties of the organ of Corti. II. Analysis including reactive elements, *Hearing Res. 14*, 281–291.

36. J. O. Pickles, S. D. Comis, and M. P. Osborne, Cross-links between ste-reocilia in the guinea pig organ of Corti, and their possible relation to sensory transduction, *Hearing Res. 15*, 103–112 (1984).

37. W. T. Peake, H. S. Sohmer, and T. F. Weiss, Microelectrode recordings of intracochlear potentials, *M.I.T. Res. Lab. Electronics Quart. Prog. Rep. 94*, 293–304 (1969).

38. I. Tasaki, H. Davis, and D. H. Eldredge, Exploration of cochlear potentials in guinea pig with a microelectrode, *J. Acoust. Soc. Amer. 26*, 765–773 (1954).

39. I. Tasaki and C. S. Spiropoulos, Stria vascularis as a source of endocochlear potential, *J. Neurophysiol. 22*, 149–155 (1959).

40. T. Konishi, R. A. Butler, and C. Fernandez, Effect of anoxia on cochlear potentials, *J. Acoust. Soc. Amer. 33*, 349–356 (1961).

41. P. Dallos, *The Auditory Periphery*, Academic Press, New York, 1973.

42. I. J. Russell and P. M. Sellick, Intracellular studies of hair cells in the mammalian cochlea, *J. of Physiology 284*, 261–290 (1978a).

43. P. Dallos, J. Santos-Sacchi, and A. Flock, Intracellular recordings from cochlear outer hair cells, *Science 218*, 582–584 (1982).

44. P. Dallos, Response characteristics of mammalian cochlear hair cells, *J. Neurosci. 5*, 1591–1608 (1985).

45. P. Dallos, Neurobiology of cochlear inner and outer hair cells: Intracellular recordings, *Hearing Res. 22*, 185–198 (1986).

46. E. G. Wever and C. W. Bray, Action currents in the auditory nerve in response to acoustic stimulation, *Proc. Natl. Acad. Sci. 16*, 344–350 (1930).

47. E. D. Adrian, The microphonic action of the cochlea: An interpretation of Wever and Bray's experiments, *J. Physiol. 71*, 28–29 (1931).

48. H. Davis, A. Derbyshire, M. Lurie, and L. Saul, The electric response of the cochlea, *Ann. Otol. 68*, 665–674 (1934).

49. E. G. Wever, Electrical potentials of the cochlea, *Physiol. Rev. 46*, 102–126 (1966).

50. T. Konishi and T. Yasuna, Summating potential of the cochlea in the guinea pig, *J. Acoust. Soc. Amer. 35*, 1448–1452 (1963).

51. P. Dallos and M. A. Cheatham, Production of cochlear potentials by inner and outer hair cells, *J. Acoust. Soc. Am. 60*, 510–512 (1976).

52. C. S. Hallpike and A. F. Rawdon-Smith, The Wever-Bray phenomenon: Origin of the cochlear effect, *Ann. Otol. 46*, 976–990 (1937).

53. H. Davis, A model for transducer action in the cochlea, *Cold Spring Harbor Symp. Quant. Biol. 30*, 181–190 (1965).

54. V. Honrubia and P. H. Ward, Dependence of the cochlear microphonic and summating potential on the endocochlear potential, *J. Acoust. Soc. Amer. 46*, 388–392 (1969).

55. A. E. Hubbard, C. D. Geisler, and D. C. Mountain, Comparison of the spectra of the cochlear microphonic and of the sound-elicited electrical impedance changes measured in scala media of the guinea pig, *J. Acoust. Soc. Am. 66*, 431–445 (1979).

56. D. C. Mountain, A. E. Hubbard, and C. D. Geisler, Voltage-dependent elements are involved in the generation of the cochlear microphonic and the sound-induced resistance changes measured in scala media of the guinea pig, *Hearing Res. 3*, 215–229 (1980).

57. Y. Katsuki, The origin of the microphonic potential, in *Hearing and Davis: Essays Honoring Hallowell Davis* (S. K. Hirsh, D. H. Eldridge, I. J. Hirsh, and S. R. Silverman, eds.), Washington Univ. Press, St. Louis, Missouri 1976, pp. 25–35.

58. Y. Tanaka, A. Asanuma, K. Yanagisawa, and Y. Katsuki, DC potential and distribution of the cochlear microphonic potential [in Japanese], *Audiol. Jpn. 18*, 241–245 (1975).

59. E. G. Wever and M. Lawrence, *Physiological Acoustics*, Princeton Univ. Press, Princeton, New Jersey, 1954.

60. J. J. Eggermont, D. W. Odenthal, P. N. Schmidt, and A. Spoor, Electrocochleography: Basic principles and clinical application, *Acta Otol., Suppl. 316* (1974).

61. G. S. Misrahy, K. M. Hildreth, E. W. Shinabarger, and W. J. Gannon, Electrical properties of the wall of endolymphatic space of the cochlea (guinea pig), *Amer. J. Physiol. 194*, 396–402 (1958).

62. I. Tasaki, H. Davis, and J. P. Legouix, The space-time pattern of the cochlear microphonic (guinea pig) as recorded by differential electrodes, *J. Acoust. Soc. Amer. 24*, 502–518 (1952).

63. H. Davis, Mechanisms of excitation of auditory nerve impulses, in *Neural Mechanisms of the Auditory and Vestibular Systems* (G. L. Rasmussen and W. F. Windle, eds.), Thomas, Springfield, Illinois, 1960, pp. 21–39.

64. V. Honrubia and P. H. Ward, Longitudinal distribution of the cochlear microphonics inside the cochlear duct (guinea pig), *J. Acoust. Soc. Amer. 44*, 951–958 (1968).

65. P. Dallos, M. S. Cheathan, and J. Ferraro, Cochlear mechanics, nonlinearities, and cochlear potentials, *J. Acoust. Soc. Amer. 55*, 597–605 (1974).

66. H. Davis, C. Fernandez, and D. R. McAuliffe, The excitatory process in the cochlea, *Proc. Natl. Acad. Sci. 36*, 580–587 (1950).

67. H. Davis, B. H. Deatherage, D. H. Eldredge, and C. A. Smith, Summating potentials of the cochlea, *Amer. J. Physiol. 195*, 251–261 (1958).

68. I. J. Russell and P. M. Sellick, Tuning properties of cochlear hair cells. *Nature 267*, 858–860 (1977a).

69. I. J. Russell and P. M. Sellick, The tuning properties of cochlear hair cells, in *Psychophysics and Physiology of Hearing* (E. F. Evans and J. P. Wilson, eds.) Academic Press, London, 1977b, pp. 71–87.

70. I. J. Russell and P. M. Sellick, Intracellular studies of cochlear hair cells: Filling the gap between basilar membrane mechanics and neural excitation, in *Evoked Electrical Activity in the Auditory Nervous System* (R. F. Naunton and C. Fernandez, eds.) Academic Press, London, 1978b, pp. 113–139.

71. H. Davis, B. Deatherage, B. Rosenblut, C. Fernandez, R. Kimura, and C. A. Smith, Modificatiaon of cochlear potentials by streptomycin poisoning and by extensive venous obstruction, *Laryngoscopy 68*, 596–627 (1958).

72. P. E. Stopp and I. C. Whitfield, Summating potentials of the avian cochlea, *J. Physiol. 175*, 45p–46p (1964).

73. N. Y.-S. Kiang and W. T. Peake, Components of electrical responses, *Ann. Otol. 69*, 448–458 (1960).

74. J. Fex, Efferent inhibition in the cochlea related to hair-cell dc activity: Study of postsynaptic activity of the crossed olivo-cochlear fibers in the cat, *J. Acoust. Soc. Amer. 41*, 666–675 (1967).

75. V. Honrubia and P. H. Ward, Properties of the summating potential of the guinea pig's cochlea, *J. Acoust. Soc. Amer. 45*, 1443–1449 (1969).

76. P. Dallos, Z. G. Shoeny, M. A. Cheatham, Cochlear summating potentials: Composition, *Science 170*, 641–644 (1970).

77. P. Dallos, Z. G. Shoeny, and M. A. Cheatham, Cochlear summating potentials: Descriptive aspects, *Acta Otol.*, Suppl. 302 (1972).

78. M. A. Cheatham, and P. Dallos, Summating potential (SP) tuning curves, *Hearing Res. 16*, 189–200 (1984).

79. R. H. Sweetman and P. Dallos, Distribution pattern of cochlear combination tones, *J. Acoust. Soc. Amer. 45*, 58–71 (1969).

80. J. Tonndorf, Cochlear nonlinearities, in *Basic Mechanisms in Hearing* (A. R. Møller, ed.), Academic Press, New York, 1973, pp. 11–47.

81. J. Tonndorf, The hydrodynamic origin of aural harmonics in the cochlea, *Ann Otol. 67*, 754–774 (1958).

82. J. Zwislocki, Discussion of cochlear nonlinearities (by Tonndorf), in *Basic Mechanisms in Hearing* (A. R. Møller, ed.), Academic Press, New York, 1973.

83. J. Tonndorf, Nonlinearities in cochlear hydrodynamics, *J. Acoust. Soc. Amer. 47*, 579–591 (1970).
84. P. Dallos, Z. G. Shoeny, D. W. Worthington, and M. A. Cheatham, Cochlear distortion: Effects of direct current polarization, *Science 164*, 449–451 (1969).
85. P. Dallos and R. H. Sweetman, Distribution pattern of cochlear harmonics, *J. Acoust. Soc. Amer. 45*, 37–46 (1969).
86. P. Dallos, Combination tone $2f_1-f_h$ in microphonic potentials, *J. Acoust. Soc. Amer. 46*, 1437–1444 (1969).
87. D. W. Worthington and P. Dallos, Spacial patterns of cochlear difference tones, *J. Acoust. Soc. Amer. 49*, 1818–1830 (1971).
88. M. C. Liberman, The cochlear frequency map for the cat: Labeling auditory-nerve fibers of known characteristic frequency, *J. Acoust. Soc. Am. 72*, 1441–1449 (1982).
89. E. F. Evans, The sharpening of cochlear frequency selectivity in the normal and abnormal cochlea, *Audiology 14*, 419–442 (1975).
90. N. Y.-S. Kiang, *Discharge Patterns of Single Nerve Fibers in the Cat's Auditory Nerve*, MIT Press, Cambridge, Massachusetts, 1965.
91. E. F. Evans and J. P. Wilson, Frequency resolving power of the cochlea: The effective bandwidth of cochlear nerve fibers, in *Proc. 7th Intl. Congr. on Acoustics*, Vol. 3, Akademiai Kiado, Budapest, 1971, pp. 453–456.
92. E. F. Evans and J. P. Wilson, Frequency selectivity of the cochlea, in *Basic Mechanisms in Hearing* (A. R. Møoller, ed.), Academic Press, New York, 1973, pp. 519–554.
93. E. F. Evans, The frequency response and other properties of single nerve fibers in the guinea pig cochlea, *J. Physiol. 226*, 263–287 (1972).
94. C. D. Geisler, W. S. Rhode, and D. T. Kenedy, Responses to tonal stimuli of single auditory nerve fibers and their relationship to basilar membrane motion in the squirrel monkey. *J. Neurophysiol. 37*, 1156–1172 (1974).
95. J. P. Wilson and J. R. Johnstone, Capacitive probe measures of basilar membrane vibration, paper at Symposium on Hearing Theory, Institute for Perception Research, Eindhoven, The Netherlands, 1972, pp. 172–181.
96. B. M. Johnstone, K. J. Taylor, and A. J. Boyle, Mechanics of the guinea pig cochlea, *J. Acoust. Soc. Amer. 47*, 504–509 (1970).
97. B. M. Johnstone and J. F. Boyle, Basilar membrane vibration examined with the Mössbauer technique, *Science 158*, 389–390 (1967).
98. J. Tonndorf and S. M. Khanna, Displacement pattern of the basilar membrane: A comparison of experimental data, *Science 160*, 1139–1140 (1968).
99. B. M. Johnstone and K. Taylor, Mechanical aspects of cochlear function, in *Frequency Analysis and Periodicity Detection in Hearing* (R. Plomp and G. F. Smoorenburg, eds.), Sijthoff, Leiden, 1970, pp. 81–93.
100. B. M. Johnstone and G. K. Yates, Basilar membrane tuning curves in the guinea pig, *J. Acoust. Soc. Amer. 55*, 584–587 (1974).
101. W. S. Rhode, Observations of the vibration of the basilar membrane in squirrel monkey using the Mössbauer technique, *J. Acoust. Soc. Amer. 49*, 1218–1231 (1971).

102. W. S. Rhode and L. Robles, Evidence from Mössbauer experiments for nonlinear vibration in the cochlea, *J. Acoust. Soc. Amer. 55*, 588–596 (1974).

103. L. Robles and W. S. Rhode, Nonlinear effects in the transient response of the basilar membrane, in *Facts and Models in Hearing* (E. Zwicker and E. Terhardt, eds.), Springer-Verlag, New York, 1974.

104. L. U. E. Kohllöfel, A study of basilar membrane vibrations, *Acoustica 27*, 49–89 (1972).

105. J. P. Wilson and J. R. Johnstone, Basilar membrane and middle ear vibration in guinea pig measured by capacitive probe, *J. Acoust. Soc. Amer. 57*, 705–723 (1975).

106. D. Robertson, Cochlear neurons: Frequency selectivity altered by perilymph removal, *Science 186*, 153–155 (1974).

107. E. F. Evans and J. P. Wilson, Cochlear tuning properties: Concurrent basilar membrane and single nerve fiber measurements, *Science 190*, 1218–1221 (1975).

108. E. L. LePage and B. M. Johnstone, Nonlinear mechanical behavior of the basilar membrane in the basal turn of the guinea pig cochlea, *Hearing Res. 2*, 183–192 (1980).

109. E. F. Evans, Does frequency sharpening occur in the cochlea? paper at Symposium on Hearing Theory, Institute for Perception Research, Eindhoven, The Netherlands, 1972.

110. E. F. Evans, The effects of hypoxia on tuning of single fibers in the cochlear nerve, *J. Physiol. 238*, 65–67 (1974).

111. G. G. Furman and L. S. Frishoff, Model of neural inhibition in the mammalian cochlea, *J. Acoust. Soc. Amer. 36*, 2194–2207 (1964).

112. E. C. Carterette, M. P. Friedman, and S. D. Lovell, Mach bands in hearing, *J. Acoust. Soc. Amer. 45*, 986–998 (1969).

113. T. Houtgast, Psychophysical evidence for lateral inhibition in hearing, *J. Acoust. Soc. Amer. 51*, 1885–1894 (1974).

114. J. Zwislocki, E. Buining, and J. Glantz, Frequency distribution of central masking, *J. Acoust. Soc. Amer. 43*, 1267–1271 (1968).

115. A. R. Møller, Studies of the damped oscillatory response of the auditory frequency analyzer, *Acta Physiol. Scand. 78*, 299–314 (1970).

116. J. P. Wilson and E. F. Evans, Grating acuity of the ear: Psychophysical and neurophysiological measures of frequency resolving power, in *Proc. 7th Intl. Congr. on Acoustics*, Vol. 3, Akademiai Kiado, Budapest, 1971.

117. H. Rainbolt and A. M. Small, Mach bands in auditory masking: An attempted replication, *J. Acoust. Soc. Amer. 51*, 567–574 (1974).

118. J. Zwislocki, A possible neuro-mechanical sound analysis in the cochlea, *Acoustica 31*, 354–359 (1974).

119. J. Zwislocki, Phase opposition between inner and outer hair cells and auditory sound analysis, *Audiology 14*, 443–455 (1975).

120. G. A. Manley, Cochlear frequency sharpening—A new synthesis, *Acta Otol. 85*, 167–176 (1978).

121. S. M. Khanna, R. E. Sears, and J. Tonndorf, Some properties of longitudinal shear waves: A study by computer simulation, *J. Acoust. Soc. Amer. 43*, 1077–1084 (1968).

122. H. Duifhuis, Cochlear nonlinearity and second filter: possible mechanisms and implications, *J. Acoust. Soc. Am. 59*, 408–423 (1976).

123. J. Zwislocki and E. J. Kletsky, Micromechanics in the theory of cochlear mechanics, *Hearing Res. 2*, 505–512 (1980).

124. A. C. Crawford and R. Fettiplace, An electrical tuning mechanism in turtle cochlear hair cells, *J. Laryngol. 312*, 377–422 (1981).

125. J. O. Pickles, *An Introduction to the Physiology of Hearing*, Academic Press, London, 1982.

126. S. A. Gelfand, *Hearing: An Introduction to Physchological and Physiological Acoustics*, Marcel Dekker, New York, 1981.

127. S. M. Khanna and D. G. B. Leonard, Basilar membrane tuning in the cat cochlea, *Science 215*, 305–306 (1982).

128. S. M. Khanna, Homodyne interferometer for basilar membrane measurements, *Hearing Res. 23*, 9–26 (1986).

129. S. M. Khanna, G. W. Johnson, and J. Jacobs, Homodyne interferometer for basilar membrane vibration measurments. II. Hardware and techniques, *Hearing Res. 23*, 27–36 (1986).

130. S. M. Khanna and D. G. B. Leonard, Measurement of basilar membrane vibrations and evaluation of the cochlear condition. *Hearing Res. 23*, 37–53 (1986).

131. S. M. Khanna and D. G. B. Leonard, Relationship between basilar membrane tuning and hair cell condition, *Hearing Res. 23*, 55–70 (1986).

132. P. M. Sellick, R. Patuzzi, and B. M. Johnstone, Measurement of basilar membrane motion in the guinea pig using the Mossbauer technique, *J. Acoust. Soc. Am. 72*, 131–141 (1982).

133. L. Robles, M. A. Ruggero, and N. C. Rich, Mossbauer measurements of the mechanical response to single-tone and two-tone stimuli at the base of the chinchilla cochlea, in *Peripheral Auditory Mechanisms* (J. B. Allen, J. L. Hall, A. Hubbard, S. T. Neely, and A. Tubis, eds.) Springer, Munich, pp. 121–128.

134. S. M. Khanna, Inner ear function based on the mechanical tuning of the hair cells, in *Hearing Science* (C. I. Berlin, ed.) College Hill, San Diego, 1984, pp. 213–240.

135. J. P. Kelly and S. M. Khanna, Ultrastructural damage in cochleas used for studies of basilar membrane mechanics, *Hearing Res. 14*, 59–78 (1984a).

136. J. P. Kelly and S. M. Khanna, The distribution of damage in the cochlea after removal of the round window membrane, *Hearing Res. 16*, 109–126 (1984b).

137. D. G. B. Leonard and S. M. Khanna, Histological evaluation of damage in cat cochleas used for measurement of basilar membrane mechanics, *J. Acoust. Soc. Am. 75*, 515–527 (1984).

138. M. C. Liberman and L. W. Dodds, Single-neuron labeling and chronic

cochlear pathology. III. Stereocilia damage and alterations of threshold tuning curves, *Hearing Res. 16,* 55–74 (1984b).

139. P. Dallos and D. Harris, Properties of auditory-nerve responses in the absence of outer hair cells, *J. Neurophys. 41,* 365–383 (1978).
140. M. C. Liberman, Single-neuron labeling and chronic cochlear pathology. I. Threshold shift and characteristic-frequency shift, *Hearing Res. 16,* 33–41 (1984).
141. M. C. Liberman and L. W. Dodds, Single-neuron labeling and chronic cochlear pathology. II. Stereocilia damage and alterations of spontaneous discharge rates, *Hearing Res. 16,* 43–53 (1984a).
142. M. C. Liberman and N. Y. S. Kiang, Single-neuron labeling and chronic cochlear pathology. IV. Stereocilia damage and alterations in rate- and phase-level functions, *Hearing Res. 16,* 75–90 (1984).
143. N. Y. S. Kiang, M. C. Liberman, W. F. Sewell, and J. J. Guinan, Single unit clues to cochlear mechanisms, *Hearing Res. 22,* 171–182 (1986).
144. M. C. Liberman, Single-neuron labeling in cat auditory nerve, *Science 216,* 1239–1241 (1982).
145. D. W. Smith, D. B. Moody, W. C. Stebbins, and M. A. Norat, Effects of outer hair cell loss on the frequency selectivity of the patas monkey auditory system, *Hearing Res. 29,* 125–138 (1987).
146. T. J. Garfinkle and J. C. Saunders, Morphological properties of inner hair cell stereocilia in C57BL/6J mouse, *J. Otol., Head and Neck Surg. 9,* 421–426 (1983).
147. R. G. Turner, A. A. Muraski, and D. W. Nielsen, Cilium length: Influence on neuronal tonotopic organization, *Science 213,* 1519–1521 (1981).
148. D. J. Lim, Cochlear anatomy related to cochlear micromechanics—A review. *J. Acoust. Soc. Am. 67,* 1686–1695 (1980).
149. L. G. Tilney and J. C. Saunders, Actin filaments, stereocilia, and hair cells of bird cochlea. I. The length, number, width, and distribution of stereocilia of each hair cell in relation to the position of the hair cell on the cochlea, *J. Cell Biol. 96,* 807–821 (1982).
150. A. Wright, Scanning electron microscopy of the human cochlea—The organ of Corti, *Arch. Oto-Rhino-Laryngol. 230,* 11–19 (1981).
151. J. C. Saunders, S. P. Dear, and M. E. Schneider, The anatomical consequences of acoustic injury: A review and tutorial, *J. Acoust. Soc. Am. 78,* 833–860 (1985).
152. D. T. Kemp. Stimulated acoustic emissions from within the human auditory system, *J. Acoust. Soc. Am. 64,* 1386–1391 (1978).
153. D. T. Kemp, Evidence of mechanical nonlinearity and frequency selective wave amplification in the cochlea, *Arch. Otol. Rhinol. Laryngol. 224,* 37–45 (1979).
154. J. P. Wilson, Model for cochlear echoes and tinnitus based on an observed electrical correlate, *Hearing Res. 2,* 527–532 (1980).
155. P. M. Zurek, Spontaneous narrow-band acoustic signals emitted by human ears, *J. Acoust. Soc. Am. 69,* 514–523 (1981).

156. E. A. Strickland, E. M. Burns, and A. Tubis, Incidence of spontaneous oto-acoustic emissions in children and infants, *J. Acoust. Soc. Am. 78*, 931–935 (1985).

157. D. McFadden and F. L. Wightman, Audition: Some relations between normal and pathological hearing, *Ann. Rev. Psychol. 34*, 95–128 (1983).

158. E. Zwicker and E. Schloth, Interrelation of different oto-acoustic emissions, *J. Acoust. Soc. Am. 75*, 1148–1154 (1984).

159. P. M. Zurek, Acoustic emissions from the ear: A summary of results from humans and animals, *J. Acoust. Soc. Am. 78*, 340–344 (1985).

160. N. J. Johnsen and C. Elberling, Evoked acoustic emissions from the human ear I. Equipment and response parameters, *Scand. Audiol. 11*, 3–12 (1982a).

161. H. P. Wit and R. J. Ritsma, Stimulated acoustic emissions from the human ear, *J. Acoust. Soc. Am. 66*, 911–913 (1979).

162. H. P. Wit and R. J. Ritsma, Evoked acoustical emissions from the human ear: Some experimental results, *Hearing Res. 2*, 253–261 (1980).

163. D. T. Kemp and R. Chum, Properties of the generator of stimulated acoustic emissions, *Hearing Res. 2*, 213–232 (1980).

164. W. L. C. Rutten, Evoked acoustic emissions from within normal and abnormal human ears: Comparison with audiometric and electrocochleographic findings, *Hearing Res. 2*, 263–271 (1980).

165. J. P. Wilson, Evidence for a cochlear origin for acoustic re-emission, threshold fine-structure, and tonal tinnitus, *Hearing Res. 2*, 233–252 (1980).

166. N. J. Johnsen and C. Elberling, Evoked acoustic emissions from the human ear II. Normative data in young adults and influence of posture, *Scand. Audiol. 11*, 69–77 (1982b).

167. R. Probst, A. C. Coats, G. K. Martin, and B. L. Lonsbury-Martin, Spontaneous, click-, and toneburst-evoked otoacoustic emissions from normal ears, *Hearing Res. 21*, 261–275 (1986).

168. S. J. Norton and S. T. Neeley, Tone-burst-evoked otoacoustic emissions from normal-hearing subjects, *J. Acoust. Soc. Am. 81*, 1860–1872 (1987).

169. S. T. Neeley, S. J. Norton, M. P. Gorga, and W. Jesteadt, Latency of otoacoustic emissions and ABR wave V using tone-burst stimuli, *J. Acoust. Soc. Am. 79*, Suppl. 1, S5 (1986).

170. E. M. Burns, E. A. Strickland, A. Tubis, and K. Jones, Interactions among spontaneous otoacoustic emissions. I. Distortion products and linked emissions. *Hearing Res. 16*, 271–278 (1984).

171. D. T. Kemp, Otoacoustic emissions, travelling waves and cochlear mechanisms, *Hearing Res. 22*, 95–104 (1986).

172. D. O. Kim, Active and nonlinear cochlear biomechanics and the role of outer-hair-cell subsystem in the mammalian auditory system, *Hearing Res. 22*, 105–114 (1986).

173. A. Flock, B. Flock, and M. Ulfendahl, Mechanisms of movement in outer hair cells and a possible structural basis, *Arch. Otorhinolaryngol. 243*, 83–90 (1986).

174. N. Slepecky, M. Ulfendahl, and A. Flock, Effects of caffeine and tetracaine

on outer hair cell shortening suggest intracellular calcium involvement, *Hearing Res. 32,* 11–32 (1988a).

175. W. E. Brownell, C. R. Bader, D. Bertrand, and Y. deRibaupierre, Evoked mechanical response of isolated cochlear outer hair cells, *Science 227,* 194–196 (1985).

176. H. P. Zenner, U. Zimmerman, and U. Schmitt, Reversible contraction of isolated mammalian cochlear hair cells, *Hearing Res. 18,* 127–133 (1985).

177. M. Ulfendahl, Motility in auditory sensory cells, *Acta Physiol. Scand. 130,* 521–527 (1987).

178. N. Slepecky, M. Ulfendahl, and A. Flock, Shortening and elongation of isolated outer hair cells in response to application of potassium gluconate, acetylcholine and cationized ferritin, *Hearing Res. 34,* 119–126 (1988b).

179. B. Kachar, W. E. Brownell, R. Altschuler, and J. Fex, Electrokinetic shape changes of cochlear outer hair cells, *Nature 322,* 365–368 (1986).

180. J. F. Ashmore, A fast motile response in guinea-pig outer hair cells: The cellular basis of the cochlear amplifier, *J. Physiol. 388,* 323–347 (1987).

181. D. O. Kim, Functional roles of the inner- and outer-hair-cell subsystems in the cochlea and brainstem, in *Hearing Science* (C.I. Berlin, ed.), College-Hill, San Diego, 1984, pp. 241–262.

182. D. O. Kim, Active and nonlinear cochlear biomechanics and the role of outer-hair-cell subsystem in the mammalian auditory system, *Hearing Res. 22,* 105–114 (1986).

183. C. D. Geisler, A model of the effect of outer hair cell motility on cochlear vibrations, *Hearing Res. 24,* 125–131 (1986).

184. D. J. Lim, Cochlear micromechanics in understanding otoacoustic emission, *Scand. Audiol. 25,* 17–25 (1986).

185. P. Dallos, Cochlear neurobiology: Revolutionary developments, *Asha 30:6/7,* 50–56 (1988).

5
Auditory Nerve

This chapter deals with the coding of information in the auditory nerve. This is done by monitoring the electrical responses of individual neurons or the compound output of the nerve "as a whole" during the presentation of various (usually acoustic) stimuli. The resulting observations suggest how various parameters of sound are represented in this primary stage of the auditory nervous system. Moreover, as we have already seen in previous chapters, responses from the auditory nerve have also been used as a window for observing cochlear processes.

Major advances in this area have been enabled by the use of intracellular recordings from individual auditory neurons labeled with horseradish peroxidase (HRP), which was introduced by Liberman [1]. This approach makes it possible to definitively identify the neuron from which recordings have been made, and to trace its course to other neurons or to the hair cells. Two fundamental and interrelated findings based upon this method must of necessity be highlighted at the outset of this chapter: First, recall from Chap. 2 that Kiang et al. [2] established the correspondence of the Type I auditory neurons (marked intracellularly) and radial fibers which synapse with the IHCs; and that the Type II neurons (marked extracellularly) continue as the outer spiral fibers to the OHCs. Second, it is now accepted that all individual auditory nerve fiber responses to date have actually been derived from the Type I auditory neurons which innervate the inner HCs [3,4].

FREQUENCY CODING

Tuning Curves

The responses of single auditory nerve fibers to acoustic stimulation at various frequencies were reported by Galambos and Davis [5], and their results were confirmed and expanded upon by many others. The response areas of single neurons as a function of frequency are shown by their tuning curves (Fig. 5.1). A narrowly tuned cell responds to a very limited range of frequencies, whereas a broadly tuned cell responds to a much wider frequency range. Since an unstimulated neuron maintains an ongoing (spontaneous) discharge rate even in the absence of any apparent stimulation, its threshold may be determined by varying the stimulus level until the lowest intensity is reached at which the neuron responds above its spontaneous rate. An alternative approach is to present the stimulus at a fixed intensity, and to measure the number of spike potentials with which the unit responds at different stimulus frequencies. The former method measures the neuron's sensitivity, and the latter its firing rate, as functions of frequency. The frequency with the

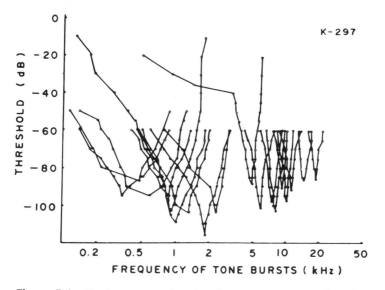

Figure 5.1 Tuning curves showing the response areas of single auditory nerve fibers in the cat. (Reprinted from *Discharge Patterns of Single Fibers in the Cat's Auditory Nerve* by N. Y.-S. Kiang with permission of The M.I.T. Press, Cambridge, Massachusetts © 1965, p. 87.)

lowest threshold (or the greatest firing rate) is the best or characteristic frequency (CF) of the neuron.

The tuning curves of various single fibers in the auditory nerve of the cat are shown in Fig. 5.1. Frequency is along the x-axis and the level needed to reach the neuron's threshold is on the y-axis. Notice that each fiber will respond to a range of frequencies if the stimulus level is high enough. This frequency range extends considerably below the CF, but is quite restricted above it. In other words, a fiber responds readily to intense stimulation below its CF, but is only minimally responsive to stimulation above it. At lower intensity levels, the fibers are quite narrowly tuned to a particular frequency, as is shown by the V-shaped troughs around each CF [6–10].

Although stimulus amplitude may be expressed in SPL, the tuning curves become sharper and more regular when stimulus level is expressed as the degree of stapes footplate displacement in the oval window. This sharpening occurs because using stapes displacement as the reference omits middle ear effects (see Chap. 3), which are included when the stimulus is expressed as the SPL at the ear canal or the voltage applied to the earphone [7,8].

The sensitivity of a particular neuron generally falls at a rate of more than 25 dB per octave below the CF and well over 100 dB per octave above it. The low-frequency "tails" of higher-CF fibers actually extend very far below the CF; and phase-locked* responses for low-frequency stimuli at high levels have been demonstrated for these fibers [9]. (These low-frequency tails should not be surprising, since we know that much of the cochlear partition is affected at high intensities.)

The tuning of the auditory nerve fibers thus appears to reflect the frequency analysis of the cochlea. Figure 5.1 also shows that there tends to be a gradation in the sharpness of neural tuning with increasing frequency. In other words, the high-frequency neural tuning curves tend to have sharper tips (as well as the above-noted low-frequency tails) than do the lower-frequency tuning curves (which do not possess low-frequency tails). The same general relationships occur in the cochlea, and are demonstrated by comparing the tuning curves for the intracellular receptor potentials of the hair cells in the first (higher-frequency) and third (lower-frequency) turns [11].

---

*"Phase locking" refers to a clear and fixed relationship between some aspect of the response and the phase (or time) of some aspect of the stimulus. The importance of this phenomenon will become clear in the following sections dealing with firing patterns.

One might recall here that the CFs of individual auditory nerve fibers are related to distance along the length of the cochlea by Liberman's [12] cochlear frequency map (see Fig. 4.29). This relationship was developed by determining the CFs of individual auditory neurons which were labeled with HRP, and then tracing these fibers back to where they innervated various IHCs along the cochlear partition. More recently, Keithley and Schreiber [13] developed a spiral ganglion frequency map for the cat in which CF is related to percentage distance from the base of Rosenthal's canal.

Firing Patterns

Single nerve fibers discharge spike potentials ("fire") in an all-or-none manner. The firing pattern is the manner in which a fiber discharges in response to a stimulus (or spontaneously in the absence of stimulation). The firing patterns of fibers can suggest how information is coded and transmitted in the auditory nervous system. The firing patterns of auditory nerve fibers also provide corroborative information about cochlear mechanics.

Various stimuli are used to provide different kinds of information about neural coding. Clicks (at least ideally) are discrete and instantaneous in time, with energy distributed equally throughout the frequency range. On the other hand, pure tones (also ideally) extend indefinitely in time, but are discrete in frequency. Thus, click stimuli lend themselves to the study of the temporal characteristics of the discharge pattern, while sinusoids can be used to study frequency-related aspects. Tone bursts can be used to investigate both frequency and temporal characteristics, since they are similar to clicks in their duration and to tones in their frequency specificity [14]. One should remember, however, that a tone burst is a compromise between the two extremes, so that it is really less discrete in time than a click and less discrete in frequency than a pure tone.

Responses to Clicks

One way to study the response of an auditory nerve fiber is to determine the probability that it will discharge under given circumstances. This is not as complicated as it sounds. Assume that we have placed a microelectrode into an auditory nerve fiber. We then present a click to the animal's ear and record the time between the click onset and the discharge of any spike potential which it may elicit. In other words, we record the time delay or latency of each spike from the start of the click. This procedure is repeated many times for the same fiber, and the number of spikes that occurrred after each latency is counted. These data are plotted on a graph called a poststimulus time (PST) histogram, in which the latencies are shown on the abscissa and the number of spikes on the ordinate (Fig. 5.2). If many spikes occurred at a latency of 2 msec, for

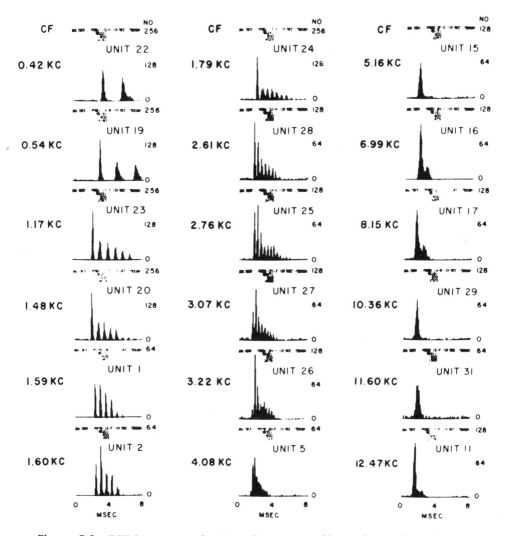

Figure 5.2 PST histograms for 18 auditory nerve fibers of a single cat in response to clicks. (Reprinted from *Discharge Patterns of Single Fibers in the Cat's Auditory Nerve* by N. Y.-S. Kiang with permission of The M.I.T. Press, Cambridge, Massachusetts © 1965, p. 28.)

example, then we can say that there is a high probability that the fiber will respond at 2 msec. If concentrations of spikes (modes) also occur at other latencies, we can say that there is a good probability that the fiber will respond at these other latencies as well as at the first one.

Figure 5.2 shows the PST histograms obtained by Kiang [6] for 18 auditory nerve fibers in one cat. The CF of each fiber is given to the left of its histogram. Note that fibers with lower CFs have multiple peaks, while those with higher CFs have single peaks. Three other observations are important. First, the latency to the first peak decreases as the CF increases. Second, the interpeak intervals (the time between successive modes) gets smaller as the CF increases. Closer scrutiny reveals that the interpeak interval corresponds to the period of the characteristic frequency of a fiber (i.e., to 1/CF) in a relationship which constitutes a linear function. Lastly, baseline activity is actually reduced between the peaks. Kiang found that these time-locked multiple peaks and the reduced baseline activity were maintained even at very low levels of stimulation. Decreased baseline activity was, in fact, the initial response noted at the lowest stimulus levels.

If the PST histograms are compared for clicks of opposite polarity, the peaks resulting from rarefaction clicks are found to occur *between* those in response to condensation clicks [6]. That is, when the click's polarity is reversed (which means that drum, and eventually basilar membrane, deflection is reversed, see Chap. 4), then so are the times at which the peaks and dips occur in the PST histogram. Furthermore, the rarefaction phase is related to increased neural activity, in accordance with the earlier findings of Davis et al. [15] for stimuli up to 2000 Hz.

The traveling wave response to an impulsive stimulus such as a click travels up the cochlea at a speed which is quite fast at the basal end and slows down toward the apex [16]. We would therefore expect the PST histogram to reflect rapid and synchronous discharges of higher-frequency fibers originating from the basal turn. This effect is shown by the short latencies of the first peak for higher CFs. The longer latencies for successively lower CFs reflect the propagation time of the traveling wave up the cochlear partition to the places from which the fiber arise. Thus, the latency to the first peak represents a neural coding of the mechanical activity in the cochlea.

The interpeak interval also reflects the activity of the cochlea, since it is a function of the period of the frequency (1/f) in the click stimulus to which the fiber responds. Since the latencies of the peaks do not change with click level, Kiang suggested that deflections of the cochlear partition in one direction result in increased neural activity, while neural activity is reduced relative to the baseline rate when the basilar membrane is deflected in the opposite direction. This interpretation is further supported by the reversal of peaks and dips for clicks of opposite polarity.

Responses to Tone Bursts

The response of eight auditory nerve fibers to tone bursts are shown in Fig. 5.3. Each PST histogram shows the response pattern beginning 5 msec after tone burst onset. Note that there is an initial peak in response to stimulus onset in each response pattern. The prominence of this peak is a function of the tone burst intensity. The peak is followed by a gradual decrease in the discharge rate until a stable level is attained. The

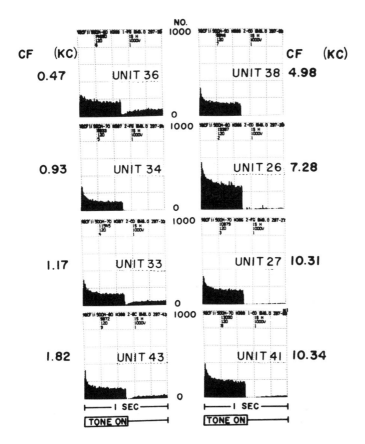

Figure 5.3   PST histograms in response to tone burst for fibers of different CFs. [Reprinted from *Discharge Patterns of Single Fibers in the Cat's Auditory Nerve* by N. Y.-S. Kiang with permission of The M.I.T. Press, Cambridge, Massachusetts (© 1965, p. 69.)

stable rate continues until the tone burst is turned off, at which time activity drops sharply to a level below the spontaneous discharge rate. The spontaneous rate is then gradually reattained. The neural discharges are time-locked to individual cycles of the tone burst for fibers up to about 5000 Hz. (This effect is not seen in the figure because of the restricted time scale.)

Responses to Tones and Tonal Complexes

Kiang [6] found that the discharges of auditory nerve fibers are time-locked to tonal stimuli up to about 4000–5000 Hz. This relation was demonstrated by the presence on the PST histogram of single peaks corresponding to individual cycles of the stimulus; and it is consistent with other evidence that auditory nerve fibers respond to the particular phase of the stimulus within this frequency range [17,18]. Furthermore, there is impressive evidence that auditory nerve fibers respond only to deflections of the basilar membrane in one direction (which is consistent with the click data), and that the timing of the firings corresponds to unilateral elevations of the partition [19,20]. (See Chap. 4.)

The relationship of the responses of single auditory nerve fibers to stimulus phase is illustrated in Fig. 5.4. These graphs are not PST histograms, instead they show the number of spikes discharged at various time intervals in response to 1 sec pure tones from 412–1600 Hz. The tones were presented at 80 dB SPL. A single fiber was monitored. It responded to frequencies between 412 and 1800 Hz, with its best responses between 1000 and 1200 Hz.

The dots under each histogram correspond to integral multiples of the period of the stimulus tone. Thus, in the upper left-hand graph of Fig. 5.4, with a frequency of 412 Hz and a period of 2427 μsec, the dots indicate 2427 μsec time intervals (2427 μsec, 4854 μsec, 7281 μsec, etc.). The spikes in each histogram cluster at a number of relatively discrete latencies, with fewer spikes at successively higher multiples of the period. Of primary significance is that the locations of the peaks closely correspond to integral multiples of the period for each stimulus frequency up to and including 1100 Hz. At higher frequencies, the period of the peaks become as low as 625 μsec (for 1600 Hz), although the latencies of the first peak stay in the 800–900 μsec range. This minimum period reflects the fiber's refractory period.

These findings suggest that, at least for pure tones, a period-time code is used to transmit frequency information in auditory nerve fibers: The discharge pattern of the neuron is in cadence with the period of the stimulus. The locking of the response pattern to the period of the sinusoid is maintained even if the stimulus frequency is not the CF of the

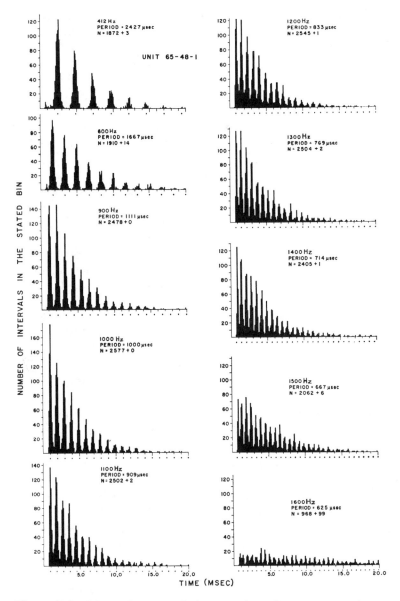

Figure 5.4 Interspike intervals for a single auditory neuron of a squirrel monkey in response to 1 sec tones at 80 dB SPL. Stimulus frequency is shown above each graph. The dots below the abscissa are integral multiples of the period of the stimulus. (N is the number of intervals plotted plus the number of intervals with values greater than shown on the abscissa.) (From Rose, Brugge, Anderson, and Hind [17], with permission of *J. Neurophysiol.*)

fiber, and regardless of stimulus intensity. When the spike discharges were studied relative to a fixed point on the stimulus cycle, phase locking of the discharge pattern was found for frequencies as high as 5000 Hz. This result is not to suggest that place coding is unfounded. On the contrary, the important of place coding is demonstrated by the tuning curves in Fig. 5.1. Both mechanisms contribute to frequency coding.

When an auditory nerve fiber is stimulated simultaneously by two relatively low-frequency tones, the resulting firing pattern will be phase locked to either: (1) the cycles of the first sinusoid, (2) the cycles of the second sinusoid, or (3) the cycles of both stimuli [18]. When the response pattern is to only one of the two original tones, the phase-locked response is the same as it would have been if that tone were presented alone. Which of the three response modes occurs is determined by the intensities of the two tones and by whether their frequencies lie within the fiber's response area. (See the section Two-Tone Inhibition.)

Brugge et al. [19] have reported the discharge patterns in response to complex periodic sounds. Their stimuli were made up of two relatively low-frequency primary tones combined in various ways, as shown in Fig. 5.5. The firing patterns are shown in period histograms, in which discharges are represented as a function of the period of the stimulus (i.e., as though they all occurred during one period of the complex wave). Again, we see clear-cut phase locking of the discharge pattern to the stimulus, reflecting neural coding of the mechanical activity along the cochlear partition in a straightforward manner. Note that the neural activity shown by the period histogram follows the shape of the stimulus waveform above and below the origin of the y-axis. These observations were associated with the concept that nerve fiber activation is linked to the upward deflections of the basilar membrane [19]. However, more recent studies have revealed that neural activation is also associated with downward deflections of the cochlear partition [21–27], reflecting a more complicated state of affairs and is the subject of some controversy.

The neural firing patterns reported by Brugge et al. were corroborated by a study by Rose, Brugge, Anderson and Hind [20]. They found that when two tones resulted in a complex wave whose peaks are not equidistant, then the spikes cluster about integral multiples of the period of the complex wave. The complex wave's period corresponds to its fundamental frequency, which, in turn, is the greatest common denominator of the two original tones. Note in this regard that when the ratio of the low to the high primary has a numerator of one less than the denominator, as for 1000 and 1100 Hz (1000/1100 = 10/11), the fundamental is the difference tone (1000 − 1000 = 100 Hz). In this case, the spike discharges correspond to a period of 100 Hz, and the listener would perceive a tone correspond-

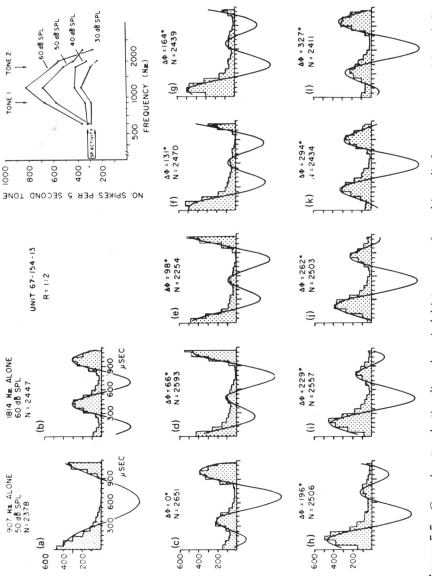

Figure 5.5 Complex tonal stimuli and period histograms of resulting discharge patterns. (a) and (b), primary tones; (c)–(l), complex tones; ϕ is phase shift between the primaries; upper right-hand graph shows the response area at various SPLs. (From Brugge, Anderson, Hind, and Rose [19], with permission of *J. Neurophysiol.*)

ing to a pitch of 100 Hz. This provides one basis for the "missing fundamental" phenomenon discussed in Chap. 12.

Two-Tone Inhibition

Assume that a single auditory nerve fiber is discharging in response to a
continuous tone at its CF (Fig. 5.6a). A second tone at a slightly different
frequency is then added to the first. The presence of the second tone will
actually cause a *decrease* in the firing rate (Fig. 5.6b). This decrease in the
unit's firing rate due to the addition of the second tone is called two-tone
inhibition, and has been repeatedly demonstrated in auditory nerve
fibers [6,18,28,29]. Many studies of two-tone inhibition (or suppression,
as it is sometimes called) have used tone bursts to inhibit a unit's response to a continuous tone at its CF, as shown schematically in Fig.
5.6b. As might be imagined, it would be cumbersome to "map out" the
inhibitory area(s) of a neuron: An excessive number of discrete tone
bursts would be needed at all of the frequencies and intensities being
tested.

Instead of tone bursts, Sachs and Kiang [29] used a sweep frequency
(SF) tone to inhibit the fiber's response to a continuous tone at its characteristic frequency (CTCF). (A sweep frequency tone is one which
changes frequency continuously over time.) Figure 5.7 shows a series of
PST histograms for a fiber with a CF of 22.2 kHz. The left column shows
the firing patterns (as a function of log frequency) for the SF (inhibiting)
tone alone. The frequency of the SF tone was smoothly changed from 6

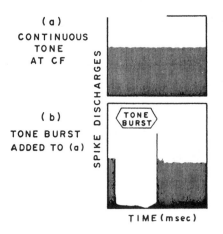

Figure 5.6   Idealized example two-tone inhibition (see text).

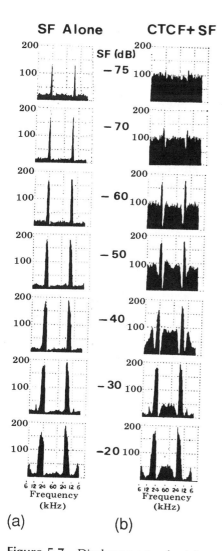

SF Alone　　**CTCF+SF**

(a)　　　(b)

Figure 5.7 Discharge rates for (a) a sweep frequency (SF) tone alone, and (b) the SF tone added to a continuous tone at its characteristic frequency (CTCF) at various levels of the SF tone. The CTCF is 22.2 kHz at −75 dB. Duration is 72 sec going from 6 kHz to 60 kHz and back to 6 kHz. Abscissa: log frequency for the SF tone; ordinate: spike rate. (From Sachs and Kiang [29], with permission of *J. Acoust. Soc. Am.*)

kHz to 60 kHz and then back down to 6 kHz. There were thus two "approaches" by the SF tone to the CF: one from below and one from above. The histograms in the right-hand column of the figure are for the ongoing CTCF combined with the SF tone. Observe that the SF tone causes a reduction in the firing rate at frequencies near the CF. The series of histograms in the right-hand column reveals that a wider range of frequencies will inhibit the discharge rate as the intensity of the SF tone is increased (from −75 to −20 dB). The data compiled at various SF tone frequencies and intensities can be plotted in a manner similar to a tuning curve. An idealized representation is given in Fig. 5.8, where the cross-hatched areas show the combinations of SF frequencies and intensities that inhibit the firing of a fiber for a CTCF. This figure illustrates several aspects of two-tone inhibition.

Two-tone inhibition can be elicited by a suppressing (SF) tone either higher or lower than the CF, as long as its intensity and frequency are appropriate. Figure 5.8 shows that the high-frequency inhibitory area extends to within 10 dB of the level of the CTCF, although the low-frequency inhibitory area does not. In other words, inhibitory tones higher in frequency than the CF are effective at lower intensities than tones whose frequencies are below the CF. It should be added that Sachs and Kiang found inhibitory areas for all 310 fibers they studied, and were able to demonstrate this effect at intensities near the threshold of

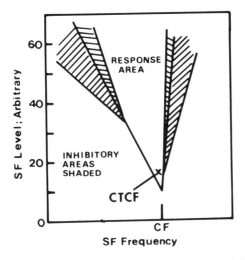

Figure 5.8 Idealized response and inhibitory areas in a two-tone inhibition experiment. (Adapted from Sachs and Kiang [29], with permission of *J. Acoust. Soc. Am.*)

the fiber. Other intensity and frequency and intensity dependencies in two-tone inhibition have been described [30,31], but are beyond the current scope. One might also note in this context that two-tone inhibition can affect auditory neuron tuning curves, although these effects are different depending upon whether the inhibitory tone is in close proximity to the CF or considerably below it [9,32,33]: For example, the sharpness of tuning is hardly affected in the former case, whereas broader tuning results from the latter.

Although two-tone inhibition certainly represents a nonlinearity in the ear's response, its origin is still not firmly established. The well-known demonstration of two-tone inhibition in auditory nerve responses makes it enticing to attribute it to a neural source. Yet, the preponderance of the evidence implies that two-tone inhibition most likely results from nonlinear processes in the cochlea. One line of evidence stems from the fact that two-tone inhibition has been shown to occur for the cochlear microphonic [34–36], which is a preneural event. Related to this, Sellick and Russell [37] demonstrated two-tone inhibition in the intracellular receptor potentials of IHCs. Moreover, it has been observed in basilar membrane vibrations at high levels [38], and has also been demonstrated in otoacoustic emissions [39]. Further, the latency of two-tone inhibition is too short to be the result of efferent feedback, which also suggests some interaction at the cochlear level [40]. All of these points suggest a cochlear source.

INTENSITY CODING

Determining how intensity is coded by the auditory neural system is a formidable problem. The most difficult aspect is to explain how the auditory nerve is able to subserve an intenstiy continuum covering 120+ dB. Although there are several ways in which intensity information might be coded, the precise mechanism is still unresolved.

The first neural responses at barely threshold intensities appear to be a decrease in spontaneous activity [6], and phase locking of spike discharges to the stimulus cycle [17]. This is not to say that the fiber will fire in response to every cycle of a near-threshold stimulus. Rather, even though the overall discharge rate may not be significantly greater than the spontaneous level, those spikes that do occur will tend to be locked in phase with the stimulus cycle [41]. Effects such as this might provide some degree of intensity coding since it has been known for some time that fibers with higher spontaneous rates have lower thresholds [6,42]. We will return to the latter relationship below.

While threshold differences are unquestionably, important, it makes sense to also consider the neuron's dynamic range, which is the intensity range over which the auditory nerve fiber continues to respond with increasing magnitude. Saturation is said to have occurred when the neuron's response no longer increases as the stimulus level is raised. Order to make this concept clear, Fig. 5.9 shows an example of the growth and saturation of an auditory neuron's firing pattern with increasing stimulus intensity. In their classic experiment, Galambos and Davis [5] found that the dynamic range of auditory nerve fibers is only about 20–40 dB. In other words, the discharge rate increases with stimulus intensity from threshold up to a level 20–40 dB above it. At higher intensities the spike rate either levels off or decreases. Obviously, a single fiber cannot accommodate the 120+ dB range from minimal audi-

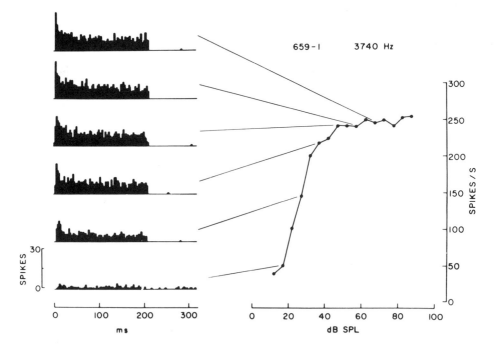

Figure 5.9 The input–output (rate-level) function on the right shows the effect of stimulus intensity on the firing rate of an auditory nerve fiber. The PST histograms on the left correspond to various points indicated on the input–output function. [From Salvi, Henderson, and Hamernick [42], Physiological bases of sensorineural hearing loss, in *Hearing Research and Theory, Vol. 2*, (Tobias and Shuber, eds.), © 1983 by Academic Press.]

bility to the upper usable limits of hearing. However, if there were a set of units with graded thresholds, they could cooperate to produce the dynamic range of the ear [43]. For example, if there were four fibers with similar CF having dynamic ranges of 0–40, 30–70, 60–100, and 90–130 dB, respectively, then they could conceivably accommodate the ear's dynamic range.

Subsequent findings have revealed a wider dynamic range in fibers with similar CFs than was previously thought, and it is now established that auditory neurons can have dynamic ranges of as much as 40 dB [1,43,46–50]. The relationship between stimulus level and firing rate is shown by the rate-level function. Several examples of rate-level functions for various fibers with similar CFs in the same cat are shown in Fig. 5.10 from the study by Sachs and Abbas [45]. In each case, the arrow

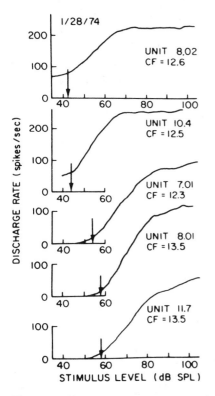

Figure 5.10 Discharge rate as a function of stimulus level for five auditory nerve fibers with similar CFs in the same cat. Arrows are fiber thresholds. (From Sachs and Abbas [45], with permission of *J. Acoust. Soc. Am.*)

indicates the fiber's threshold. Notice that whereas the lower threshold fibers tend to saturate about 20 dB above threshold, the units with higher thresholds tend to have dynamic ranges that can be roughly 40 dB wide.

Considerable insight into this area was provided by the identification of three relatively distinct groups of auditory nerve fibers with respect to their spontaneous rates and thresholds by Liberman [51] in 1978. The groups described by Liberman included units covering an overall threshold range as great as about 80 dB for fibers with similar CFs in the same cat. The relationship between auditory neuron thresholds and spontaneous rates also been reported by Kim and Molnar [52]. Figure 5.11 shows the three groups of auditory nerve fibers in terms of the relationship between their spontaneous firing rates and their relative threshold sensitivities. The fibers that had high spontaneous rates (over 18 spikes/sec) had the lowest thresholds of the three groups. These are indicated as group c in the figure. Within this high spontaneous rate (SR) group, the thresholds were essentially the same regardless of the actual spontaneous rate. That is, thresholds were within ±5 dB whether the spontaneous rate was 20 spikes/sec or 100 spikes/sec. These high-SR fibers made up about 61% of those sampled.

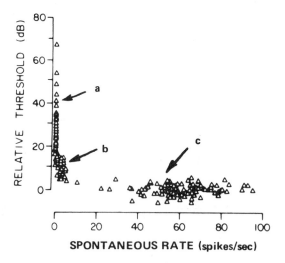

Figure 5.11   Relationship between spontaneous rate and relative thresholds for fibers with low (a), medium (b), and high (c) spontaneous firing rates. (From Liberman [51], with permission of *J. Acoust. Soc. Amer.*)

The second group included fibers with medium spontaneous rates (between 0.5 and 18 spikes/sec). These medium-SR units comprised approximately 23% of the fibers and are shown as group b in the figure. The remaining 16% had low spontaneous rates (under 0.5 spikes/sec). Not only did these low-SR units have the highest thresholds of the three groups, but they also had a threshold range covering about 50 dB (group c).

It is now established that they are all radial units innervating the IHCs, and that each IHC receives all three types of fibers [1]. They are also distinguished on the basis of size, morphology and where they attach to the IHCs [1,2,12,50,51–56]. The high-SR fibers have the largest diameters and the greatest number of mitochondria. On the other hand, the low-SR units have the smallest diameters and relatively fewest mitochondria. Figure 2.33 shows the attachments of the three types of fibers to a typical IHC. Notice that the thick, high-SR fiber synapses on the side of the hair cell which faces toward the tunnel and OHCs (toward the right in the figure). In contrast, low-SR and medium-SR fibers attach on the surfaces facing the modiolus (toward the left). Of the three groups, the low-SR fibers appear to have the greatest association with the efferent neurons.

The individual rate-level functions of a larger number of high-SR, medium- and low-SR fibers are shown in Fig. 5.12 from a recent study by Liberman [50]. Because these rate-level functions have been normalized in terms of both spike rates and stimulus levels, it is possible to directly compare the dynamic ranges. These functions revealed that high-SR and medium-SR auditory nerve fibers reached saturation about 25 dB above their thresholds; however, this did not occur for any of the fibers with low spontaneous rates. Instead, the spike rates of the low-SR units continued to increase with stimulus level through 40 dB above threshold, and some achieved continuing growth of magnitude as high as 60 dB above threshold.

To recapitulate, it appears that type 1 auditory nerve fibers with similar CFs have a considerable range of thresholds and dynamic ranges, and both of these parameters are correlated with the spontaneous rates of the fibers. In turn, these spontaneous rate characteristics tend to categorize themselves into three groups, which are also distinguishable on the bases of their size, morphology and the locations of their synapses. Moreover, each sensory receptor cell (IHC) synapses with all three types of fibers. It would thus appear that there is a reasonable basis for the coding of intensity on the basis of the auditory nerve fibers and their responses, at least to a first approximation.

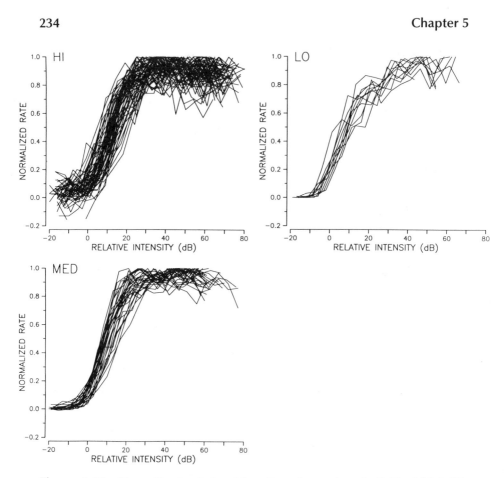

Figure 5.12 Normalized rate-level functions for various individual high-SR, medium-SR and low-SR auditory nerve fibers (cat). (Modified from Liberman [50], with permission of *Hearing Research*.)

An complementary if not alternative explanation based on several on several things we already know is also consistent with the factors already covered. For example, we know that auditory nerve fiber activity reflects the pattern of cochlear excitation in a rather straightforward manner. Figure 5.13 shows the effect of stimulus intensity on the response area of a single auditory neuron whose CF is 2100 Hz. Note that as intensity is increased, the number of spikes per second also increases, as does the frequency range to which the fiber responds. Also, the frequency range over which the fiber responds tends to increase more below than above the CF.

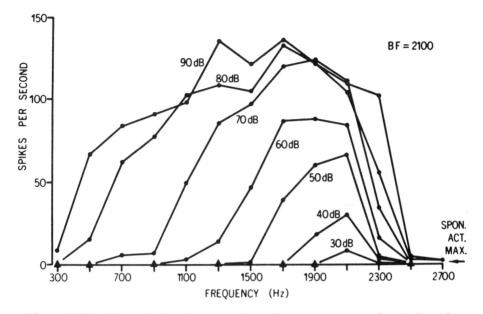

Figure 5.13   Effect of stimulus intensity on the response area of a single auditory neuron (CF = 2100 Hz). (From Rose, Hind, Anderson, and Brugge [43], with Permission of *J. Neurophysiol.*)

Keeping this in mind, recall also that the basilar membrane may be conceived of as an array of elements which are selectively responsive to successively lower frequencies going from base to apex. Now refer to Fig. 5.14 by Whitfield [57]. Frequency is represented along the horizontal axis from left to right; the ordinate respresents spike rate. The hypothesis for neural coding is as follows. Figure 5.14a represents the response area resulting from stimulation at a given frequency. Figure 5.14b shows the discharge pattern for equivalent stimulation at a higher frequency. The frequency change is represented as a simple displacement of the hypothetical response area long the frequency axis, and is analogous to the movement of the traveling wave along the basilar membrane. Figure 5.14c represents the effect of increasing the stimulus level at the same frequency as in Fig. 5.14a. The position of the response area stays the same, but the number of responding fibers increases. Here is what hypothetically occurs: A particular number of fibers are responding in Fig. 5.14a. As the stimulus level increases, the fibers increase their spike rates (until saturation is reached). Although some fibers saturate, other fibers with similar CFs but different thresholds continue to increase their dis-

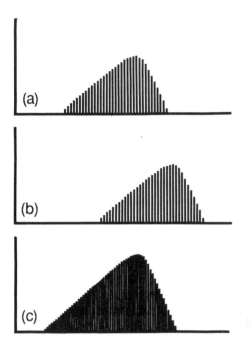

Figure 5.14 Hypothetical changes in the array of auditory nerve responses (see text). (Courtesy of I. C. Whitfield [57].)

charge rates as the level increases. As intensity continues to increase, the stimulus enters the excitatory areas of other fibers which respond to that frequency only at higher intensities. The overall effect, then, is for the intensity increment to be coded by increased overall firing rates, among more fibers, over a wider frequency range. (We shall see in the next section that increasing the stimulus level also results in greater synchrony of the individual neural discharges, so that the whole-nerve action potential has a shorter latency and greater magnitude.)

Such a model could employ all of the preceding factors in arriving at the overall change in the excitation pattern between Fig. 5.14a and Fig. 5.14c, and could account for the wide dynamic range of the ear. It does not, however, account for the observation in Fig. 4.13 that the peak of a fiber's response curve shifts in frequency as the stimulus level is increased [43]. The implication is that phase-locking to the stimulus cycle would be particularly important in maintaining frequency coding when the intensity increment is encoded by increases in density of discharges per unit time and by widening of the array of active fibers.

WHOLE-NERVE ACTION POTENTIALS

So far we have examined individual auditory nerve fibers. In this section we shall review some aspects of the whole-nerve, or compound, action potential (AP) of the auditory nerve. In addition to its contribution to an understanding of the auditory system, the whole-nerve AP is also clinically useful in the procedure called electrocochleography [58,59]. The whole-nerve AP, as its name suggests, is a composite of many individual fiber discharges. These more or less synchonous discharges are recorded by an extracellular electrode as a negative deflection. Recall from Chap 4 that the AP must be separated from the cochlear microphonic (CM), which is generally accomplished by an averaging procedure. (Recall that the CM is in opposite phase in the scalae vestibuli and tympani, whereas the AP is always negative. Thus, averaging the responses from the two scalae cancels the CM and enhances the AP.)

The AP is also frequently recorded from other locations than the inside of the cochlea, for example at the round window in animals, and at the promontory and even from the ear canal in humans. In these cases, averaging the responses has the important effect of enhancing the AP and reducing the random background noise (see Chap. 6 for a discussion of signal averaging).

As shown in Fig. 5.15a, the AP appears as a negative amplitude peak (N_1) at some latency following stimulus onset, and then as one or more smaller peaks (N_2, N_3, etc.). Whole-nerve APs are elicited by transient stimuli with fast rise times, such as clicks or tone bursts. It is generally accepted that the transient stimulus leads to the synchronous firing of many fibers [61] exclusively from the basal turn of the cochlea [62]. The AP is attributed to the basal turn because the high speed of the traveling wave in this part of the cochlea causes a large number of receptors to be stimulated almost simultaneously, leading to the synchrony of the neural discharges. More apical parts of the cochlea are not thought to contribute because the longer travel time up the partition would cause firings from these regions to be nonsynchronous. However, there is some evidence that other parts of the cochlea may also contribute to the AP response [63].

The origin of the N_2 peak has been the subject of some controversy. Teas et al. [64] pointed out that the diphasic waveform (a negative deflection followed by a positive one) would result in the N_1 and N_2 peaks. Other suggested sources of these peaks have included more apical areas of the cochlea [65], repeated firings of the auditory nerve fibers [62], and discharges from the second-order neurons of the cochlear nucleus [66]. Eggermont [67] found that the distinct N_2 peaks found in the guinea pig

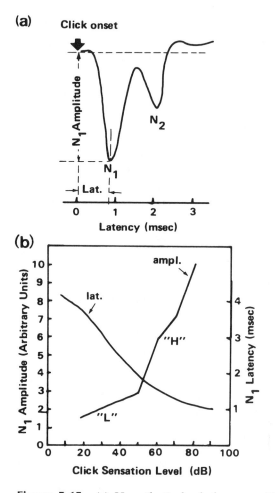

Figure 5.15 (a) Hypothetical whole-nerve AP response. (b) Amplitude and latency functions of the AP response based on Yoshie's [60] data. Amplitude is in arbitrary units where 10 is the amplitude of the response to a click at 80 dB SPL.

response were absent in the human response. He attributed this to differences in the electroanatomy of the human and guinea pig, and suggested that the source of the peak might be cochlear nucleus discharges, which are more readily recorded in the guinea pig than in man. Experimental data, however, have shown that it is the positive deflection of the diphasic response which separates the AP into N_1 and N_2 peaks; and that this separation occurs within the internal auditory meatus

[63,68]. These studies showed that when the central end of the auditory nerve (in the internal auditory canal) was deactivated chemically or mechanically, the result was a change in the AP wave so that the N_2 peak was absent. This loss is apparently due to the removal of the positive deflection of the diphasic response, which normally separates the N_1 and N_2 peaks.

Figure 5.15b shows that both the magnitude and latency of the AP depend on stimulus intensity [60,61]: Increasing the level of the stimulus increases the amplitude of the response and decreases its latency. This relationship is actually not a simple one-to-one correspondence between stimulus level and AP amplitude and latency. Notice that the amplitude curve in Fig. 5.15b is made up of two rather distinct line segments rather than of a single straight line. There is a portion with a shallow or low ("L") slope at lower stimulus levels, and a segment which becomes abruptly steep or high ("H") in slope as stimulus intensity continues to increase. Furthermore, the function is not necessarily monotonic; i.e., the relationship between stimulus level and AP amplitude is not always in the same direction for all parts of the curve. A small dip in AP amplitude has been reported to occur at about the place where the L and H segments meet, before the curve resumes increasing with stimulus level [69].

In the past, it has been proposed that the source of the two-part amplitude function might be the two population of receptor cells in the cochlea [44,59]. That is, the L segment was interpreted as reflecting the output of the OHCs and the H portion was seen as derived from the IHCs. This concept was based upon contemporary interpretations of the different innervation patterns of the two hair cell populations, and the subsequently disproven notion that the OHCs are more sensitive than the IHCs. As discussed in Chaps. 2 and 4, these suppositions are now known to be erroneous. There are other experimental data which also contradict the previously held idea that the different sets of receptor cells cause the two segments of the AP amplitude function. In particular, the amplitude function has been found to have a single slope over its entire length when the central end of the nerve within the internal auditory meatus is deactivated [68]. Deactivation of this part of the auditory nerve changes the shape of the AP waveform, also, by removing the positive deflection that separates the N1 and N2 peaks.

Alternative models to explain the two segments of the AP amplitude function, which have obvious implications for intensity coding in general, have been proposed by Evans [70–72] and by Özdamar and Dallos [73]. These similar models explain the shape of the amplitude function on the basis of single-fiber tuning curves. Recall that the typical tuning curve has two parts: a narrowly tuned area around the CF at low levels, and a more widely tuned area extending downward in frequency as stimulus intensity is raised. This shape is shown in Fig. 5.16a. The important point is that the low-frequency tails make a neu-ron responsive to a wide frequency range provided the intensity is great enough. Consider the responses of various fibers to a 1000 Hz

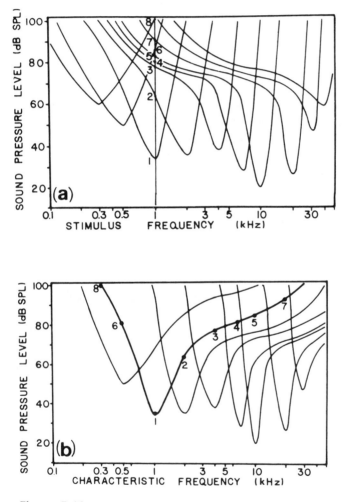

Figure 5.16 (a) Auditory nerve fibers tuning curves. (b) Across-fiber tuning curves (From Özdamar and Dallos [73], with permission of *J. Acoust. Soc. Amer.*)

tone, represented by the vertical line at 1000 Hz in the figure. Point 1 represents the lowest level at which a 1000 Hz CF fiber responds. The remaining points (2 through 8) show the levels at which the 1000 Hz tone activates fibers with other CFs.

The 1000 Hz tone primarily crosses the low-frequency tails of the higher-CF tuning curves, but it also crosses the higher-frequency portions of some lower-CF tuning curves (e.g. point 6). Thus, a 1000 Hz tone activates more and more fibers with different CFs as its level increases. This situation is plotted in Fig. 5.16b, which shows *across*-fiber tuning curves. The numbers correspond to those in Fig. 5.16a. Across-fiber tuning curves show the levels at which fibers with various CFs respond to a particular frequency (1000 Hz here). The tip of the across-fiber tuning curve represents the lowest level at which *any* fiber responds to that frequency. The width of the across-fiber tuning curve shows the *range* of neurons with different CFs that respond at a given stimulus level. For example, only the 1000 Hz CF fiber responds to 1000 Hz at 35 dB SPL; but fibers with CFs between about 500 and 10,000 Hz may respond when the same tone is presented at 80 dB SPL (i.e., between points 6 and 5).

Across-fiber tuning curves have high-frequency tails instead of the low-frequency tails of individual fiber tuning curves. This situation occurs because the low-frequency tails of an increasing number of high-frequency fibers respond as the intensity is raised (Fig. 5.16a).

How might this effect account for the two segments of the AP amplitude function? The insert in Fig. 5.17 shows the width of a hypothetical across-fiber tuning curve. Line a shows the width of the across-fiber tuning curve within the narrowly tuned segment. The width of the tuning curve at 90 dB SPL is shown by line b, which is in the widely tuned part of the curve. The main figure shows the width of the across-fiber tuning curve on the y-axis as a function of SPL. Lines a and b correspond to those in the insert. Only a small population of fibers with CFs close to the stimulus frequency respond at low intensity levels. At higher levels there is a dramatic increase in the number of responding fibers, as the stimulus level reaches the low-frequency tails of the other neurons. There is thus a slow increase in the width of the across-fiber tuning curve followed by a sharp increase as intensity rises. Comparison of Fig. 5.17 with Fig. 5.15b shows that this curve is remarkably similar to the AP amplitude function. The portion of the curve in the vicinity of line a corresponds to the L portion of the AP amplitude funtion, while the part around line b corresponds to the steeper H segment. This correspondence provides a mechanism which might underlie the two segments of the compound AP ampli-

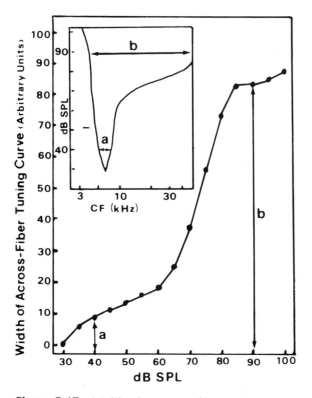

Figure 5.17 Width of an across-fiber tuning curve as a function of SPL. Insert: across-fiber tuning curve upon which the figure is based. Lines a and b correspond on both curves. (Adapted from Özdamar and Dallos [73], with permission of *J. Acoust. Soc. Amer.*)

tude function. (One might also consider this mechanism with respect to excitation models like the one in Fig. 2.33). Physiological findings by Özedamar and Dallos [74] support this mechanism.

REFERENCES

1. M. C. Liberman, Single-neuron labeling in cat auditory nerve, *Science 216*, 1239–1241 (1982a).
2. N. Y. S. Kiang, J. M. Rho, C. C. Northrop, M. C. Liberman, and D. K. Ryugo, Hair-cell innervation by spiral ganglion cells in adult cats, *Science 217*, 175–177 (1982).
3. M. C. Liberman and D. D. Simmons, Applications of neuronal labeling

techniques to the study of the peripheral auditory system, *J. Acoust. Soc. Am. 78*, 312–319 (1985).

4. N. Y. S. Kiang, M. C. Liberman, W. F. Sewell, and J. J. Guinan, Single unit clues to cochlear mechanisms, *Hearing Res. 22*, 171–182 (1986).

5. R. Galambos and H. Davis, The response of single auditory nerve fibers to acoustic stimulation, *J. Neurophysiol 6*, 39–57 (1943).

6. N. Y.-S. Kiang, Discharge Patterns of Single Fibers in the Cat's Auditory Nerve, M.I.T. Press, Cambridge, Mass., 1965.

7. N. Y.-S. Kiang, M. B. Sachs, and W. T. Peake, Shapes of tuning curves for single auditory-nerve fibers, *J. Acoust. Soc. Amer. 42*, 1341–1342 (1967).

8. N. Y.-S. Kiang. A survey of recent developments in the study of auditory physiology, *Ann. Otol. 77*, 656–675 (1968).

9. N. Y.-S. Kiang and E. C. Moxon, Tails of tuning curves of auditory-nerve fibers, *J. Acoust. Soc. Amer. 55*, 620–630 (1974).

10. N. Y. S. Kiang, and E. C. Moxon, Physiological considerations in artificial stimulation of the inner ear. *Annals Otol. 81*, 714–731 (1972).

11. P. Dallos, Response characteristics of mammalian cochlear hair cells, *J. Neurosci. 5*, 1591–1608 (1985).

12. M.C. Liberman, The cochlear frequency map for the cat: Labeling auditory-nerve fibers of known characteristic frequency, *J. Acoust. Soc. Am. 72*, 1441–1449 (1982b).

13. E. M. Keithley, and R. C. Schreiber, Frequency map of the spiral ganglion in the cat, *J. Acoust. Soc. Am. 81*, 1036–1042 (1987).

14. N. Y.-S. Kiang, Stimulus representation in the discharge patterns of auditory neurons, in *The Nervous System* (D. B. Tower and E. L. Eagles, eds.), Vol. 3: *Human Communication and Its Disorders*, Raven, New York, 1975, pp. 81–96.

15. H. Davis, C. Fernandez, and D. R. McAuliffe, The excitatory process in the cochlea, *Proc. Natl. Acad. Sci.* 580–587 (1950).

16. G. Bekesy, *Experiments in Hearing*, McGraw-Hill, New York, 1960.

17. J. E. Rose, J. F. Brugge, D. J. Anderson, and J. E. Hind, Phase-locked response to low-frequency tones in single auditory nerve fibers of the squirrel monkey, *J. Neurophysiol, 30*, 769–793 (1967).

18. J. E. Hind, D. J. Anderson, J. F. Brugge, and J. E. Rose. Coding of information pertaining to paired low-frequency tones in single auditory nerve fibers of the squirrel monkey, *J. Neurophysiol. 30*, 794–816 (1967).

19. J. F. Brugge, D. J. Anderson, J. E. Hind, and J. E. Rose, Time structure of discharges in single auditory nerve fibers of the squirrel monkey in response to complex periodic sounds, *J. Neurophysiol. 32*, 386–401 (1969).

20. J. E. Rose, J. F. Brugge, D. J. Anderson, and J. E. Hind, Some possible neural correlates of combination tones, *J. Neurophysiol. 32*, 402–423 (1969).

21. T. Konishi and D. W. Nielsen, The temporal relationship between basilar membrane motion and nerve impulse inhibition in auditory nerve fibers of guinea pigs, *Japan J. Physiol. 28*, 291–307 (1973).

22. W. G. Sokolich, R. P. Hamernick, J. J. Zwislocki, and R. A. Schmiedt,

Inferred response polarities of cochlear hair cells, *J. Acoust. Soc. Am. 59*, 963–974 (1976).

23. P. M. Sellick, R. Patuzzi, and B. M. Johnstone, Modulation of responses of spiral ganglion cells in the guinea pig by low frequency sound. *Hearing Res. 7*, 199–221 (1982).

24. M. A. Ruggero and N. C. Rich, Chinchilla auditory-nerve responses to low-frequency tones, *J. Acoust. Soc. Am. 73*, 2096–2108 (1983).

25. J. Zwislocki, How OHC lesions can lead to neural cochlear hypersensitivity, *Acta Otol. 97*, 529–534 (1984).

26. J. Zwislocki, Cochlear function—An analysis, *Acta Otol. 100*, 201–209 (1985).

27. J. Zwislocki, Analysis of cochlear mechanics, *Hearing Res. 22*, 155–169 (1986).

28. M. Nomoto, N. Suga, and Y. Katsuki, Discharge pattern and inhibition of primary auditory nerve fibers in the monkey, *J. Neurophysiol, 27*, 768–787 (1964).

29. M. B. Sachs and N. Y. S. Kiang. Two-tone inhibition in auditory nerve fibers, *J. Acoust. Soc. Amer. 43*, 1120–1128 (1968).

30. P. J. Abbas and M. B. Sachs, Two-tone suppression in auditory-nerve fibers: Extension of a stimulus-response reslationship, *J. Acoust. Soc. Amer. 59*, 112–122 (1976).

31. M. B. Sachs and P. J. Abbas, Phenomenological model for two-tone inhibition, *J. Acoust. Soc. Amer. 60*, 1157–1163 (1976).

32. E. Javell, J. McGee, E. J. Walsh, G. R. Farley, and M. P. Gorga, Suppression of auditory nerve responses. II. Suppression threshold and growth, iso-suppression contours, *J. Acoust. Soc. Am. 74*, 801–813 (1983).

33. R. Patuzzi and P. M. Sellick, The modulation of the sensitivity of mammalian cochlea by low frequency tones. II. Inner hair cell receptor potentials, *Hearing Res. 13*, 9–18 (1984).

34. R. R. Pfeiffer and C. E. Molnar, Cochlear nerve fiber discharge patterns: Relationship to cochlear microphonic, *Science 167*, 1614–1616 (1970).

35. J. P. Legouix, M. C. Remond, and H. B. Greenbaum, Inteference and two-tone inhibition, *J. Acoust. Soc. Amer, 53*, 409–1419 (1973).

36. P. Dallos and M. A. Cheatham, Cochlear microphonic correlates of cubic difference tones, in *Facts and Models in Hearing* (E. Zwicker and E. Terhardt, eds.), Springer-Verlag, New York, 1974.

37. P. M. Sellick and I. J. Russell, Two-tone suppression in cochelar hair cells, *Hearing Res. 1*, 227–236 (1979).

38. W. S. Rhode, Some observations on two-tone interaction measured with the Mossbauer effect, in *Psychophysics and Physiology of Hearing* (E. F. Evans and J. P. Wilson, eds.), Academic Press, London, 1977, pp. 27–38.

39. D. T. Kemp and R. A. Chum, Observations on the generator mechanism of stimulus frequency acoustic emissions—two tone suppression, in *Physiological and Behavioral Studies in Hearing* (G. van den Brink and F. A. Bilsen, eds.), Delft Univ. Press, Delft, The Netherlands, 1980, pp. 34–42.

40. G. G. Furman and R. R. Frishkopf, Model for neural inhibition in the mammalian cochlea, *J. Acoust. Soc. Amer. 36*, 2194–2201 (1964).

41. J. E. Hind, Physiological correlates of auditory stimuius periodicity, *Audiology 11*, 42–57 (1972).
42. R. Salvi, D. Henderson, and R. Hamernick, Physiological bases of sensorineural hearing loss, in *Hearing Research and Theory*, Vol. 2 (J. V. Tobias and E. D. Schubert, eds.), Academic Press, New York, 1983, pp. 173–231.
43. J. E. Rose, J. E. Hind, D. J. Anderson, and J. F. Brugge, Some effects of stimulus intensity on response of auditory nerve fibers in the squirrel monkey, *J. Neurophysiol, 34*, 685–699 (1971).
44. H. Davis, Peripheral coding of auditory information, in *Sensory Communication* (W. A. Rosenblith, ed.), M.I.T. Press, Cambridge, Massachusetts, 1961, pp. 119–141.
45. M. B. Sachs and P. J. Abbas, Rate versus level functions for auditory-nerve fibers in cats: Tone-burst stimuli, *J. Acoust. Soc. Amer. 56*, 1835–1847 (1974).
46. T. B. Schalk and M. B. Sachs, Nonlinearities in auditory-nerve fiber responses to bandlimited noise, *J. Acoust. Soc. Am. 67*, 903–913 (1980).
47. E. F. Evans and A. R. Palmer, Relationship between the dynamic range of cochlear nerve fibers and their spontaneous activity, *Exp. Brain Res. 240*, 115–118 (1980).
48. N. Y. S. Kiang, Peripheral neural processing of auditory information, In *Handbook of Physiology: The Nervous System*, Vol. III, Part 2 (J. M. Brookhart and V. B. Mountcastle, eds.), Amer. Physiol. Soc., Bethesda, 1984, pp. 639–674.
49. M. C. Liberman and N. Y. S. Kiang, Single-neuron labeling and chronic cochlear pathology. IV. Stereocilia damage and alterations in rate- and phase-level functions, *Hearing Res. 16*, 75–90 (1984).
50. M. C. Liberman, Physiology of cochlear efferent and afferent neurons: Direct comparisons in the same animal, *Hearing Res. 34*, 179–192 (1988).
51. M. C. Liberman, Auditory-nerve response from cats raised in a low-noise chamber, *J. Acoust. Soc. Amer. 63*, 442–455 (1978).
52. D. O. Kim and C. E. Molnar, A population study of cochlear nerve fibers: Comparison of spacial distributions of average-rate and phase-locking measures of responses to single tones, *J. Neurophysiol. 48*, 16–30 (1979).
53. M. C. Liberman, Morphological differences among radial afferent fibers in the cat cochlea: An electron microscopic study of serial sections, *Hearing Res. 3*, 45–63 (1980a).
54. M. C. Liberman, Efferent synapses in the inner hair cell area of the cat cochlea: An electron microscopic study of serial sections, *Hearing Res. 3*, 189–204 (1980b).
55. M. C. Liberman and M. E. Oliver, Morphometry of intracellularly labeled neurons of the auditory nerve: Correlations with functional properties, *J. Comp. Neurol. 223*, 163–176 (1984).
56. M. C. Liberman and M. C. Brown, Physiology and anatomy of single olivocochlear neurons in the cat, *Hearing Res. 24*, 17–36 (1986).
57. I. C. Whitfield, *The Auditory Pathway*, Arnold, London, 1967.
58. J. J. Eggermont, D. W. Odenthal, P. H. Schmidt, and A. Spoor, Electrocochleography: Basic principles and clinical applications, *Acta Otol.*, Suppl. 316 (1974).

59. J. J. Eggermont, Electrocochleography, in *Handbook of Sensory Physiology* (W. D. Keidel and W. D. Neff, eds.), Vol. 3, Springer-Verlag, Berlin, 1976, pp. 625–705.

60. N. Yoshie, Auditory nerve action potential responses to clicks in man, *Laryngoscope 78*, 198–213 (1968).

61. M. H. Goldstein and N. Y.-S. Kiang, Synchrony of neural activity in electrical responses evoked by transient acoustic clicks, *J. Acoust. Soc. Amer. 30*, 107–114 (1958).

62. I. Tasaki, Nerve impulses in individual auditory nerve fibers, *J. Neurophysiol. 17*, 97–122 (1954).

63. J. P. Legouix and A. Pierson, Investigations on the source of whole-nerve action potentials from various places in the guinea pig cochlea, *J. Acoust. Soc. Amer. 56*, 1222–1225 (1974).

64. D. C. Teas, D. H. Eldredge, and H. Davis, Cochlear responses to acoustic transients: An interpretation of whole nerve action potentials, *J. Acoust. Soc. Amer. 34*, 1438–1459 (1962).

65. J. E. Pugh, Jr., D. J. Anderson, and P. A. Burgio, The origin of N_2 of the cochlear whole-nerve action potential, *J. Acoust. Soc. Amer. 53*, 325(A) (1973).

66. I. Tasaki, H. Davis, and R. Goldstein, The peripheral organization of activity, with reference to the ear, *Cold Spring Harbor Symp. Quant. Biol. 17*, 143–154 (1952).

67. J. J. Eggermont, Analysis of compound action potential responses to tone bursts in the human and guinea pig cochlea, *J. Acoust. Soc. Amer. 60*, 1132–1139 (1976).

68. J. P. Legouix, D. C. Teas, H. A. Beagley, and M. C. Remond, Relation between the waveform of the cochlear whole nerve action potential and its intensity function, *Acta Otol. 85*, 177–183 (1978).

69. N. Y.-S. Kiang, M. H. Goldstein, and W. T. Peake, Temporal coding of neural responses to acoustic stimuli, *Inst. Radio Eng. Trans. Inform. Theory IT-8*, 113–119 (1962).

70. E. F. Evans, The sharpening of cochlear frequency selectivity in the normal and abnormal cochlea, *Audiology 14*, 419–442 (1975).

71. E. F. Evans, The effects of bandwidths of individual cochlear nerve fibers from pathological cochleas in the cat, in *Disorders of Auditory Function* (S. D. G. Stephens, ed.), Academic Press, London, 1976, pp. 99–110.

72. E. F. Evans, Peripheral auditory processing in normal and abnormal ears: Physiological considerations for attempts to compensate for auditory deficits by acoustic or electrical prostheses, *Scand. Audiol. Suppl. 6*, 9–47 (1978).

73. Ö. Özdamar and P. Dallos, Input-output function of cochlear whole-nerve action potentials: Interpretation in terms of one population of neurons, *J. Acoust. Soc. Amer. 59*, 143–147 (1976).

74. Ö. Özdamar and P. Dallos, Synchronous responses of the primary auditory fibers to the onset of tone burst and their relation to compound action potentials, *Brain REs. 155*, 169–175 (1978).

6
Auditory Pathways

STIMULUS CODING

Tuning to best or characteristic frequencies (CFs) has been observed at all levels of the auditory system. This tuning is implicit in the tonotopic organization of these pathways; i.e., in the orderly arrangement of frequency by place. Such tuning curves have been reported for the cochlear nuclei [1], the superior olivary complex and trapezoid body [2–5], the inferior colliculus and medial geniculate [4,6], and the auditory cortex [7,8]. Particularly sharp tuning curves resembling those of the cochlear nerve have been reported at levels up to the superior olivary complex, while some nuclei even at these relatively low levels show broad tuning [5]. Both narrowly and broadly tuned fibers have been observed at higher levels. Although there is debate as to whether there is sharper tuning in individual auditory nerve fibers than in the cochlea (see Chaps. 4 and 5), it does not appear likely that further sharpening occurs at higher levels in the auditory system.

Auditory nerve firing patterns were discussed in some detail in the previous chapter. These primary units are exclusively excitatory. In other words, they always respond to stimulation. As we shall see, this and other characteristics of the response of auditory nerve fibers are not seen in all neurons at higher levels. In fact, discharge patterns drastically divergent from those of auditory nerve units are seen as low as the cochlear nuclei.

The nature of stimulus coding in the cochlear nuclei in the cat has been described in great detail [1,9–14]. These studies have revealed a variety of discharge patterns, which are in turn associated with neurons differing in terms of their morphologies, and which are variously distributed within the cochlear nuclei. Several examples of these descriptively named firing patterns are shown in Fig. 6.1. These patterns are often called peristimulus time histograms (PSTHs) because they indicate spike rates (vertically) as a function of the time while a stimulus is on. Figure 6.2 shows examples of several of the cells associated with these firing patterns.

The "primary-like" units have firing patterns that are like those of auditory nerve fibers. This firing pattern is associated with bushy cells. They are found in the interstitial nucleus (IN) and in posteroventral cochlear nucleus (PVCN).

The second category of neurons, described as "onset" units are found almost exclusively in the IN and PVCN, although several are observed in the anteroventral cochlear nucleus (AVCN) and in the dorsal cochlear nucleus (DCN). Onset units have been associated with octopus cells, as well as with small stellate and large monopolar cells. These

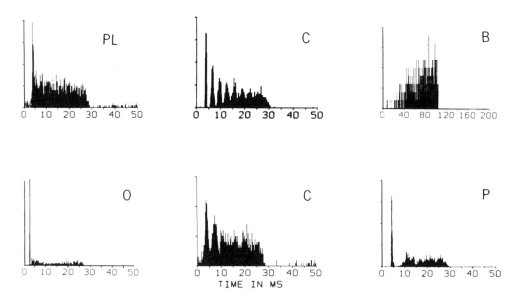

Figure 6.1 Examples of peristimulus time histograms (spike rate as a function of time from stimulus onset) recorded from the cochlear nucleus. The firing patterns represented here are "primary-like" (PL), "onset" (O), "chopper (C), "build-up" (B), and "pauser" (P). (From Rhode [14], with permission of *J. Acoust. Soc. Am.*)

fibers are particularly interesting because they respond to the onset of a tone burst with a momentary discharge of spikes, but do not respond to the remainder of the tone burst or to continuous tones.

The third group, found primarily in the IN and PVCN, but also observed in the DCN, are called "choppers." This firing pattern is associated with stellate cells. They are labeled as such because of the chopped appearance in their peristimulus time histograms, which look as though segments have been chopped out. The chopping itself is probably due to the presence of preferred discharge times which are regularly spaced over time; the rate of chopping is related to the tone burst's level, duration, and rate. The response is greatest at onset of the tone burst, and decreases over the time that the stimulus is left on.

"Build-up" units are associated with fusiform cells, and are characterized by a graduate increase in their firing rates until they achieve a steady-state discharge rate for the remainder of the tone burst. These are often encountered in the DCN.

The fifth major classification of units represented in Fig. 6.1 are "pausers," and appear to be found only in the DCN. Like build-up units, pausers are also associated with fusiform cells. They take on this name because they respond after longer latencies than the other cells. At higher stimulus levels pausers have an initial discharge peak, then a silent interval followed by discharges that last for the rest of the tone burst.

These five major categories are by no means the only types, nor are these firing patterns mutually exclusive: there are cells with combinations of these "basic" categories, as well as other types. The AVCM encompasses cells whose discharge patterns differ from other units in that their responses decay at an exponential rate.

A central point being made is that responses at higher levels are more variable than the exclusively excitatory firing patterns of the auditory nerve fibers. For example, some superior olivary complex fibers respond to clicks with a single discharge, others with two, and still others with a train of firings [15,16]. Moreover, onset units, pausers, and fibers responding to the duration of a tone burst have been identified in the inferior colliculus [9]. Similarly, many fibers in the medial geniculate are onset units, while others are pausers, cells which fire upon stimulus offset, and cells that respond as long as the stimulus is present [17–19].

The responses of single neurons in the auditory cortex demonstrate the importance of stimulus novelty. That is, cortical neurons are more interested in change than in ongoing stimulation. For example, they yield few discharges in response to a continuous background noise [20]. In contrast, auditory neurons tend to respond to the onset and to the

(a)

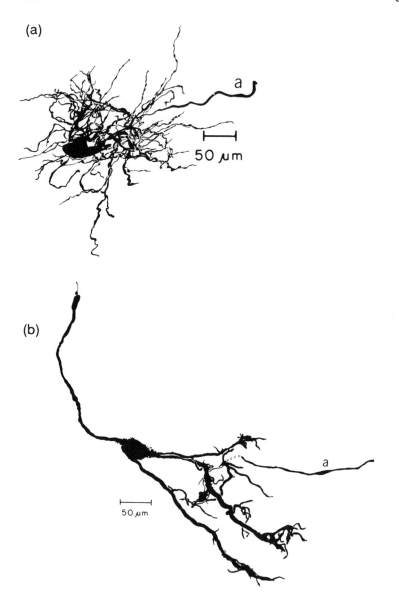

(b)

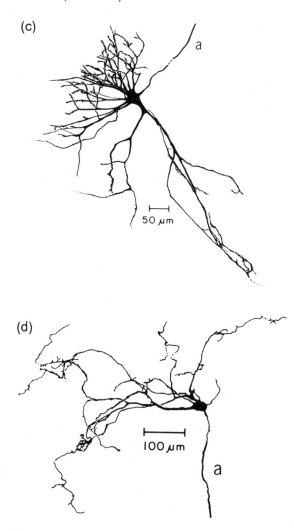

Figure 6.2   Examples of (a) bushy cell, (b) octopus, (c) fusiform, and (d) stellate cells. (From Rhode [14], with permission of *J. Acoust. Soc. Am.*)

offset of stimuli [7,8]. While auditory cortical neurons will not respond to steady-state tones, but they will respond to tones that are modulated in frequency [21]. Furthermore, many of these cells will respond only to a rise or fall in frequency; while other cortical neurons are responsive to movements of a sound source around the head [22].

Cortical auditory neurons are considerably affected by anesthesia. For example, Hind [7] has reported that the typical response from cortical auditory neurons in anesthetized animals is composed perhaps only one to four spikes rather than a sustained discharge. On the other hand, Brugge and Merzenich [23] have indicated that the typical response of an *un*anthesthetized animal is a high rate of spike discharges which adapts to a lower rate in under a second.

BINAURAL CODING

A variety of auditory functions depend upon information from both ears, or binaural hearing. For example, the ability to localize a sound source is dependent upon differences in the intensity and time of arrival of the sound at the two ears. This topic will be discussed further in Chap. 13. The current question is how the auditory system encodes and uses information from the two ears.

Superior Olivary Complex

Inputs from both ears must obviously be available to a neural center if binaural information is to be processed. Referring back to Fig. 2.36, recall that the superior olivary complex (SOC) is the lowest level at which binaural information is available in a single way station. This binaural convergence is particularly observed at the medial superior olive (MSO), whose connections with the cochlear nuclei (CN) of both sides make it well suited for this function. Consider a representative cell in the MSO. It synapses on its medial surface with a fiber from the opposite CN and on its lateral surface with a fiber from the CN on the same side [24]. These connections are represented in Fig. 6.3. Thus, neurons in the right MSO receive primarily projections from the left CN on their left (medial) sides and inputs from the right CN on their right (lateral) surfaces.

Hall [25] found that most SOC neurons responded to click stimulation of the opposite ear only. Stimulation of the ipsilateral ear did not yield a response unless the opposite ear also was stimulated. Such cells might be called excitatory-inhibitory (EI), since a signal from one side causes an increase in the firing rate (excitation) while an input from the other side decreases the discharge rate (inhibition). If the ipsilateral (in-

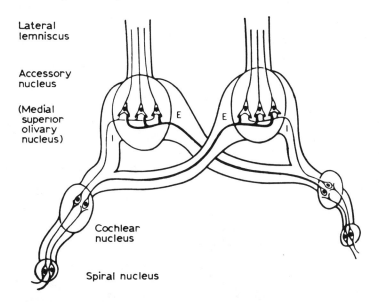

Lateral
lemniscus

Accessory
nucleus

(Medial
superior
olivary
nucleus)

E   E

I   I

Cochlear
nucleus

Spiral nucleus

Figure 6.3   Schematic representation of the bilateral projections to MSO cells. The existence of only excitatory (E) contralateral inputs and inhibitory (I) ipsilateral ones is questioned by subsequent research (see text). (From van Bergeijk [26], with permission of *J. Acoust. Soc. Amer.*)

hibitory) click preceded the click from the other (excitatory) side, then the firing rate decreased. The firing rate also decreased if the click intensity was greater at the ipsilateral ear. Thus, excitation and/or inhibition of the cell was controlled by the relative intensities and times of stimulus arrival at the two ears.

Figure 6.3 reflects Hall's finding that contralateral stimulation is excitatory and ipsilateral stimulation is inhibitory. However, this situation was not observed for every fiber; and Moushegian et al [27] found that the opposite situation occurred in some click-stimulated fibers. They also found ipsilateral as well as contralateral excitation in response to tones [28]. More recently, they reported that ipsilateral and contralateral inputs each excite roughly half of the MSO neurons, while binaural clicks are inhibitory [29]. Using tone bursts, Goldberg and Brown [30] found two groups of SOC neurons responsive to high frequencies. One group was excitatory–excitatory (EE)—it responded to inputs from either ear. The second group was excitatory–inhibitory (EI), responding to one ear and being suppressed by the other. The EE neurons were sensitive to the average intensity of the tones at both ears, but not to a difference between the intensities at the two ears. The EI cells were sensitive to interaural intensity differences (IIDs), but not to the average binaural level.

Interestingly, Goldberg and Brown observed a different effect at low frequencies. Here, cells responded in a manner which was synchronized with the phase of the stimulus tone when there was a certain characteristic delay, or interaural time difference (ITD), between the ears. In other words, the discharge rate was related to the relative timing of the low-frequency tones at each ear. The cell's responses were maximized when the inputs arrived in phase and were minimized when they were out of phase. This result is consistent with other studies which found that SOC cells fire in a probabilistic manner that is in cadence with multiples of the period of the stimulus tone [29,31]. Thus, the phase locking of neural responses to stimulus cycle (period) seen at the cochlear nerve is maintained as high as the SOC; and it appears that these phase-locked volleys contribute to binaural analysis as well as to frequency coding.

In summary, SOC neurons code binaural information through an interaction of excitatory and inhibitory inputs, which are the results of intensity and time (phase) differences in the stimuli at the two ears.

Inferior Colliculus

Binaural information is also available to the inferior colliculus (IC). Rose et al. [32] found cells in the IC that are sensitive to ITDs at characteristics delays. In other words, the neuron responded maximally at a particular ITD independent of the intensity or frequency of the tone. Figure 6.4 shows the spike counts of a single IC neuron in response to various stimulus frequencies as a function of the ITD. Note that the number of discharges is greatest at an interaural time delay of about 140 μsec regardless of the frequency. If the time scale were extended, one would see additional peaks repeated at intervals equal to the period of the frequency of the stimulus tones. Thus, the peaks for the 2100 Hz tone would recur at 476 μsec intervals, while the period of the function for 1400 Hz would be 715 μsec. This period/spike function for ITDs is observed throughout the auditory system.

Other cells were found that were sensitive to IIDs. Rose et al. [32] suggested the ITD-sensitive cells play a role in low frequency localization, and that IID-sensitive cells are involved in high frequency localization (see Chap. 13).

The findings of Rose et al. have been essentially confirmed for tonal, click, and noise stimuli [33–35], with the general finding that contralateral inputs are excitatory and ipsilateral signals are inhibitory. In addition to IID- and ITD-sensitive cells, Benevento and Coleman [34] found

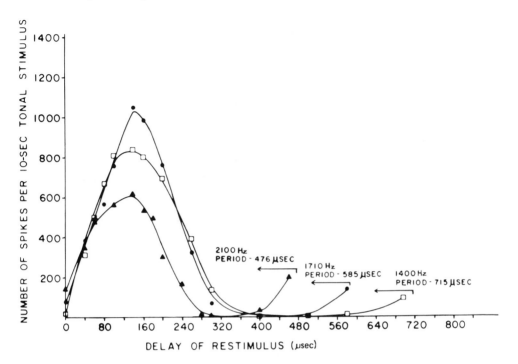

Figure 6.4 Responses of a single IC neuron with a characteristic delay of approximately 140 μsec to binaural stimulation at various low frequencies. The function shows a peak at the characteristic delay regardless of frequency. (From Rose et al [32], with permission of *J. Neurophysiol.*)

IC neurons sensitive to both IID and ITD, as well as units not sensitive to either one. This result is also evidence that certain IC cells are particularly responsive to a sound source which is moved around the head [30].

In summary, neurons in the inferior colliculus respond to interaural intensity and time differences. These differences between the ears result in excitatory and inhibitory inputs to IC neurons, whose firing depends upon the interaction of these inputs. The IC and SOC thus respond to binaural stimulation in similar ways. However, there is an interesting distinction that should be added here. Although phase locking to low frequencies is the rule in the SOC, it occurs for less than a third of the cells in the IC [33].

Other Subcortical Nuclei

Most of the work on binaural coding has been concentrated upon the SOC and IC. However, responses to interaural time-of-arrival and intensity differences have also been found in the dorsal nucleus of the lateral lemniscus [37] and in the medial geniculate body [38,39]. Findings in the dorsal nucleus of the lateral lemniscus have been similar to those for the SOC. Medial geniculate neurons tend to respond with short-latency initial discharges (up to about 30 msec) and/or a late discharge (over 500 msec). These units may be EE or EI, and some fibers respond to the direction of sound source movement. The longer-latency fibers may play a role in maintaining a short-term memory for interaural differences [39].

Auditory Cortex

The responses to single units to monaural and binaural stimulation in the auditory cortex [in the primary (AI) and secondary (AII) areas] have been studied in laboratory animals [23,40—42]. It has been demonstrated that auditory cortex cells tend to exhibit onset or offset responses to clicks and tone or noise bursts, although some units yield a sustained discharge during tone bursts. Most units are excitatory-inhibitory. The cells tend to respond to contralateral but not to ipsilateral stimulation; and the response to a stimulus at the opposite ear is generally inhibited by ipsilateral stimulation. Cells in the auditory cortex are responsive to interaural intensity differences (but not to changes in the binaural level), as well as to interaural time differences.

In addition to single-cell responses, evoked surface (gross) potentials also reflect the resonses of the auditory cortex to ITDs [43]. For lower frequencies (below roughly 3 kHz), cortical auditory neurons respond maximally to ITDs at characteristic delays, and with a periodic function that is repeated at the period of the stimulus frequency. This situation is similar to the one seen at lower levels. There are also cells at AI that respond to the direction of sound source movement [22].

A very interesting study of directional sensitivity of neurons in the cat's primary auditory cortex was reported by Middlebrooks and Pettigrew [44]. They found that about half of the units they sampled responded differentially according to the location of a sound source around the cat's head. Some of these units were sensitive to sounds from the opposite side and others responded to circumscribed areas in space.

In summary, it appears that the interaction of excitatory and inhibitory inputs contributes to the processing of binaural information (particularly with regard to localization) at all levels for which binaural inputs are represented up to and including the cortex. This constellation of findings is consistent with the localization difficulties demonstrated by animals whose auditory cortices have been ablated (as discussed later in this chapter).

TONOTOPIC ORGANIZATION

One of the most interesting aspects of the auditory pathways is the relatively systematic representation of frequency at each level. That is, there is a virtual "mapping" of the audible frequency range within each nuclear mass; neurons most sensitive to high frequencies are in one area, those sensitive to lows are in another part, and those sensitive to intermediate frequencies are located successively between them. This orderly representation of frequency according to place is called tonotopic organization.

It is generally accepted that high frequencies are represented basally in the cochlea, tapering down to low frequencies at the apex. This tonotopic arrangement is continued in the eighth nerve, where apical fibers are found toward the core of the nerve trunk and basal fibers on the outside and of the inferior margin [44], as shown in Fig. 6.5. Moreover, as pointed out in Chaps. 4 and 5, frequency maps have been developed which relate auditory nerve fiber CFs to distance along the the cochlear duct and to distance from the base of Rosenthal's canal [45,46]. Keithley and Schreiber [46] used these two sets of data to establish the relationship of the relative distances (from the base to apex) along the organ of Corti and Rosenthal's canal (Fig. 6.6).

Lewy and Kobrak [47] found that basal axons enter the dorsal part of the dorsal cochlear nucleus, and apical fibers enter the ventral cochlear nucleus (VCN) as well as part of the DCN. The ventrolateral terminations of the fibers from the apical turn and the dorsomedial insertions of the basal fibers were confirmed by Sando's [44] degeneration studies.

Experimenting on cats, Rose and colleagues [9,48] used microelectrodes to study the frequency sensitivity of the cochlear nuclei. They advanced the microelectrode through the cochlear nuclei of an anesthetized cat, and measured the number of neural discharges in response to tone pips of various frequencies. At a given intensity, a neuron responds with the greatest number of spikes at its characteristic frequency (CF). Rose et al. found that each of the three nuclear groups of the cochlear nuclear complex has a complete frequency mapping in a dorsoventral direction; i.e., low frequencies ventrally and high frequencies dorsally in each division of the cat's CN (Fig. 6.7).

Rose [48] hypothesized that the three complete representations of frequency in each part of the CN could be subserved by an arrangement in which each axon distributes to each of the nuclei. Sando's [44] findings are particularly interesting in this regard (Fig. 6.5). He found that eighth nerve axons bifurcate into an anterior branch to the VCN and a

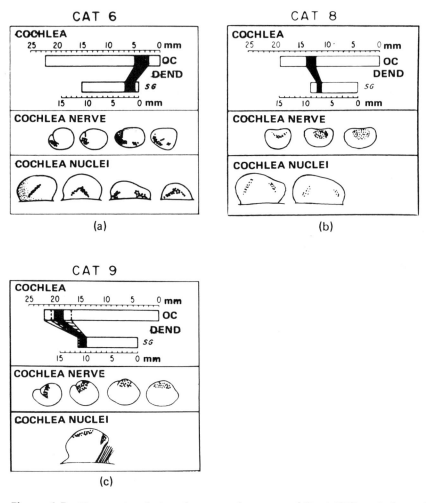

Figure 6.5 Tonotopic relations between the organ of Corti (OC), spiral ganglia (SG), cochlear nerve, and cochlear nuclei based on degeneration observed after selective lesions of the OC and SG. Solid lines indicate the induced lesions; crosshatched and dotted areas are resulting degenerations: (a) basal, (b) middle, and (c) apical turns of different cats. (From Sando [44], with permission of *Acta Otol.*)

posterior branch to the DCN. Fibers from the basal turn distribute dorsomedially in the CN, while fibers with more apical origins in the cochlea distribute ventrolaterally. Furthermore, the apical fibers of the posterior branch were found more inferiorly in the DCN than the corre-

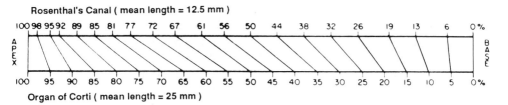

Rosenthal's Canal (mean length = 12.5 mm)

Organ of Corti (mean length = 25 mm)

Figure 6.6 Relationship of distances (in percent) along the organ of Corti and Rosenthal's canal. (From Keithley and Schreiber [46], with permission of *J. Acoust. Soc. Am.*)

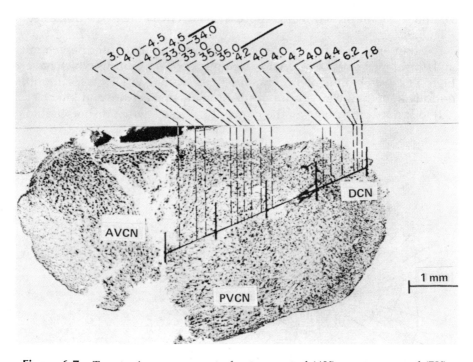

Figure 6.7 Tonotopic arrangement of anteroventral (AV), posteroventral (PV), and dorsal (DC) cochlear nuclei of a cat (saggital section on left side). Each nuclear group has its own sequence from low- to high-frequency representation. (From Rose, Galambos, and Hughes [9], Microelectrode studies of the cochlear nuclear nuclei of the cat, *Bull. Johns Hopkins Hosp. 104,* 211–251, © 1959. Johns Hopkins University Press.)

sponding fibers of the anterior branch of the VCN. On the other hand, the basally derived fibers in the posterior branch are distributed more superiorly in the DCN than the corresponding anterior branch fibers in the VCN. Middle turn fibers in both branches terminate at similar levels in each nucleus. Thus, Rose's hypothesis appears to be borne out.

Tsuchitani and Boudreau [49] studied the responses of single neurons in the S-shaped lateral nucleus of the cat's superior olivary complex (SOC). This structure appears as a backward "S" (Fig. 6.8). The higher CFs were found in the curve lying downward toward the dorsomedial curve of the S. Goldberg and Brown [50] studied the distribution of CFs in the dog's medial SOC. By advancing a microelectrode through the U-shaped nucleus, they found that the neurons with higher CFs are in the ventral leg of the structure and those with lower CFs are in the dorsal leg (Fig. 6.9).

Aitkin et al. [51] found a tonotopic organization in both the ventral and dorsal nuclei of the cat's lateral lemniscus (LL). Neurons which have high CFs were found ventrally and those with low CFs were found dorsally in both nuclei. It is interesting to note that Ferraro and Minckler [52] found that the nuclei of the human LL are somewhat dispersed into

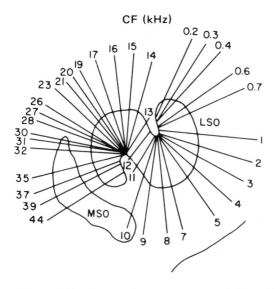

Figure 6.8 Tonotopic arrangement of the cells in the lateral superior olivary complex of the cat. Characteristic frequencies (kHz) taper from high ventro-medially to low dorsomedially. (From Tsuchitani and Boudreau [49], with permission of *J. Neurophysiol.*)

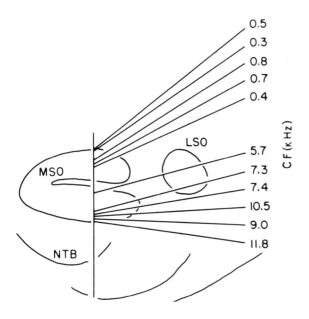

0.5
0.3
0.8
0.7
0.4

CF (кHz)

LSO

5.7
7.3
7.4
10.5
9.0
11.8

MSO

NTB

Figure 6.9 Distribution of neurons with high (ventral) and low (dorsal) characteristic frequencies in the medial superior olivary nucleus of the dog. (From Goldberg and Brown [50], with permission of *J. Neurophsiol.*)

scattered cell clusters among the lemniscal fibers, and that a clear-cut demarcation between them could not be found. However, the effect (if any) of this dispersed nuclear arrangement upon the tonotonicity of the human LL is not yet determined.

The tonotopic arrangement of the cat's inferior colliculus (IC) was studied by Rose et al. [6]. They inserted a microelectrode into the dorsomedial surface of the IC, and advanced it in a ventromedial direction (Fig. 6.10). The electrode thus passed through the external nucleus and into the central nucleus. Within the central nucleus, cells with increasing CFs were encountered as the electrode proceeded ventromedially into the nucleus. The opposite arrangement was observed in the external nucleus, i.e., the CFs went from high to low as the electrode was advanced ventromedially. However, the high-to-low frequency organization was found in only 9 out of 17 external nuclei. Thus, while there is most likely a tonotopic arrangement in the external nucleus, it is not as consistent as in the central nucleus of the IC.

The existence of a tonotopic organization in the medial geniculate body (MGB) was confirmed by Aitkin and Webster [53]. They found that

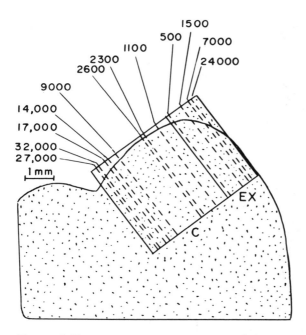

Figure 6.10 Tonotopic representation of characteristic frequencies in the central nucleus (C) and external nucleus (EX) of the inferior colliculus of the cat. (Based on Rose et al. [6]).

lateral units in the pars principalis of the cat responded to low frequencies, while medial neurons were responsive to high. This was a significant finding because there was very little to support tonotonicity in the MGB prior to their report [54].

Tonotopic Organization of the Cortex

Woolsey and Walzl [55] measured the electrical potentials of the cat's cortex in response to stimulation of the auditory nerve. They found two auditory areas in each hemisphere, each with its own projection of the auditory nerve. A primary auditory area (AI) was identified in the middle ectosylvian area, and a secondary auditory area (AII) was found just ventral to AI. Stimulating the basal fibers of the auditory nerve resulted in response in the rostral part of AI, whereas stimulation of fibers from the apical turn yielded responses from the caudal part. The opposite arrangement was observed in AII, i.e., the basal fibers were projected caudally and the apical fibers rostrally. This arrangement was essentially confirmed by Tunturi [56], who studied the cortical responses to tone burst stimuli in the dog. He later reported a third auditory area (AIII) under the anterior part of the suprasylvian gyrus.

Rose [57] described the cytoarchitecture (arrangement by cell types) of the cat's auditory cortex (Fig. 6.11). Rose identified AI as essentially triangular, with AII placed somewhat ventrally, and a posterior ectosylvian area (Ep) posteriorly. This result apparently contradicted Woolsey and Walzl's findings, since their electrophysiologic data had shown high-frequency responses from AII extending posteriorly to the place where this area ends anatomically [58]. This apparent discrepancy was resolved by the finding that both of these areas (AII and Ep) actually respond separately to apical stimulation, rather than just as one larger area (the original AII), as was previously supposed [59,60]. Furthermore, findings by Sindberg and Thompsen [61] suggested that the Ep also responds to low frequencies ventral to the part that responds to basal (high-frequency) stimulation. Several studies make it appear that the responses of AII and the Ep are mediated by the primary area, AI [60,62–64].

Woolsey [60] proposed a general summary of the tonotopic organization of the cortex based upon these and other experiments. This summary is shown in Fig. 6.12, and continues to be the accepted representation [65]. The figure shows complete representations of the cochlea in four cortical areas; as well as several other areas also responsive to auditory stimulation.

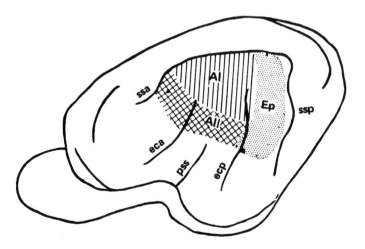

Figure 6.11 Cytoarchitecture (arrangement by cell types) of the auditory cortex of the cat (see text). (From Rose [57], with permission of The Wistar Press.)

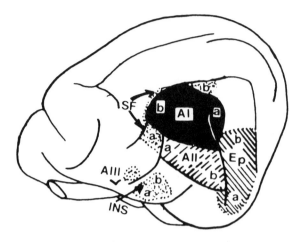

Figure 6.12 Summary of the tonotopic organization of the cortex. a indicates the projection of the apical part of the cochlea (low frequencies) on the cortex, and b indicates the basal projections (high frequencies). See text for details. [Adapted from Woolsey [60], in *Neural Mechanisms of the Auditory and Vestibular Systems* (G. L. Rasmussen and W. F. Windle, eds.), 1960. Courtesy of Charles C Thomas, Publisher.]

   In AI, the tonotopic organization is from high frequencies rostrally in this area to low frequencies caudally. Area AII lies ventral to AI. Its frequency representation is less distinct than that of the primary area, and is also in the opposite direction. The ectosylvian area Ep has a frequency representation in which the basal part of the cochlea is projected above and the apical cochlea is projected below. Organized fiber connections between AI and the MGB have been observed in the cat [58,66] and monkey [67]. It appears that, while the MGB sends essential projections to AI, only sustaining projections are received by AII and the Ep [58,66,68].
   The fourth cortical area with a complete projection of the cochlea is the syvian fringe area [SF], which has a posterior representation of high frequencies and an anterior representation of low. Note in Fig. 6.12 that the SF lies on the surface on the anterior ectosylvian gyrus, sinks deep into the suprasylvian sulcus, and then reappears on the surface above the posterior ectosylvian sulcus. Woolsey [60] noted that the thalamic connection of the SF is possibly with the pars principalis of the MGB, but that the specific relationship is not known.
   Tunturi's AIII is situated in the head subdivision of somatic sensory area II, and is apparently connected with the posterior medial geniculate

of the thalamus. Some degree of frequency representation has been identified in the insular area (INS) [69,70]. Woolsey [60] considers the thalamic connections of the INS to be undetermined.

Cortical tonotopic organization has also been demonstrated in primates. After removing the portions of parietal cortex covering this area, Merzenich and Brugge [71] exposed AI on the supratemporal gyrus of the monkey. Their electrophysiologic results showed that in this area high frequencies are represented caudomedially and lows rostrally. The secondary auditory cortex is made up of a belt of cortex around AI. As shown in Fig. 6.13 for the owl monkey [72] this belt includes a number of fields shown electrophysiologically to be responsive to auditory stimulation. Mesulam and Pandya [67] have demonstrated that the MGB sends a tonotopically arranged projection to the primary auditory cortex of the rhesus monkey.

Based upon findings that the somesthetic and visual cortices are organized in vertical columns. Abeles and Goldstein [73] undertook a study to determine whether the cat's primary auditory cortex is organized in columnar fashion, and whether it is organized by depth. They reported that neurons narrowly tuned to the same or similar frequencies are found in clusters. They also found that the auditory cortex is not organized by depth; i.e., the cells in a given vertical column of cortex show the same

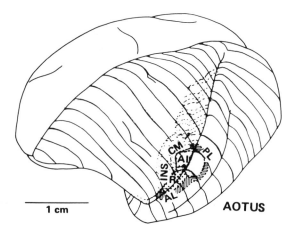

Figure 6.13 Primary (AI) and secondary auditory fields in the owl monkey *Aotus*, obtained by Imig et al. [72]. (CM, caudomedial field; PL, posterolateral field; AL, anterolateral field; R, rostrolateral field.) [From Brugge [65], in *The Nervous System, Vol 3: Human Communication and Its Disorders* (D. B. Tower and E. L. Eagles, eds.), © 1975, Raven Press.]

CFs as a microelectrode is advanced deeper into the cortex. Thus, the tonotopic organization of AI has cells with essentially similar CFs arranged in vertical columns, and in bands horizontally. These isofrequency bands widen as stimulus intensity is increased [65]; i.e., as a stimulus gets more intense a wider band of cortex responds to it.

Most of the auditory areas of each cerebral hemisphere are connected by commissural pathways with their counterparts on the other side. This arrangement has been shown in both cats [74] and monkeys [75]. Also, most of the auditory areas on the same side are interconnected in both animals [41,75,76].

AVERAGED EVOKED AUDITORY POTENTIALS

Until now we have been primarily concerned with the responses of single cells, measured by inserting microelectrodes directly into the neural material. It is also possible to measure the neural responses evoked by sound stimulation by using electrodes placed on the surface of the brain or, more often, on the scalp. While this approach does not allow one to focus upon the activity of single neurons, it does permit the study of aggregate responses of various nuclei. The major advantage is that surface electrodes allow noninvasive study, and hence may readily be applied to diagnostic audiology. This section provides a brief description of these evoked responses.

Two problems are readily apparent when measuring evoked auditory responses. One is the very low intensity of any one response, and the other is the excessive noise in the form of ongoing neural activity. Both problems are overcome by obtaining an averaged response from many stimulus repetitions.

Suppose we measure the ongoing electrical response of the brain, or the electroencephalographic response (EEG). In the absence of stimulation, the EEG will be random at any particular moment. That is, if we randomly select and line up a large number of segments from an ongoing EEG, there will be about as many positive as negative values at the points being compared. The algebraic sum of these random values will be zero. Alternatively, suppose a group of cells fire at a given time (latency) after the onset of a click. If we always measure the activity at the same latency, then we would find that the responses at that point are always positive- (or negative-) going. Instead of averaging these responses out, algebraic summation will exaggerate them, since positives are always added to positives and negatives to negatives. Thus, the averaging (or summation) process improves the signal-to-noise ratio by averaging out the background activity (noise) and summating the real responses which are locked in time to the stimulus.

Auditory evoked responses are commonly described with regard to their response latencies. The earliest are the evoked brainstem responses (or "Jewett bumps") occurring within the first 8 msec of stimulus onset in both cats [77,78] and humans [79,80]. These appear as about seven successive peaks, the largest and most stable of which is peak V (Fig. 6.14a). The various peaks have been attributed on the basis of their latencies to successive nuclei in the auditory pathways [77,78]. Peak I is

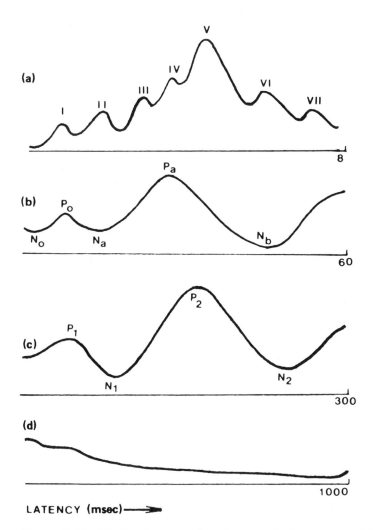

LATENCY (msec)——➤

Figure 6.14 Idealized averaged auditory evoked responses: (a) brainstem response, (b) middle response, (c) late response, (d) contingent negative variation.

the negative compound action potential of the auditory nerve. The remaining peaks are positive. The second peak (II) is most likely due to activity of the cochlear nuclei, and possibly also to some double firings of the eighth nerve. Wave III has been attributed to the superior olive. The lateral lemniscus and/or inferior colliculus appear to elicit peak IV; and the inferior colliculus (and possibly higher centers) contribute to peak V. Peak VI may possibly be related to the medial geniculate. Actually, however, one should not attribute each peak to a single neural center. For example, Jewett and Williston [80] have pointed out that the peaks beyond the first two almost definitely result from multiple generators. One should consult the review by Møller and Jannetta [81] for a comprehensive discussion of these neural generators.

The "middle response" (Fig. 6.14b) occurs at latencies between about 8 and 60 msec [82,83]. It appears that this response is neurogenic [83,84], but the locus of its origin is not apparent. R. Goldstein has been cited [84] as suggesting that the response may arise from the subcortical alerting (reticular) system.

The "late response" (Fig. 6.14c) is observed between roughly 70 and 300 msec [85–87], and has been the subject of extensive study. Although it is a diffuse response, there is reason to believe that it is derived from the primary auditory cortex [88,89].

The "contingent negative variation" (Fig. 6.14d) appears as a slow shift in the DC baseline after a latency of about 300 msec [90,91]. Unlike the other potentials, the contingent negative variation requires a mental or motor task. The response begins prefrontally and sweeps back toward the motor cortex.

EFFECTS OF CORTICAL ABLATION

Which auditory functions are subserved at a cortical level? Equivalent to this question is the more testable one of which functions can still be accomplished (or relearned) after the auditory cortex has been removed, and which ones can be carried out only when the cortex is intact. This question has been investigated extensively in laboratory animals, particularly cats. Although the specific experimental paradigms have differed somewhat, the fundamental approach has been fairly consistent. This approach has been to bilaterally ablate the auditory cortex, and then to test the animal's ability to perform (or relearn) various sound discrimination tasks. The assumption is that discriminations unaffected by the ablations are subserved by subcortical and/or nonauditory cortical centers, whereas discriminations impaired after ablation must require processing in the auditory cortices. Figure 6.15, by Neff [92], shows those

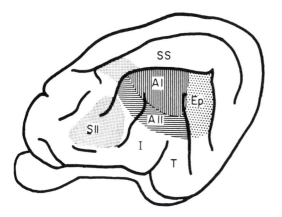

Figure 6.15 Cortical projection areas (in the cat) which were subjected to bilateral ablation in various sound discrimination studies: AI, auditory area I; AII, auditory area II; Ep, posterior ectosylvian area; I, insular area; T, temporal area; SSII, somatosensory area II; SS, suprasylvian area. [From Neff [92], in *Neural Mechanisms of the Auditory and Vestibular Systems* (G. L. Rasmussen and and W. F. Windle, eds.), 1960 Courtesy of Charles C Thomas, Publisher.]

auditory projection areas of the cat's cortex that have been ablated in various sound discrimination studies. Comparison with Fig. 6.12 reveals that these are essentially the same as the ones revealed by electrophysiologic and cytoarchitectural studies of the auditory cortex.

It is well established that certain sound discriminations can be accomplished after bilateral ablation of the auditory cortices, while others cannot. The bilaterally ablated animal *can* discriminate (1) and onset of a sound [93,94], (2) changes in tonal intensity [92,95,96], and (3) changes in the frequency of a tonal stimulus [94,97,98]. However, the type of frequency discrimination is critical, especially when the discrimination is between sequences of tones. Diamond et al. [99] presented bilaterally ablated animals with discrimination tasks between two sequences of three tones each. One sequence contained three lowfrequency tones (LO-LO-LO), and the other group had two low tones separated by a higher frequency (LO-HI-LO). The LO-HI-LO sequence could be discriminated from the LO-LO-LO group, but the discrimination could no longer be performed when the task was reversed (i.e., when all low tones was the positive stimulus to be discriminated from the LO-HI-LO sequence).

Bilaterally ablated animals *cannot* discriminate (1) changes in tonal duration [100], (2) changes in the temporal pattern of a tonal sequence [101], or (3) sound localizations in space [102]. Masterton and Diamond

[103] presented bilaterally ablated cats with a series of pairs of clicks separated by 0.5 msec, in which the first click of each pair went to one ear and the second click went to the other ear. If the first click is directed to the right ear (R-L) then the clicks are lateralized to the right; if the first click goes to the left ear (L-R) they are lateralized left (see Chap. 13). These workers found that bilaterally ablated cats could not discriminate the change from a series of L-R click pairs to R-L click pairs. In this regard, Neff [104] suggested that the auditory cortex plays an important role in the accurate localization of sounds in space.

Cats with bilateral ablations of the auditory cortex evince a startle response to sound, but do not exhibit the orientation response of reflexive head turning in the direction of the sound source found in normal cats [104]. Also, bilaterally ablated animals do appear to be able to push a response lever indicating whether a sound came from the right or left, but cannot approach the sound source (to get a reward) [105,106]. Neff and Casseday [107] suggested that the right-left distinction may be based upon different perceptual cues than spatial location. However, they explained that the auditory cortex is essential if the animal is to perceive spatial orientations and the relationships of its own body to the environment. In light of this fact, Strominger [108] found that localization is particularly mediated by area AI: and Sovijärvi and Hyvärinen [22] found that there are cells in the cat's primary auditory cortex that respond to the movement of a sound source in space.

There is evidence that localization ability is impaired by unilateral ablation of the auditory cortex [109]. An experiment by Neff and Casseday [107] is especially interesting in this regard. They surgically destroyed one cochlea each in a group of cats, and then trained these unilaterally hearing animals to make sound localizations. Following this procedure, half of the animals were subjected to unilateral ablations of the auditory cortex opposite the good ear, and half were ablated ipsilateral to the good ear (opposite the deaf ear). Those with cortical ablations on the same side as the hearing ear were essentially unaffected in localization ability. The animals whose cortical ablations were contralateral to the good ear could not relearn the localization task. These findings demonstrate that localization behavior is affected by destruction of the auditory cortex opposite to a functioning ear. This result also suggests that excitation of the auditory cortex on one side serves as a cue that the opposite ear is stimulated. These results are consistent with single-cell data suggesting that contralateral stimulation is excitatory to cells in the auditory cortex.

Most studies on humans with central auditory lesions have employed speech tests. However, tests using nonverbal materials are particularly valuable since they are directly comparable with the results of animal studies [110]. Bilateral temporal lobe damage in humans has been shown to result in impaired ability to make temporal pattern discriminations [111–113]. Temporal lobe damage in humans has also been reported to result in impaired sound localization in space [106,111]. These results essentially confirm the animal studies. Clinical data also tend to support Neff and Casseday's [107] position that neural activity at the contralateral cortex provides a "sign" of the stimulated ear. For example, patients who underwent unilateral temporal lobectomies have reported localization difficulties on the side opposite to the removed cortex [114]; and electrical stimulation of the auditory cortex has resulted in hallucinations of sounds or hearing loss at the ear opposite to the stimulated cortex [115,116].

Neff [92,104] has proposed that in order for sound discriminations to be accomplished after bilateral ablation of the auditory cortex, it is necessary for the positive stimulus to excite neural units that were not excited by the previous (neutral) stimulus. Thus, stimulus onset, as well as intensity and frequency changes, are discriminated because new neural units are excited by the changes in each case. The same is true when the sequence LO-HI-LO is discriminated from LO-LO-LO. However, LO-LO-LO is not discriminated from LO-HI-LO because there is nothing new in the LO-LO-LO sequence that was not already present in LO-HI-LO; so that no new neural units are excited by the change. These functions may be processed below the level of the auditory cortex, or by other cortical areas. On the other hand, discriminations that involve the processing of serial orders or time sequences (i.e., discriminations in the temporal domain) are subserved by the auditory cortex. Thus, they are obliterated when the auditory cortex is bilaterally removed.

OLIVOCOCHLEAR BUNDLE

The fundamental approach to studying the effects of the olivocochlear bundle (OCB) has been to electrically stimulate the crossed olivocochlear bundle (COCB) where it crosses the floor of the fourth ventricle, and then to measure how this has affected some aspect of the afferent system. Early studies revealed that electrical stimulation of the COCB results in a reduced auditory nerve action potential (N1) and a slight increase in the cochlear microphonic (CM) [117,118]. On the other hand, stimulation of the uncrossed olivocochlear bundle (UOCB) yielded a drop in the action potential without affecting the CM [119]. These findings, of course, reflect the inhibitory action of the OCB. They are also consistent with the anatomical findings: The COCB principally involves the medial system terminating directly upon the OHCs; whereas the UOCB entails mainly the lateral system terminating on the afferent nerve fibers of the IHCs, rather than on the hair cells themselves (Chap. 2). Further, they are consistent with the point that the OHCs are the principal contributors to the CM (Chap. 4). One might also note in this context that activation of the COCB has been shown to result in a drop in the endocochlear potential [120].

The inhibitory effect of COCB activation is reflected as a reduction in the firing rate of the afferent auditory neurons which occurs after a relatively long latency of 15 msec or more, and is often found to be greater on the afferent response to higher frequency sounds than to lower ones [121–124]. Recall from the previous chapter that an auditory neuron's firing rate (the number of spikes that are generated per second) increases as the sound level of the stimulus is raised. If firing rate is expressed as a function of the sound pressure level of the stimulus, then the inhibitory effect of COCB activation observed as a shift to the right of this function (Fig. 6.16). This effect is often on the order of roughly 20 dB for low to moderate sound pressure levels. The primary effects of COCB stimulation occurs at the sharply tuned tip of the auditory neuron's tuning curve, with little affect upon its low frequency tail [125]. This phenomenon is depicted in Fig. 6.17, where we see that it is tantamount to a reduction in sensitivity in the vicinity of the tip of the tuning curve. The rightward movement of the rate-level function and the sensitivity decrement at the tip of the tuning curve are often on the order of approximately 20 dB.

The findings just discussed clearly reveal that the OCB provides a mechanism for central feedback to and control of activity at the auditory periphery. An enticing interface by which this control might be achieved

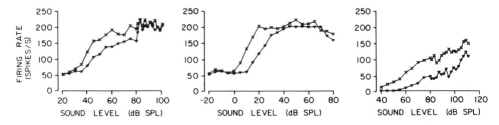

Figure 6.16   Rate-level functions of individual cat auditory neurons showing the rightward shift of the functions during stimulation of the COCB. (Xs, without COCB stimulation; triangles, with COCB stimulation). (From Gifford and Guinan [124], with permission of *J. Acoust. Soc. Am.*)

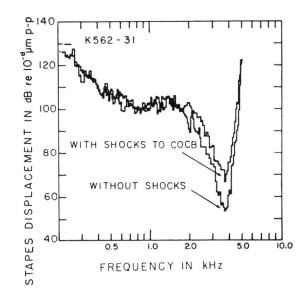

Figure 6.17   Effect of COCB stimulation on the tuning curve of the auditory neuron tuning curve. [From Kiang, Moxon, and Levine [125]. Auditory-nerve activity in cats with normal and abnormal cochleas, in *Sensorineural Hearing Loss* (G.E.W. Wolstenholme and J. Knight, eds.), CIBA Foundation Symposium, Churchill, London, 1970.]

is provided by the peculiar anatomical and functional relationships of the OHCs with the efferent system and the architecture of the organ of Corti. While this idea may still be debated, it is noteworthy that the supportive evidence is impressive and growing: We have already discussed the concept of mechanical influences over sensory activities via the OHCs in Chapter 4. One must note in this context that Brown et al. [126] demonstrated that COCB activation causes a reduction of intracellular receptor potential magnitudes and a drop of sensitivity at the tip of the tuning curves for the *inner* hair cells. This is, of course similar to what was described above for afferent auditory neurons. Moreover, the efferent neurotransmitter, acetylcholine has been shown to induce contraction [127,128] and even elongation [128] of isolated OHCs. Further, stimulation of the efferent system as also been shown to result in changes in the distortion products observed in otoacoustic emissions [129,130].

Some further insight into the nature and potential practical implications of the efferent system is gained when one examines the effects of

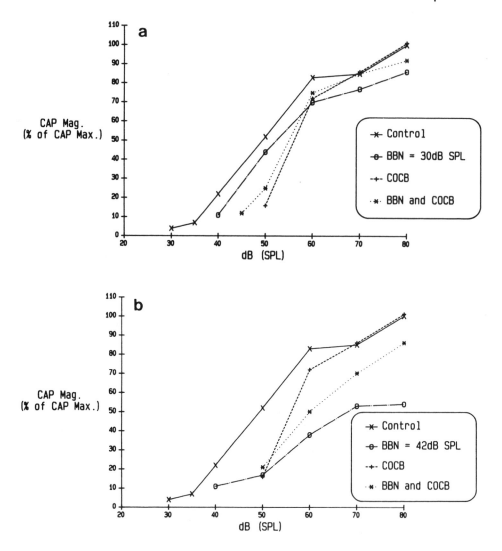

COCB stimulation in the presence of masking noise [131–133]. Figure 6.18 from a recent study by Dolan and Nuttall [133] shows how COCB stimulation affects the responses to are different levels of a stimulus (10 kHz tone bursts) is presented with and without various levels of masking noise (see Chap. 10). The response is the magnitude of the guinea pig's auditory nerve compound action potential (CAP). Notice first that the effect upon the CAP of COCB stimulation alone is very much like

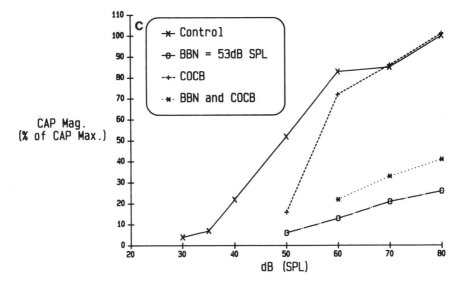

Figure 6.18 Effects of combining COCB stimulation with various masking noise (BBN) levels upon the compound action potential response to 10 kHz tone bursts presented at low to high sound pressure levels (see text). (From Dolan and Nuttall [133], with permission of *J. Acoust. Soc. Am.*)

what we have already seen for individual neuron rate-level functions: The response magnitude is reduced considerably at lower stimulus levels and less so (or not at all) at the highest levels of the tone burst. This effect (seen by comparing the "control" and "COCB" curves) is the same in each frame of the figure. Also, see how CAP magnitude is reduced more and more as the masker is increased from 30 dB (frame a) to 42 dB (frame b) to 53 dB (frame c).

The effect of COCB stimulation upon masking can be seen by comparing the curves for the masker alone ("BBN") with those for COCB combined with the noise ("BBN and COCB"). Combining COCB stimulation with the low level masker (frame a) causes a smaller response (compared to the masker alone) at low stimulus levels, and a slight improvement at high levels. For the higher-level maskers (frames b and c), adding COCB stimulation to the masker increases the response magnitude over what it was for the masker alone for all conditions where the comparison is made. The role of this "unmasking" effect of COCB stimulation may be to improve the signal-to-noise ratio of signals to the auditory system [133].

REFERENCES

1. N. Y.-S. Kiang, R. R. Pfeiffer, W. B. Warr, and A. S. Backus, Stimulus coding in the cochlear nucleus, *Ann Otol. 74*, 463–485 (1965).
2. J. D. Boudreau and C. C. Tsuchitani, Cat superior olivary S segment cell discharge to tonal stimulation, in *Contributions to Sensory Physiology* (W. D. Neff, ed.), Academic Press, New York, 1970, pp. 143–213.
3. J. J. Guinan, B. E. Norris, and S. S. Guinan. Single auditory units in the superior olivary complex II: Locations of unit categories and tonotopic organization, *Intl. J. Neurosci. 4*, 147–166 (1972).
4. Y. Katsuki, Neural mechanisms of auditory sensation in cats, in *Sensory Communication* (W. A. Rosenblith, ed.), MIT Press, Cambridge, Massachusetts, 1961, pp. 561–583.
5. N. Y.-S. Kiang, D. K. Morest, D. A. Godfrey, J. J. Guinan, and E. C. Kane, Stimulus coding at caudal levels of the cat's auditory nervous system: I. Response characteristics of single units, in *Basic Mechanisms in Hearing* (A. R. Møller, ed.), Academic Press, New York, 1973, pp. 455–478.
6. J. E. Rose, D. D. Greenwood, J. M. Goldberg, and J. E. Hind. Some discharge characteristics of single neurons in the inferior colliculus of the cat. I. Tonotopical organization, relation of spike-counts to tone intensity, and firing patterns of single elements, *J. Neurophysiol. 26*, 294–320 (1963).
7. J. E. Hind, Unit activity in the auditory cortex, in *Neural Mechanisms of the Auditory and Vestibular Systems* (G. L. Rasmussen and W. F. Windle, eds.), Thomas, Springfield, Illinois, 1960, pp. 201–210.
8. Y. Katsuki, N. Suga, and Y. Kanno, Neural mechanisms of the peripheral and central auditory systems in monkeys, *J. Acoust. Soc. Amer. 32*, 1396–1410 (1962).
9. J. E. Rose, R. Galambos, and J. R. Hughes, Microelectrode studies of the cochlear nuclei of the cat, *Bull. Johns Jopkins Hosp. 104*, 211–251 (1959).
10. D. A. Godfrey, N. Y. S. Kiang, and B. E. Norris, Single unit activity in the posteroventral cochlear nucleus of the cat, *J. Comp. Neurol. 162*, 247–268 (1975a).
11. D. A. Godfrey, N. Y. S. Kiang, and B. E. Norris, Single unit activity in the dorsal cochlear nucleus of the cat, *J. Comp. Neurol. 162*, 269–284 (1975b).
12. W. S. Rhode, P. H. Smith, and D. Oertel, Physiological response properties of cells labeled intracellularly with horseradish peroxidase in cat dorsal cochlear nucleus, *J. Comp. Neurol., 213*, 426–447 (1983a).
13. W. S. Rhode, P. H. Smith, and D. Oertel, Physiological response properties of cells labeled intracellularly with horseradish peroxidase in cat ventral cochlear nucleus, *J. Comp. Neurol., 213*, 448–463 (1983b).
14. W. S. Rhode, The use of intracellular techniques in the study of the cochlear nucleus, *J. Acoust. Soc. Am. 78*, 320–327 (1985).
15. R. Galambos, J. Schwartzkopff, and A. L. Rupert, Microelectrode study of superior olivary nuclei, *Amer. J. Physiol. 197*, 527–536 (1959).
16. A. L. Rupert, G. M. Moushegian, and M. A. Whitcomb, Superior olivary

complex response patterns to monaural and binaural clicks, *J. Acoust. Soc. Amer. 39,* 1069–1076 (1966).

17. R. Galambos, Microelectrode studies on medial geniculate body of cat. III. Response to pure tones, *J. Neurophysiol. 15,* 381–400 (1952).

18. Y. Katsuki, T. Watanabe, and N. Maruyama, Activity of auditory neurons in upper levels of brain of cat, *J. Neurophysiol. 22,* 343–359 (1959).

19. I. M. Aitkin, C. W. Dunlop, and W. R. Webster, Click evoked response patterns in single units in the medial geniculate body of the cat, *J. Neurophysiol. 29,* 109–123 (1966).

20. D. P. Phillips and S. E. Hall, Spike-rate intensity functions of at cortical neurons studies with combined tone-noise stimuli, *J. Acoust. Soc. Am. 80,* 177–187 (1986).

21. I. C. Whitfield and E. F. Evans, Responses of auditory cortical neurons to stimuli of changing frequency, *J. Neurophysiol. 28,* 655–672 (1965).

22. A. R. A. Sovijärvi and J. Hyvärinen, Auditory cortical neurons in the cat sensitive to the direction of sound source movement, *Brain Res. 73,* 455–471 (1974).

23. J. F. Brugge and M. M. Merzenich, Patterns of activity of single neurons of the auditory cortex in monkey, in *Basic Mechanisms in Hearing* (A. R. Møller, ed.), Academic Press, New York, 1973.

24. W. A. Stotler, An experimental study of the cells and connections of the superior olivary complex of the cat, *J. Comp. Neurol. 98,* 401–431 (1953).

25. J. L. Hall, Binaural interaction in the accessory superior olivary nucleus of the cat: An electrophysiological study of single neurons, *MIT Res. Lab. Electron,* Tech. Rept. 416, Cambridge, Mass, 1964.

26. W. A. van Bergeijk, Variation on a theory of Bekesy: A model of binaural interaction, *J. Acoust. Soc. Amer. 34,* 1431–1437 (1962).

27. G. M. Moushegian, A. L. Rupert, and M. A. Whitcomb, Medial-superior-olivary unit response patterns to monaural and binaural clicks, *J. Acoust. Soc. Amer. 36,* 196–202 (1964).

28. G. M. Moushegian, A. L. Rupert, and M. A. Whitcomb, Brainstem neuronal response patterns to monaural and binaural tones, *J. Neurophysiol. 27,* 1174–1191 (1964).

29. G. M. Moushegian, A. L. Rupert, and M. A. Whitcomb, Processing of auditory information by medial superior-olivary neurons, in *Foundations of Modern Auditory Theory* (J. V. Tobias, ed.), Vol. 2, Academic Press, New York, 1972, pp. 263–299.

30. J. M. Goldberg and P. B. Brown, Response of binaural neurons of dog superior olivary complex to dichotic tonal stimuli: Some physiological mechanisms of sound localization, *J. Neurophysiol. 32,* 613–636 (1969).

31. G. M. Moushegian, A. L. Rupert, and T. L. Langford, Stimulus coding by medial superior olivary neurons, *J. Neurophysiol. 30,* 1239–1261 (1967).

32. J. E. Rose, N. B. Gross, C. D. Geisler, and J. E. Hind, Some neural mechanisms in the inferior colliculus of the cat which may be relevant to localization of a sound source, *J. Neurophysiol. 29,* 288–314 (1966).

33. C. D. Geisler, W. S. Rhode, and D. W. Hazelton, Responses of inferior colliculus neurons in the cat to binaural acoustic stimuli having wide-band spectra, *L. Neurophysiol. 32*, 960–974 (1969).

34. L. A. Benevento and P. D. Coleman, Responses of single cells in cat inferior colliculus to binaural click stimuli: Combinations of intensity levels, time differences and intensity differences, *Brain Res. 17*, 387–405 (1970).

35. F. Flammino and B. M. Clopton. Neural response in the inferior colliculus of albino rat to binaural stimuli, *J. Acoust. Soc. Amer. 57*, 692–695 (1975).

36. J. A. Altman, Are there neurons detecting direction of sound source motion? *Exp. Neurol. 22*, 13–25 (1968).

37. J. F. Brugge, D. J. Anderson, and L. M. Aitkin, Responses of neurons in the dorsal nucleus of the lateral lemniscus of cat to binaural tonal stimulation, *J. Neurophysiol, 33*, 441–458 (1970).

38. I. M. Aitkin and C. W. Dunlop, Interplay of excitation and inhibition in the cat medial geniculate body, *J. Neurophysiol. 31*, 44–61 (1968).

39. J. A. Atlman, J. Syka, and G. N. Shmigidina, Neuronal activity in the medial geniculate body of the cat during monaural and binaural stimulation, *Exp. Brain Res. 10*, 81–93 (1970).

40. J. F. Brugge, N. A. Dubrovsky, L. M. Aitkin, and D. J. Anderson, Sensitivity of single neurons in auditory cortex of cat to binaural tonal stimulation: Effects of varying interaural time and intensity, *J. Neurophysiol. 32*, 1005–1024 (1969).

41. J. L. Hall and M. H. Goldstein, Representation of binaural stimuli by single units in primary auditory cortex of unanesthetized cats, *J. Acoust. Soc. Amer. 43*, 456–461 (1968).

42. D. P. Phillips, and D. R. F. Irvine, Responses of single neurons in physiologically defined area AI of cat cerebral cortex: Sensitivity to interaural intensity differences, *Hearing Res. 4*, 299–307 (1981).

43. J. E. Hirsch, Effect of interaural time delay on amplitude of cortical responses evoked by tones, *J. Neurophysiol. 31*, 916–927 (1968).

44. I. Sando, The anatomical interrelationships of the cochlear nerve fibers, *Acta Otol. 59*, 417–436 (1965).

45. M. C. Liberman, The cochlear frequency map for the cat: Labeling auditory-nerve fibers of known characteristic frequency, *J. Acoust. Soc. Am. 72*, 1441–1449 (1982).

46. E. M. Keithley, and R. C. Schreiber, Frequency map of the spiral ganglion in the cat, *J. Acoust. Soc. Am. 81*, 1036–1042 (1987).

47. F. H. Lewy and H. Kobrak, The neural projection of the cochlear spirals of primary acoustic centers, *Arch. Neurol. Psychiat. 35*, 839–852 (1936).

48. J. E. Rose, Organization of frequency sensitive neurons in the cochlear nuclear complex of the cat, in *Neural Mechanisms of the Auditory and Vestibular Systems* (G. L. Rasmussen and W. F. Windle, eds.), Thomas, Springfield Illinois, 1960, pp. 116–136.

49. C. Tsuchitani and J. D. Boudreau, Single unit analysis of cat superior olive S segment with tonal stimuli, *J. Neurophysiol, 29*, 684–697 (1966).

50. J. M. Goldberg and P. B. Brown, Functional organization of the dog superior olivary complex: An anatomical and physiological study, *J. Neurophysiol. 31*, 639–656 (1968).

51. I. M. Aitkin, D. J. Anderson, and J. F. Brugge, Tonotopic organization and discharge characteristics of single neurons in nuclei of the lateral lemniscus of the cat, *J. Neurophysiol. 33*, 421–440 (1970).

52. J. A. Ferraro and J. Minckler, The human auditory pathways: A quantitative study: The human lateral lemniscus and its nuclei, *Brain Language 4*, 277–294 (1977).

53. I. M. Aitkin and W. R. Webster, Tonotopic organization in the medial geniculate body of the cat, *Brain Res. 26*, 402–405 (1971).

54. I. C. Whitfield, *The Auditory Pathway*, Arnold, London, 1967.

55. C. N. Woolsey and E. M. Walzl, Topical projection of nerve fibers from local regions of the cochlea to the cerebral cortex of the cat, *Bull. Johns Hopkins Hosp. 71*, 315–344 (1942).

56. A. R. Tunturi, Audio frequency localization in the acoustic cortex of the dog, *Amer, J. Physiol, 141*, 397–403 (1944).

57. J. E. Rose, The cellular structure of the auditory region of the cat, *J. Comp. Neurol. 91*, 409–439 (1949).

58. J. E. Rose and C. N. Woolsey, The relations of thalamic connections, cellular structure and evokable electrical activity in the auditory region of the cat, *J. Comp. Neurol. 91*, 441–466 (1949).

59. C. B. Downman, C. N. Woolsey, and R. A. Lende, Auditory areas I, II and Ep: Cochlear representation, afferent paths and interconnections, *Bull. Johns Hopkins Hosp. 106*, 127–146 (1960).

60. C. N. Woolsey, Organization of cortical auditory system: A review and a synthesis, in *Neural Mechanisms of the Auditory and Vestibular Systems* (G. L. Rasmussen and W. F. Windle, eds.), Thomas, Springfield, Illinois, 1960, pp. 165–180.

61. R. M. Sindberg and R. F. Thompsen, Auditory responses in the ventral temporal cortex of cat, *Physiologist 2*, 108–109 (1959).

62. A. H. Ades, A secondary acoustic area in the cerebral cortex of the cat, *J. Neurophysiol. 6*, 59–63 (1943).

63. A. H. Ades, Functional relationships between the middle and posterior ectosylvian areas in the cat, *Amer. J. Physiol. 159*, 561 (1949).

64. J. L. Arteta, V. Bonnet, and F. Bremer, Répercussions corticales de la réponse d'aire acoustique primaire: L'aire acoustique secondaire, Arch. Intl. Physiol. 57, 425–428 (1950).

65. J. F. Brugge, Progress in neuroanatomy and neurophysiology of auditory cortex, in *The Nervous System* (D. B. Tower, ed.), Vol. 3: *Human Communication and Its Disorders*, Raven, New York, 1975, pp. 97–111.

66. J. E. Rose and C. N. Woolsey, Cortical connections and functional organization of the thalamic auditory system of the cat, in *Biological and Biochemical Bases of Behavior* (H. F. Harlow and C. N. Woolsey, eds.), University of Wisconsin Press, Madison, Wisc., 1958, pp. 127–150.

67. M. M. Mesulam and D. N. Pandya. The projections of the medial geniculate complex within the Sylvian fissure of the rhesus monkey, *Brain Res. 60*, 315–333 (1973).

68. I. T. Diamond, K. L. Chow, and W. D. Neff, Degeneration of caudal medial geniculate body following cortical lesion ventral to auditory area II in the cat, *J. Comp. Neurol. 109*, 349–362 (1958).

69. J. D. Loeffler, An investigation of auditory responses in insular cortex of cat and dog, Thesis, University of Wisconsin, Madison, Wisc., (1958).

70. J. E. Desmedt and K. Michelse, Corticofugal projections from temporal lobe in cat and their possible role in acoustic discrimination, *J. Physiol. (London) 147*, 17–18 (1959).

71. M. M. Merzenich and J. F. Brugge, Representation of the cochlear partition on the superior temporal plane of the macaque monkey, *Brain Res. 50*, 275–296 (1973).

72. T. J. Imig, M. A. Ruggero, L. M. Kitzes, and J. F. Brugge, Organization of auditory cortex in the owl monkey (*Aotus trivirgatus*), *J. Acoust. Soc. Amer. 56*, S523 (1974).

73. M. Abeles and M. H. Goldstein, Functional architecture in cat primary auditory cortex: Columnar organization and organization according to depth. *J. Neurophysiol. 33*, 172–187 (1970).

74. I. T. Diamond, E. G. Jones, and T. P. S. Powell, Interhemispheric fiber connections of the auditory cortex of the cat. *Brain Res. 11*, 177–193 (1968).

75. D. N. Pandya, M. Hallett, and S. K. Mukherjee, Intra- and interhemispheric connections of the neocortical auditory system in the rhesus monkey, *Brain Res. 14*, 49–65 (1969).

76. I. T. Diamond, E. G. Jones, and T. P. S. Powell, The association connections of the auditory cortex of the cat, *Brain Res. 11*, 560–579 (1968).

77. D. L. Jewett, Volume-conducted potentials in response to auditory stimuli as detected by averaging in the cat, *EEG Clin. Neurophysiol. 28*, 609–618 (1970).

78. J. S. Buchwald and C.-M. Huang. Far-field acoustic response: Origins in the cat, *Science 189*, 382–384 (1975).

79. D. L. Jewett, M. N. Romano, and J. S. Williston, Human auditory evoked potentials: Possible brainstem components detected on the scalp. *Science 167*, 1517–1518 (1970).

80. D. L. Jewett and J. S. Williston, Auditory-evoked far fields averaged from the scalp of humans, *Brain 94*, 681–696 (1971).

81. A. R. Møller, and P. J. Jannetta, Neural generators of the auditory brainstem response, in *The Auditory Brainstem Response* (J. T. Jacobson, ed.), College-Hill, San Diego, 1985, pp. 13–31.

82. C. Geisler, L. Frishkopf, and W. Rosenblith, Extracranial responses to acoustic clicks in man, *Science 128*, 1210–1211 (1958).

83. H. Ruhm, E. Walker, and H. Flanigin, Acoustically evoked potentials in man: Mediation of early components, *Laryngoscope 77*, 806–822 (1967).

84. D. C. Hood, Evoked cortical response audiometry, in *Physiological Measures*

of the Audio-Vestibular System (L. J. Bradford, ed.), Academic Press, New York, 1975, pp. 349–370.

85. H. Davis, Some properties of the slow cortical response in humans, *Science* 146, 434 (1964).

86. G. McCandless and L. Best, Evoked response to auditory stimulation in man using a summating computer, *J. Speech Hearing Res. 7*, 193–202 (1964).

87. G. McCandless and L. Best, Summed evoked responses using pure tone stimuli, *J. Speech Hearing Res. 9*, 266–272 (1966).

88. H. G. Vaughan, The relationship of brain activity to scalp recordings of event-related potentials, in *Average Evoked Potentials: Methods, Results and Evaluation* (E. Donchin and D. Lindsay, eds.), NASA, SP191, Washington, D. C., 1969.

89. H. G. Vaughan and W. Ritler, The sources of auditory evoked responses recorded from the human scalp, *EEG Clin. Neurophysiol. 28*, 360–367 (1970).

90. W. G. Walter, the convergence and interaction of visual, auditory and tactile responses in human nonspecific cortex, *Ann. N.Y. Acad. Sci. 112*, 320–361 (1964).

91. W. G. Walter, Effects on anterior brain responses of an expected association between stimuli, *J. Psychosomat. Res. 9*, 45–49 (1965).

92. W. D. Neff, Role of the auditory cortex in sound discrimination, in *Neural Mechanisms of the Auditory and Vestibular Systems* (G. L. Rasmussen and W. F. Windle, eds.), Thomas, Springfield, Illinois, 1960, pp. 221–216.

93. K. D. Kryter and H. W. Ades, Studies on the function of the higher acoustic nerve centers, *Amer. J. Psych. 56*, 501–536 (1943).

94. D. R. Meyer and C. N. Woolsey. Effects of localized cortical destruction on auditory discriminative conditioning in cat, *J. Neurophysiol. 15*, 149–162 (1952).

95. D. H. Raab and H. W. Ades, Cortical and midbrain mediation of a conditioned discrimination of acoustic intensities, *Amer. J. Psych. 59*, 59–83 (1946).

96. M. R. Rosenzweig. Discrimination of auditory intensities in the cat, *Amer. J. Psych. 59*, 127–136 (1946).

97. R. A. Butler, I. T. Diamond, and W. D. Neff, Role of auditory cortex in discrimination of changes in frequency, *J. Neurophysiol. 20*, 108–120 (1957).

98. J. M. Goldberg and W. D. Neff, Frequency discrimination after bilateral ablation of auditory cortical areas, *J. Neurophysiol 24*, 119–128 (1961).

99. I. T. Diamond, J. M. Goldberg, and W. D. Neff, Tonal discrimination after ablation of auditory cortex, *J. Neurophysiol, 25*, 223–235 (1962).

100. D. P. Scharlock, W. D. Neff, and N. L. Strominger, Discrimination of tonal duration after ablation of cortical auditory areas, *J. Neurophysiol. 28*, 673–681 (1965).

101. I. T. Diamond and W. D. Neff, Ablation of temporal cortex and discrimination of auditory patterns, *J. Neurophysiol. 20*, 300–315 (1957).

102. W. D. Neff, J. F. Fisher, I. T. Diamond, and M. Yela, Role of auditory cortex

in discrimination requiring localization of sound in space, *J. Neurophysiol.* *19*, 500–512 (1956).

103. R. B. Masterton and I. T. Diamond, Effects of auditory cortex ablation on discrimination of small binaural time differences, *J. Neurophysiol. 27*, 15–36 (1964).

104. W. D. Neff, Auditory discriminations affected by cortical ablations, in *Sensorineural Hearing Processes and Disorders* (A. B. Graham, ed.), Little, Brown, Boston, Massachusetts, 1967, pp. 201–210.

105. H. E. Heffner and R. B. Masterton, The contributions of auditory cortex to sound localization in the monkey, *J. Neurophysiol. 38*, 1340–1358 (1975).

106. W. D. Neff, I. T. Diamond, and J. H. Casseday, Behavioral studies of auditory discrimination: Central nervous system, in *Handbook of Sensory Physiology* (W. D. Keiday and W. D. Neff, eds.), Vol. 5: *Auditory System*, Springer-Verlag, New York, 1975, pp. 307–400.

107. W. D. Neff and J. H. Casseday, Effects of unilateral ablation of auditory cortex on monaural cat's ability to localize sounds, *J. Neurophysiol 40*, 44–52 (1977).

108. N. L. Strominger, Subdivisions of auditory cortex and their role in localization of sound in space, *Exp. Neurol. 24*, 348–362 (1969).

109. I. C. Whitfield, J. Cranford, R. Ravizza, and I. T. Diamond, Effects of unilateral ablation of auditory cortex in cat on complex sound localization, *J. Neurophysiol. 35*, 718–731 (1972).

110. W. D. Neff, The brain and hearing: Auditory discriminations affected by brain lesions, *Ann. Otol. 86*, 500–506 (1977).

111. J. Jerger et al., Bilateral lesions of the temporal lobe, *Acta Otol.*, Suppl. 258 (1969).

112. F. Lhermitte et al., Etude de troubles perceptifs auditifs dans les lesions temporales bilaterales, *Rev. Neurol. 124*, 329–351 (1971).

113. T. A. Karaseva, The role of the temporal lobe in human auditory perception, *Neuropsychology, 10*, 227–231 (1972).

114. W. Penfield and J. Evans, Functional deficits produced by cerebral lobectomies, *A. Res. Nerv. Ment. Dis. Proc. 13*, 352–377 (1934).

115. W. Penfield and T. Rasmussen, *The Cerebral Cortex: A Clinical Study of Localization of Function*, MacMillan, New York, 1950.

116. W. Penfield and H. Jasper, Epilepsy and the Functional Anatomy of the Human Brain, Little, Brown, Boston, 1954.

117. R. Galambos, Suppression of auditory activity by stimulation of efferent fibers to cochlea, *J. Neurophysiol, 19*, 424–437 (1959).

118. J. Fex, Augmentation of the cochlear microphonics by stimulation of efferent fibers to the cochlea, *Acta Otol. 50*, 540–541 (1959).

119. H. Sohmer, A comparison of the efferent effects of the homolateral and contralateral olivo-cochlear bundles, *Acta Otol. 62*, 74–87 (1966).

120. J. Fex, Efferent inhibition in the cochlea related to hair-cell dc activity: Study of postsynaptic activity of the crossed olivocochlear fibers in the cat, *J. Acoust. Soc. Am. 41*, 666–675 (1967).

121. M. L. Wiederhold and N. Y. S. Kiang, Effects of electrical stimulation of the crossed olivo-cochlear bundle on single auditory nerve fibers in the cat, *J. Acoust. Soc. Am. 48*, 950–965 (1970).

122. M. L. Wiederhold, Variations in the effects of electrical stimulation of the crossed olivo-cochlear bundle on cat single auditory nerve fiber responses to tone bursts, *J. Acoust. Soc. Am. 48*, 966–977 (1970).

123. D. C. Teas, T. Konishi, and D. W. Neilsen, Electrophysiological studies on the spacial distribution of the crossed olivocochlear bundle along the guinea pig cochlea, *J. Acoust. Soc. Am. 51*, 1256–1264 (1972).

124. M. L. Gifford, and J. J. Guinan, Effects of crossed-olivocochlear-bundle stimulation on cat auditory nerve fiber responses to tones, *J. Acoust. Soc. Am. 74*, 115–123 (1983).

125. N. Y. S. Kiang, E. C. Moxon, and R. A. Levine, Auditory-nerve activity in cats with normal and abnormal cochleas, in *Sensorineural Hearing Loss* (G.E.W. Wolstenholme and J. Knight, eds.), (CIBA Foundation Symposium) Churchill, London, 1970, pp. 241–273.

126. M. C. Brown, A. L. Nuttall, and R. I. Masta, Intracellular recordings from cochlear inner hair cells: Effects of the crossed olivocochlear efferents, *Science 222*, 69–72 (1983).

127. W. E. Brownell, C. R. Bader, D. Bertrand, and Y. deRibaupierre, Evoked mechanical response of isolated cochlear outer hair cells, *Science 227*, 194–196 (1985).

128. N. Slepecky, M. Ulfendahl, and A. Flock, Shortening and elongation of isolated outer hair cells in response to application of potassium gluconate, acetylcholine and cationized ferritin, *Hearing Res. 34*, 119–126 (1988).

129. D. C. Mountain, Changes in endolymphatic potential and crossed olivo-cochelar bundle stimulation alter cochlear mechanics, *Science 210*, 71–72 (1980).

130. J. H. Siegel and D. O. Kim, Efferent neural control of cochlear mechanics? Olivocochlear bundle stimulation affects cochlear biomechanical nonlinearity, *Hearing Res. 6*, 171–182 (1982).

131. P. Nieder and I. Nieder, Antimasking effect of crossed olivocochlear bundle stimulation with loud clicks in guinea pig. *Exp. Neurol. 28*, 179–188 (1970a).

132. P. Nieder and I. Nieder, Stimulation of efferent olivocochlear bundle causes release from low level masking, *Nature 227*, 184–185 (1970b).

133. D. F. Dolan, and A. L. Nuttall, Masked cochlear whole-nerve response intensity functions altered by electrical stimulation of the crossed olivo-cochlear bundle, *J. Acoust. Soc. Am. 83*, 1081–1086 (1988).

7
Psychoacoustic Methods

Psychophysics is concerned with how we perceive the physical stimuli impinging upon our senses. The branch of psychophysics that deals with the perception of sound is psychoacoustics. In defining this term we make a sharp distinction between the physical stimulus and the psychological response to it. We may think of the sound presented to our ears as the stimulus and of what we hear as the response. For example, what we hear as loudness is the perceptual correlate of intensity. Other things being equal, a rise in intensity is perceived as an increase in loudness. Pitch corresponds to sound frequency: Other things being equal, pitch gets higher as frequency increases.

If there were a single one-to-one correspondence between the physical parameters of sound and how they are perceived, then we could quantify what we hear directly in terms of the attributes of the sound. That would mean that all physically existing sounds could be heard, that all changes in them would be discriminable, and that any change in stimulus magnitude would result in a perceptual change of the same magnitude. This is not the case. It is thus necessary to describe the manner in which sound is perceived, and to attempt to explain the underlying mechanisms of the auditory press. This is the province of psychoacoustics.

MEASUREMENT METHODS

Establishing relationships between the sound presented and how the subject perceives it is a primary goal. To accomplish this goal, the experi-

284

menter contrives a special situation designed to home in on the relation of interest. An experimental situation is used to avoid the ambiguities of presenting a stimulus and, in effect, asking the open-ended question "what did you hear?" Instead, the stimulus and response are clearly specified, and then some aspect of the stimulus (intensity, frequency, etc.) is manipulated. The subject's task is to respond in a predetermined manner so that the experimenter can get an unambiguous idea of what was heard. For example, one may vary the intensity of a tone and ask the subject whether it was heard during each presentation. The lowest level at which the sound is heard (the transition between audibility and inaudibility) might be considered an estimate of absolute sensitivity. Alternatively, two tones might be presented, one of which is varied in frequency. The subject is asked whether the varied tone is higher (or lower) in pitch, and the smallest perceivable frequency difference—the just noticeable difference (jnd)—might be considered an estimate of differential sensitivity.

We must also distinguish between what the subject actually hears and the manner in which he responds. The former is *sensory capability* (or *sensitivity*), and the latter is *response proclivity*. For the most part, we are interested in sensory capability. Response proclivity reflects not only the subject's sensitivity, but also the biases and criteria that affect how he responds. We therefore try to select measurement methods and techniques which minimize the effects of response bias. An excellent discussion of the many details to be considered in psychacoustic experiments is given in Robinson and Watson [1]. In this chapter, we shall be concerned with classical psychophysical methods, adaptive techniques, and some aspects of scaling. Chapter 8 covers signal detection.

Classical Methods

There are three classical psychophysical methods: limits, adjustment, and constant stimuli. Each has its individual advantages and disadvantages, as well as sharing some pros and cons with the other methods.

Method of Limits

In the method of limits, the stimulus is under the experimenter's control and the subject simply responds after each presentation. Suppose we are interested in the absolute sensitivity (threshold) for a particular sound. The sound is presented at a level expected to be well above threshold. Since it is clearly audible, the subject responds by saying that he heard the sound (+ in Fig. 7.1). The level of the sound is then decreased by a discrete amount (2 dB in Fig. 7.1) and presented again. This process is repeated until the subject no longer perceives the sound (−), at which

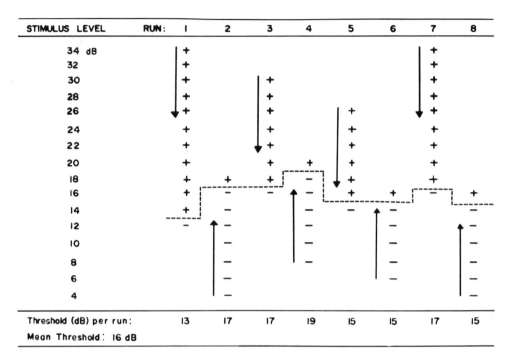

Figure 7.1   Method of limits.

point the series (or run) is terminated. This example involves a descending run. In an ascending series, the sound is first presented at a level known to be below the threshold and is increased in magnitude until a positive (+) response is obtained. The odd-numbered runs in Fig. 7.1 are descending series and the even-numbered runs are ascending. Since the crossover between "hearing" and "not hearing" lies somewhere between the lowest audible level and the highest inaudible one, the "threshold" for each series may be taken as the halfway point between them. The subject's threshold is obtained by averaging the threshold levels across runs. This average is 16 dB for the data in Fig. 7.1.

Several forms of response bias are associated with the method of limits. Since a series either ascends or descends, and is terminated by a change in response, the subject may anticipate the level at which his response should change from "no" to "yes" in an ascending run and from "yes" to "no" in a descending series. Anticipation thus results in a lower (better) ascending threshold because the subject anticipates hearing the stimulus, and a higher (poorer) descending threshold since he anticipates not hearing it. An opposite affect is caused by habituation.

INERTIA

Here, the subject does not change his response from "no" to "yes" during an ascending run until the actual threshold is exceeded by a few trials (raising the measured threshold level); and he continues to respond "yes" for one or more descending trials after the sound has actually become inaudible (lowering the measured threshold level). These biases may be minimized by using an equal number of ascending and descending test runs in each threshold determination. These runs may be presented alternatively (as in the figure) or randomly. A second way to minimize these biases is to vary the starting levels for the runs. Both tactics are illustrated in Fig. 7.1.

The method of limits is also limited in terms of step size and inefficiently placed trials. Too large a step size reduces accuracy because the actual threshold may lie anywhere between two discrete stimulus levels. For example, a 10 dB step is far less precise than a 2 dB increment; and the larger the increment between the steps, the more approximate the result. Too large a step size may place the highest inaudible presentation at a level with a 0% probability of response, and the lowest audible presentation at a level with a 100% probability of response. The 50% point (threshold) may be *anywhere* between them! To make this point clear, consider the psychometric functions in Fig. 7.2. A psychometric function shows the probability (percentage) of responses for different stimulus levels. Figure 7.2a shows the psychometric function for a particular sound. It is inaudible (0% responses) at 13 dB and is always heard (100% responses) at 21 dB. It is customary to define the threshold as the level at which the sound is heard 50% of the time (0.5 probability). The threshold in Fig. 7.2a is thus 17 dB. Suppose we try to find this threshold using a 10 dB step size, with increments corresponding to 14 dB, 24 dB, etc. Notice that this step size essentially includes the whole psychometric function, so that we do not know where the responses change from 0% to 100%; nor do we know whether they do so in a rapid jump (a step function) or along a function where gradual changes in the proportion of "yes" responses correspond to gradual changes in stimulus level. The result is low precision in estimating the location of the 50% point. However, a large step size is convenient in that it involves fewer presentations (and thus shorter test time), since responses go from "yes" to "no" in very few trials, each of which is either well above or well below threshold.

A smaller step size permits a more precise estimate of threshold because the reversals from "yes" to "no" (and vice versa) are better placed (closer) in relation to the 50% point. The relationship of a 2 dB step to the psychometric function is shown in Fig. 7.2c, which gives the probability of a response in 2 dB intervals. Notice that these points are

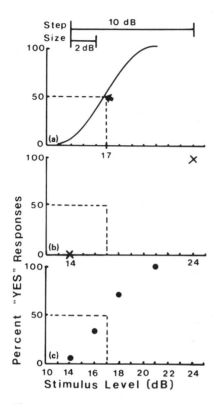

Figure 7.2   (a) Psychometric function showing 50% threshold at 17 dB (arrow). (b) Responses (x's) of 0% at 14 dB and 100% at 24 dB with a 10 dB step size. (c) Percent responses at various levels with a 2 dB step. The 50% threshold is shown on each graph. The 2 dB and 10 dB step sizes are illustrated at the top of the figure.

better placed than those for the 10 dB step size in Fig. 7.2b. For this reason, even though there may be "wasted" presentations due to test levels well above or below the threshold, the method of limits with an appropriate step size is still popular. This is particularly true in pilot experiments and in clinical evaluations, both of which take advantage of the speed with which thresholds are estimated by the method of limits. The clinical method of limits [2], however, is actually a hybrid technique with characteristics of the staircase method, discussed below.

The method of limits may also be used to determine differential thresholds. In this case, two stimuli are presented in each trial, and the subject is asked whether the second is greater than, less than, or equal to the first with respect to some parameter. The first stimulus is held constant, and the second is varied by the experimenter in discrete steps. The procedure is otherwise the same as for determining thresholds, although the findings are different. Suppose the subject is to make an equal loudness judgment. The method of limits would result in a range of intensities in which the second stimulus is louder than the first, a range in which the second is softer, and a range in which the two sounds appear equal. In Table 7.1 the averge upper limen (halfway between "higher" and "equal") is 57 dB, and the average lower limen (between "equal" and "lower") is 53.5 dB. The range between these values is an interval of uncertainty that is 3.5 dB wide. Although there is a range of "equal" judgments, we may estimate the "equal" level to lie halfway between the upper and lower limens, at 55.25 dB. This level is commonly referred to as the point of subjective equality (PSE). The jnd or difference limen (DL) is generally estimated as one-half of the uncertainty interval, or 1.75 dB for the data in Table 7.1.

Method of Adjustment

The adjustment method differs from the method of limits in two ways. First, the stimulus is controlled by the subject instead of by the experimenter. In addition, the level of the stimulus is varied continuously rather than in discrete steps. As in the method of limits, the level is adjusted downward from above threshold until it is just inaudible, or increased from below threshold until it is just audible. Threshold is

Table 7.1 Results of Method of Limits in a Hypothetical Discrimination Experiment

Stimulus level (dB)	Run			
	1	2	3	4
60	Louder			
59	Louder		Louder	
58	Louder		Louder	Louder
57	Equal	Louder	Louder	Equal
56	Equal	Equal	Equal	Equal
55	Equal	Equal	Equal	Equal
54	Equal	Equal	Equal	Softer
53	Softer	Equal	Softer	Softer
52		Softer		Softer
51		Softer		Softer
50		Softer		

taken as the average of the just audible and just inaudible levels. To obtain an estimate of differential sensitivity, the subject adjusts the level of one sound until it is as loud as a standard sound, or adjusts the frequency of one sound until it has the same pitch as the other.

The stimulus control (generally a continuous dial) must be unlabeled and should have no detents that might provide tactile cues that could bias the results. Furthermore, it is common practice to insert a second control between the subject's dial and the instrumentation, allowing the experimenter to vary the starting point of a test series by an amount unknown to the subject. This procedure avoids biases due to positioning of the response dial and to the use of dial settings as "anchors" from one series to the next. Even with these precautions, however, it is difficult for the experimenter to exercise the same degree of control over the procedure as in the method of limits. Furthermore, the subject may change his criterion of audibility during test runs, introducing another hard-to-control bias into the method of adjustment.

Just as anticipation and habituation affect the results obtained with the method of limits, stimulus persistence (perseveration) biases the results from the method of adjustment. Persistence of the stimulus means that a lower threshold is obtained on a descending run because the subject continues to turn the level down below threshold as though the sound were still audible. Thus, we may think of this phenomenon as persistence of the stimulus, or as perseveration of the response. In an ascending trial, the absence of audibility persists, so that the subject keeps turning the level up until the true threshold is passed by some amount, which has the opposite effect of raising the measured threshold level. These biases may be minimized by using both ascending and descending series in each measurement. Another variation is to have the subject "bracket" his threshold by varying the level up and down until a just audible sound is perceived. After the ending point is recorded, the experimenter may use the second stimulus control discussed above to change the starting level by an amount unknown to the subject, in preparation for the next trial.

Method of Constant Stimuli

The method of constant stimuli (or constants) involves the presentation of various stimulus levels to the subject in random order. Unlike the methods of limits and adjustments, the method of constants is a nonsequential procedure. In other words, the stimuli are not presented in an ascending or descending manner. A range of intensities is selected which, based upon previous experience or a pilot experiment, encompasses the threshold level. A step size is selected, and the stimuli are then presented to the subject in random order. During the experiment, an equal number of stimuli are presented at each level. The subject states whether there are a stimulus presentation during each test trial. (In a differential sensitivity experiment, the task would be to say whether the two items are same or different.)

In an experiment to determine the threshold for a tone by using the method of constant stimuli, one might randomly present tones in 1 dB increments between 4dB and 11 dB, for a total of 50 trials at each level. Sample results are tabulated in Table 7.2. When these data are graphed in the form of a psychometric function (Fig. 7.3), the 50% point corresponds to 7.5 dB, which is taken as the threshold.

Table 7.3 shows the results of an experiment using the method of constants to find differential sensitivity for intensity. Two tones are

Table 7.2   Threshold of a Tone Using the Method of Constant Stimuli

Stimulus level (dB)	Number of responses	Percent of responses
11	50	100
10	50	100
9	47	94
8	35	70
7	17	34
6	3	6
5	0	0
4	0	0

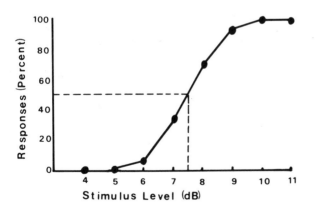

Figure 7.3   Psychometric function for method of constant stimuli. Threshold corresponds to 7.5 dB (Data from Table 7.2.)

Table 7.3   Data from an Experiment on Differential Sensitivity
for Intensity Using the Method of Constant Stimuli

Level of second tone (dB)	Percentage of louder judgments
70	100
68	95
66	85
64	70
62	55
60	35
58	20
56	10
54	8
52	5
50	0

presented and the subject is asked whether the second tone is louder
or softer than the first. The intensity of the second tone is changed so
that the various stimulus levels are presented randomly. Table 7.3
shows the percentage of presentations in which the subject judged the
second tone to be louder than the first tone at each of the levels used.
(The percentage of "softer" judgments is simply obtained by subtracting the percentage of "louder" judgments from 100%. Thus, the 60 dB
presentations of the second tone were "softer" 100% − 35% = 65% of
the time.) Figure 7.4 shows the psychometric function for these data.
Since the intensity at which the second tone is judged louder 50% of
the time is also the tone for which it was judged softer half of the time,
the 50% point is where the two tones were perceived as equal in loudness. This is the PSE. In experiments of this kind, the 75% point is
generally accepted as the threshold for "louder" judgments. (If we had
also plotted "softer" judgments, then the 75% point on that psychometric function would constitute the "softer" threshold.) The DL is
taken as the difference in stimulus values between the PSE and the
"louder" threshold. For the data in Fig. 7.4 this difference is 64.8 dB −
61.5 dB = 3.3 dB.

The method of constant stimuli enables the experimenter to include
"catch" trials over the course of the experiment. These are intervals
during which the subject is asked whether a tone was heard, when no
tone was really presented. Performance on catch trials provides a estimate of guessing, and performance on real trials is often corrected to
account for this effect (see Chap. 8). This correction reduces, but does
not completely remove, response biases from the results.

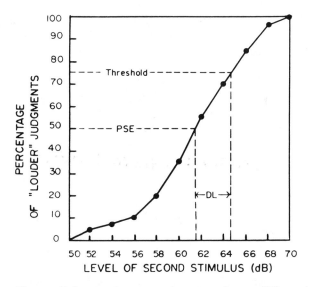

Figure 7.4 Psychometric function for a differential-sensitivity experiment showing the point of subjective equality (PSE), "higher" threshold, and difference limen (DL). (Data from Table 7.3.)

The method of constants has the advantage over the methods of limits and adjustments of greater precision of measurement; and as just mentioned has the advantage of allowing direct estimation of guessing behavior. However, it has the disadvantage of inefficiency, because a very large number of trials are needed to obtain the data. Most of these trial points are poorly placed relative to the points of interest (generally the 50% and 75% points), so that the method of constants costs heavily in time and effort for its accuracy. The prolonged test time increases the effects of subject fatigue and the difficulty of maintaining motivation to respond.

Adaptive Procedures

In an adaptive procedure, the level at which a particular stimulus is presented to the subject depends upon how the subject responded to the previous stimuli [3–6]. Broadly defined, even the classical method of limits may be considered an adaptive method because of its sequential character and the rule that stimuli are presented until there is a reversal in the subject's responses from "yes" or "no" or vice versa. However, the term adaptive procedures has come to be associated with methods that tend to *converge* upon the threshold level (or some other target point), and then place most of the observations around it. This procedure, of course, maximizes the efficiency of the method, because most of the test trials are close to the threshold rather than being "wasted" at some distance from it. It also has the advantage of not requiring prior knowledge of where the threshold level is located, since adaptive methods tend to home in on the threshold regardless of the starting point, and often include step sizes which are large at first and then become smaller as the threshold level is approached. As a result, both efficiency and precision are maximized.   BEKESY : PUSH BUTTON CONTROL

Bekesy's Tracking Method   CONTINUOUS CHANGE (ANALOG)

Bekesy [7] devised a tracking method which shares features both with the classical methods of adjustment and limits and with adaptive procedures. The level of the stimulus changes at a fixed rate (e.g. 2.5 dB/sec) under the control of a motor-driven attenuator, and the *direction* of level change is controlled by the subject via a pushbutton switch. The motor is also connected to a recorder which shows the sound level as a function of time (Fig. 7.5) or frequency. The pushbutton causes the motor to decrease the sound level when it is depressed and to increase the level when it is up. The subject is asked to press the button whenever he hears the tone and to release it whenever the tone is inaudible. Thus, the sound level is increased toward threshold from below when the tone is inaudible, and decreased toward threshold from above when the sound is heard. The threshold is thus tracked by the subject, and its value is the

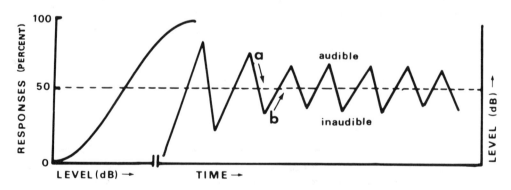

Figure 7.5 Bekesy's tracking method: (a) Intensity decreases as subject depresses the button when he hears the sound. (b) Intensity increases as subject releases the button when he cannot hear the sound. Excursion midpoints (50% level) correspond to the psychometric function at the left.

average of the midpoints of the excursions on the recording (once they are stabilized).

Tracking has the advantages of speed and reasonable precision. It is, of course, subject to several sources of response bias. At fast attenuation rates (intensity change speeds) the subject's reaction time can substantially affect the width of the tracking excursions and the precision of measurement. For example, if the tone increases and decreases in level at 5 dB/sec and a subject has a 2 sec reaction time, then the motor will have advanced the stimulus level (and pen position on the recorder) 10 dB above theshold before the button is finally depressed. Precision is improved and reaction time becomes less critical at reasonably slower attenuation rates, although the tracking may meander somewhat on the recording as the subject's criterion for threshold varies.

The tracking method has gained wide acceptance in clinical audiology. Bekesy audiometry has been used extensively in hearing screening programs, in the diagnosis of lesions in the auditory system, and in the identification of functional (nonorganic) hearing loss.

Up–Down (Staircase) Method   DISCRETE (QUANTITIZED) CHANGE

The simple up–down (or staircase) method [4,6,8] involves increasing the stimulus level when the subject does not respond to a presentation and decreasing the intensity when there is a response. It differs from the method of limits in that testing does not stop when the responses change from "yes" to "no" or vice versa. As in the method of limits, the stimuli are varied in discrete steps.

Figure 7.6 shows the first six runs of a staircase procedure using a 2 dB step size. A "run" is a group of stimulus presentations between two response reversals. In other words, a descending run starts with a positive response and continues downward until there is a negative re-

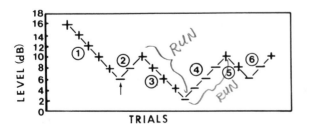

Figure 7.6 Simple up–down (staircase) method. Six runs are shown. Odd numbers are descending runs and even numbers are ascending runs. The first reversal (arrow) is generally omitted from the threshold calculation.

sponse; while an ascending run begins with a negative response and ends with a positive one. Since stimulus intensity is always increased after a negative (−) response and decreased after a positive (+) response, the staircase method converges upon the 50% point on the psychometric function. The procedure is continued through at least six to eight reversals (excluding the first one), and the threshold value is then calculated as the average of the midpoints of the runs, or as the average of their peaks and troughs [3,9]. The latter method appears to give a somewhat better estimate. The precision of the method can be increased by first estimating the threshold with a larger step size, and then using a smaller step size (generally half that of the previous one) to locate the threshold in the vicinity of the first estimate [9]. For example, if the average of six runs using a 4 dB step is 10 dB, a second group of runs using a 2 dB step might begin at 10 dB in order to obtain a more precise estimate of the threshold.

The simple up–down method has several advantages and limitations [4]. It quickly converges upon the 50% point so that most trials are efficiently placed close to the point of interest. It also has the advantage of being able to follow changes (drifts) in the subject's responses. On the other hand, the subject may bias his responses if he realized that the stimuli are being presented according to a sequential rule which depends on the way he responds. As with the method of limits, if the step size is too small a large number of trials are wasted, and if the step is too large they are badly placed for estimating the 50% point. Another limitation is that only the 50% point can be converged upon with the simple up-down rule.

PEST Procedure

Parameter estimation by sequential testing (PEST) is an adaptive procedures which uses changes in both the direction and step size of the stimulus to home in on a targeted level of performance [10,11]. The experimenter may set the target value to any location on the psychometric function he chooses (for example, 50% or 80%). However, we will concentrate here only on the 50% point in order to make clear the salient features which distinguish the PEST procedure. As in the simple up–down method, positive responses are followed by decreases in stimulus level because the threshold is probably lower, and negative responses are followed by increases in intensity since the threshold is probably higher. The difference is that PEST includes a series of rules for doubling and halving the stimulus level depending upon the previous sequence of responses.

At each stimulus level, PEST in effect asks whether the threshold has been exceeded. The level is then changed so that the maximum amount of information is obtained from the next trial. To do this, the step size is varied in the manner specified in Fig. 7.7. Although it is most efficient to know the approximate location of the threshold range in advance, it is not essential. Suppose we begin testing at some value below threshold corresponding to point A in Fig. 7.7. Since the subject gives a negative response, the stimulus is presented at a higher level (B). This level also produces no response and the stimulus is raised by the same amount as previously, and is presented again (C). Since there is still no response, the stimulus level is again increased. However, PEST has a rule which states that if there is a negative response on two successive presentations in the same direction, then the step size is doubled for the next presentation. Thus, the next stimulus is presented at level D. The doubling rule insures that a minimal number of trials are wasted in finding the range of interest.

A positive response at level D indicates that the threshold has been exceeded. As in the staircase method, the direction of the trials is changed after a response reversal. However, the PEST procedure also halves the step size at this point. The halving rule causes the stimuli to

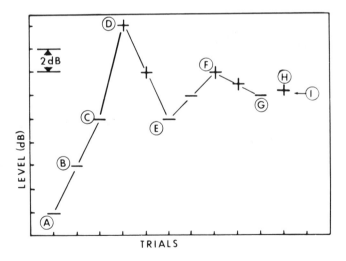

Figure 7.7   Obtaining threshold with PEST. (+) Positive response, (−) negative response. Letters are points discussed in the text. Point I is the estimate of threshold.

be presented closer to the threshold value. Thus, precision is improved as the threshold is converged upon. Since D is followed by another positive response, the stimulus is then presented at a lower level (E). A negative response at E causes the direction of stimulus change to be changed again, and the step size is halved compared to the previous one. The stimulus is heard again at the next higher level (F), so the direction is changed again and the step size is again halved. Stimuli are now presented in a descending run until there is a negative response (G). Halving the step size and changing direction results in a positive response at H, indicating that the threshold lies somewhere between points G and H. Since this interval represents an acceptable degree of precision, the procedure is terminated. The level at which the *next* stimulus would have been presented is taken as the threshold. This level is point I, which lies halfway between levels G and H. Note on the scale for Fig. 7.7 that the step size between E and F is 2 dB, between F and G is 1 dB, and between G and H is 0.5 dB. This observation highlights the rapidity with which PEST results in a precise threshold estimate.

BUDTIF Procedure

Suppose we are interested in the 75% point of psychometric function. One way to converge upon the point is to modify the simple up–down procedure by replacing the single trial per stimulus level with a block of several trials per level. Then, by adopting three out of four positive responses (75%) as the criterion per level, the strategy will home in on the 75% point. If blocks of five were used with a four out of five criterion, then the 80% point would be converged upon. The procedure may be further modified by changing the response from yes-no to a two-alternative forced choice. In other words, the subject is presented with two stimulus intervals during each trial, and must indicate which of the intervals contains the stimulus. This is the block up–down temporal interval forced-choice (BUDTIF) procedure [12]. (Using the two-interval forced choice allows the experimenter to determine the proportion of responses to the no-stimulus interval—the "false alarm" rate. We shall see when the theory of signal detection is discussed in the next chapter that this distinction is important in separating sensitivity from bias effects.)

The BUDTIF procedure is illustrated in Fig. 7.8. Note that each block is treated as though it were one trial in a staircase procedure. Since the target point has been preselected as 75%, stimulus intensity is raised whenever there are less than three out of four correct responses in a block, and is decreased when all four are correct. Testing is terminated when three out of four correct responses are obtained. The last level is

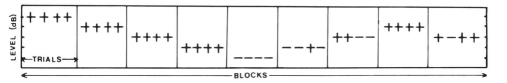

Figure 7.8 Convergence of the psychometric function upon the 75% point using BUDTIF.

the target level (75% in this case). Notice that since blocks of trials are presented at each level, poor placement of the initial test level will cause many wasted trials in converging upon the target range. ①*WASTED TRIALS*

A modification of BUDTIF replaces the two-alternative forced-choice paradigm with the familiar yes-no response. This adaptation is called the block up–down yes–no (BUDYEN) method [13]. However, it is less satisfactory than its forced-choice predecessor because an estimate of false alarms is not obtained [14].

Transformed Up–Down Procedures

The simple up–down method converges on the 50% point of the psychometric function because each positive response leads to a decrease in stimulus level and each negative response leads to an intensity increase. If the up—down rule is modified so that stimulus level is changed only after *certain sequences* have occurred, then the procedure will home in on other points of the psychometric function [3,4,6,15]. These other targets points depend upon the particular set of sequences chosen by the experimenter.

When the target is 50% on the psychometric function, as in the simple up–down method, the chances of a positive response to stimuli below the 50% point are very small. Similarly, it is likely that stimuli presented at levels well above the 50% point will frequently be heard. However, as the intensity corresponding to 50% is approached, the chances of positive and negative responses become closer and closer. At the 50% point, the probability of a positive response is the same as of a negative one. This is, of course, exactly what we mean by 50%. Now, suppose that the total probability of all responses is 1.00. If we call the probability of a positive response P, then the probability of a negative response would be (1 − P). At the 50% point

$$P = (1 - P) = 0.5$$

In other words, the probability of a positive response at the 50% point is 0.5, which is also the probability of a negative response. In effect, the simple up–down rule forces the intensity to the point on the psychometric function where the probabilities of positive and negative responses are equal (0.5 each).

Other target levels can be converged upon by changing the up–down rule so that the probabilities of increasing and decreasing stimulus intensity are unequal. This is done by setting the criteria for increasing stimulus level (the "up rule") to be a certain response sequence, and those for decreasing stimulus level (the "down rule") to be other response sequences. An example will demonstrate how the tranformed up–down method works.

Suppose we are interested in estimating a point above 50% on the psychometric function, say 70%. To accomplish this, we would increase the stimulus level after a negative response ($-$) or a positive response followed by a negative one, ($+,-$); and lower stimulus level after two successive positives ($+,+$). In other words, we have established the following rules for changing stimulus level:

$$\text{Up rule:} \qquad (-) \qquad \text{or} \qquad (+,-)$$
$$\text{Down rule:} \qquad (+,+)$$

As with the simple staircase rule, levels well above the target will often yield ($+,+$) responses, and those well below will frequently have ($-$) or ($+,-$) responses. However, at the target level, the probability of increasing the stimulus level will be

$$(1 - P) \qquad + \qquad P(1 - P)$$
$$\text{Probability} \qquad\qquad \text{Probability}$$
$$\text{of } (-) \qquad\qquad\quad \text{of } (+,-)$$

and the probability of two successive positive responses ($+,+$) will be

$$P \times P \qquad \text{or} \qquad P^2$$

The up–down strategy will converge on the point where the up and down rules have the same probabilities (0.5). In other words, the probability of the transformed positive response ($+,+$) at the target is

$$P^2 = 0.5$$

Since we are interested in the probability P of a single positive response, which is the square root of P^2, we simply find the square root of $P^2 = 0.5$, and we obtain

$$P = 0.707$$

Converting to percent, the transformed procedure just outlined homes in on the 70.7% point of the psychometric function, which is a quite acceptable estimate of the 70% point.

To converge on the 29.3% of the psychometric function (which is a reasonable estimate of the 30% point), we might choose to increase the stimulus after a sequence of two successive negative responses $(-,-)$, and to decrease stimulus level after a positive response $(+)$ or a negative response followed by a positive one $(-,+)$.

The 70.7% and 29.3% transformed up–down strategies are illustrated in Fig. 7.9. As for the simple up–down method, each strategy would be continued through six to eight reversals, and the average of the peaks and valleys would be taken as the target level. Since these two points are on the rising portion of the psychometric function and are equidistant from 50%, a reasonably good estimate of the 50% point can be obtained by averaging the levels from 70.7% and 29.3%. To increase efficiency, one might start with a large step size, and then halve it in the target range for increased precision.

Other target points can be converged upon by various sequences of positive and negative responses; and different sequences may be used to converge upon the same target points [3,6,15]. Transformed up–down procedures can also be used in the measurement of subjective judgments, such as for loudness balances [16]. In addition, both simple and transformed up–down procedures are particularly applicable to testing various aspects of speech recognition functions under a variety of conditions [5,6,15,17–21].

A good approach to minimizing biases is to interleaf different test strategies [22]. In other words, two points on the psychometric function are converged upon during the same test session by switching in an

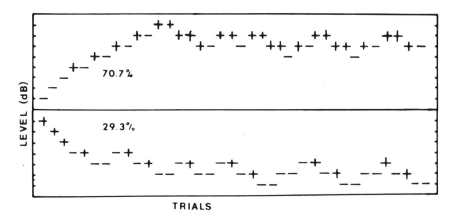

Figure 7.9 Transformed up–down strategies converging upon the 70.7% and 29.3% points of the psychometric function.

approximately random manner between their two test strategies. For example, two reversals on the 29.3% strategy might be followed by a few reversals on the 70.7% strategy, then the experimenter would return to where he left off on the 29.3% sequence, and so forth. Such interleaving can also be applied to other psychoacoustic methods.

The transformed up–down procedure is made relatively simple to administer through the use of control charts [23]. These charts have the sequence of events for each strategy printed on them, so that all the experimenter needs to do is mark down whether the response was positive or negative, and otherwise simply "follow the dotted lines." Control charts also simplify tremendously the process of interleaving test strategies, by indicating whether the experimenter should stay on the current task or switch to the other one. Of course, greater flexibility and ease of measurement is made possible when the procedure is automated [24]; and, almost needless to say, computerized administrations of these procedures have now become the norm.

Modifications, Other Procedures, and Comparisons

As one might expect, many experimenters vary the "pure" procedures in order to accommodate their specific needs. For example, levels in up–down procedures are sometimes changed in proportional steps rather than by fixed intervals.

Also, adaptive procedures are combined with various approaches regarding how the stimuli are presented and responses are obtained. These might include "yes/no" formats, and forced choices among two or more alternatives. In the latter approaches, the subject is presented with two or more alternatives from which he must choose a response. Suppose, for example, that we want to find out whether a subject can hear a tone in the presence of a noise. In a yes/no experiment the subject hears one presentation of either a noise or a tone-plus-noise, and must indicate whether the tone was there or not ("yes" or "no"). In a two-alternative forced choice (2AFC) method, the subject is presented with two noises in succession, one of which also has the tone. After listening to both stimuli, he must decide whether the tone was present for first one or the second. Similarly, in a 4AFC experiment the subject must decide which of four successive stimuli includes the tone. Because the two or more presentations occur as successive intervals, we could also say that the subject must decide which interval contains the stimulus. Therefore, these experiments are often called 2– (or more) interval forced choice methods (hence, 2-IFC, 3-IFC, etc.). These topics are covered further in the context of the theory of signal detection in the next chapter.

Several approaches have been proposed that either modify the more well-known methods to a greater or lesser extent, and/or combine adaptive procedures with maximum-likelihood (or other) methods [25–33]. The particulars of maximum likelihood methods go far beyond the current scope; however, the salient feature for our purposes is as follows: Using the history of the subject's responses combined with certain assumptions about the nature of the psychometric function, an estimate is made about where the threshold (actually the midpoint of the function) lies after each response. This estimated value then becomes the level of the next stimulus presentation. Hall's [28,29] hybrid procedure, which combines aspects of maximum likelihood methods with features of PEST, is probably the most well-known of these approaches.

A new adaptive method which assumes a step function (where the value of the step is 0 below threshold and 1 above it) and a least-squares fitting approach was recently introduced by Simpson [33]. He reasoned that if the experimenter is interested in only one point, then a step function may be assumed in order to avoid any effects associated with the slope of the psychometric functions which are involved in the other methods. He reported that the results of this approach are quite similar to those for a somewhat similar method [30] which uses maximum likelihood estimates.

Several studies [11,33–40]* have made comparisons between various adaptive methods and between adaptive and more traditional approaches. Generally speaking, thresholds obtained with the various adaptive approaches tend to be quite close to each other. For example, Shelton et al. [35] found that thresholds were nearly the same when obtained using the transformed up–down, PEST, and maximum likelihood procedures. An interesting observation has been that adaptive and forced choice methods seem to result in somewhat lower thresholds than do non-forced choice and fixed-level methods [11,37,38,40]. Differences in efficiency are noted in the various studies, and some approaches are more appropriate to given problems than others. For example, Kollmeier et al. [40] found that, among the comparison they made, the most efficient approach was to use a the 3AFC method combined with a 1-up/3-down adaptive rule. One should consult these papers when deciding upon the most appropriate approach for a given experiment. An interesting finding was reported by Simpson [33,34], who

---

*Kollmeier, et al. [40] present a review of many of the comparisons, which were based upon simulations.

found that the method of constant stimuli was essentially as efficient as his own adaptive method [33] and the one proposed by Pentland [30].

SCALES OF MEASUREMENT

Scaling is an important area in psychoacoustics. Stevens [41–44] described four scales of measurement which are now accepted as classical. These are descriptively named (1) nominal, (2) ordinal, (3) interval, and (4) ratio scales.

Nominal scales are the least restrictive, in the sense that the observations are simply assigned to groups. This is the lowest order of scaling because the nominal label does not tell us anything about the relationship among the groups other than that they are different with respect to some parameter. For example, the nominal scale "sex" enables us to separate people into two categories, "male" and "female." All we know is that the two categories are differentiable, and that we can count how many cases fill into each one. The same would apply to the number of subcompact cars made by different manufacturers. We know that there are so many Fords, Toyotas, etc.; but we have no idea of their relative attributes. A nominal scale, then, makes no assumptions of the order among the classes; thus, it is the least restrictive and least informative of the levels of scaling.

Ordinal scales imply that the observations have values which can be rank-ordered, so that one class is greater or less than another with respect to the parameter of interest. However, an ordinal scale does not tell us how far apart they are. Consider the relative quality of artistic reproductions. Painter A may produce a better reproduction of the Mona Lisa than Painter B, who in turn makes a better copy than Painter C, and so on. However, there may be one magnitude of distance between A and B, a second distance between B and C, and still a third distance between C and D. An ordinal scale thus gives the rank-order of the categories (A > B > C . . .), but does not specify the distances between them. Whereas the nominal scale allows us to express the *mode* of the data (which category contains more cases than any other), ordinal scales permit the use of the *median* (the value with the same number of observations above and below it). Sometimes the nature of the categories enables some of them to be rank-ordered, but not others. This constitutes a *partially ordered scale* [45], which lies between the nominal and ordinal scales.

An *interval scale* specifies both the order among categories and the fixed distances among them. In other words, the distance between any two successive categories is equal to the distance between any other successive pair. Interval scales, however, do not imply a true zero reference point. Examples are temperature (in Celsius or Fahrenheit) and the dates on a calendar. Since the distances between categories are equal, the central tendency of interval data may be expressed as a *mean* (average); however, interval data cannot be expressed as proportions (ratios) of one another because a true zero point is not assumed. It is also possible to rank the categories in such a way that there is an ordering of the distances between them. For example, the distances between successive categories may become progressively longer: *ORDERED METRIC SCALE (i.e. log scale?)*

A-B- -C- - -D- - - -E- - - - -F- - - - - -G . . .

This is an *ordered metric scale* [45]. An ordered metric scale actually falls between the definitions of ordinal and interval scales, but may often be treated as an interval scale [46].

Ratio scales include all the properties of interval scales as well as an inherent zero point. The zero point permits values to be expressed as ratios, and hence the use of decibels in the expression of relationships. *RATIO* As the most restrictive level, ratio scales give the most information about the data and their interrelationships. Examples are length, time intervals, and temperature (in Kelvins), as well as loudness (sone) and pitch (mel) scales.

We might also think of three classes of scaling procedures [43,47]. *discriminability (or confusion)* scales are generated by asking the subject to discriminate small differences among stimuli. For example, the subject might be required to detect small differences in intensity between otherwise equivalent tones. The smallest discriminable difference is the jnd or DL. The relationship between the magnitude of a sound (intensity) and the psychoacoustic response to it (loudness) may be indirectly inferred from the jnd's.

The other two scaling procedures ask the subject to make direct estimates of perceptual differences between stimuli. *Category* (or *partition*) scales are generated when the subject's task is to divide a range of stimuli (e.g. an intensity or frequency range) into equally spaced or sized categories. *Magnitude* (or *ratio*) scales are obtained when the subject is asked to estimate ratio (or proportional) relationships among the stimuli. For example, the subject may be asked to adjust the frequency of one tone or that it sounds twice as high in pitch as another tone. The measurement approaches in the following sections may be thought of in these terms. In general, the classical psychophysical methods discussed earlier in the chapter are discriminability scales, while those that follow are direct scaling procedures of the ratio type.

Direct Scaling

As mentioned above, direct scaling procedures ask the subject to establish a relationship between a standard stimulus and a comparison stimulus. In other words, the subject must specify a perceptual continuum that corresponds to a physical continuum. Two types of continua may be defined [43]. Prothetic continua, such as loudness, have the characteristic of *amount* (or intensity). They are additive in that the excitation due to an increase in stimulus level is added to the excitation caused by the intensity which was already present. On the other hand, pitch has the characteristic of *kind* and azimuth has the characteristic of *location*. These are metathetic continua, and are substantive rather than additive. In other words, a change in the pitch corresponds to a substitution of one excitation pattern, as it were, for another.

Ratio Estimation and Production

In ratio estimation the subject is presented with two stimuli differing in terms of some parameter, and is asked to express the subjective magnitude of one stimulus as a ratio of the other. Subjective values are thus scaled as a function of the physical magnitudes. Suppose two 1000 Hz tones with different intensities are presented to a subject, who must judge the loudness of the second tone as a ratio of the first. He might report that the intensity of the second tone sounds one-half, one-quarter, twice, or five times as loud as the first tone.

Ratio production, or fractionalization, is the opposite of ratio estimation in that the subject's task is to adjust the magnitude of a variable stimulus so that it sounds like a particular ratio (or fraction) of the magnitude of a standard stimulus. For example, the subject might adjust the intensity of a comparison tone so that it sounds half as loud as the standard, twice as loud, etc. Fractionalization has been used in the development of scales relating loudness to intensity [48] and pitch to frequency [49,50].

Magnitude Estimation and Production

In magnitude estimation (ME) the subject assigns to physical intensities numbers that correspond to their subjective magnitudes. This may be done in general two ways [44,51]. In the first method, the subject is given a standard or reference stimulus and is told that its intensity has a particular value (modulus). He is then presented with other intensities and must assign numbers to these which are ratios of the modulus. Consider a loudness scaling experiment in which the subject compares the loudness of variable tones to a standard tone of 80 dB. If the 80 dB standard is called 10 (modulus) then a magnitude estimate of 1 would be assigned to the intensity ⅒ as loud, 60 would be assigned to the one which is 6 times at loud, etc. The relationship between these magnitude estimates and intensity is shown by the circles in Fig. 7.10.

An alternative approach is to omit the modulus. Here, the subject is presented with a series of stimuli and is asked to assign numbers to them reflecting their subjective levels. The results of such an experiment are shown by the x's in Fig. 7.10. As the figure shows, magnitude estimates obtained with and without a modulus result in similar findings.

The reverse of magnitude estimation is magnitude production (MP). In this approach, the subject is presented with numbers and must adjust the magnitude of the stimulus to correspond to the numbers.

Absolute magnitude estimation and production (AME and AMP) involves the performance of magnitude estimates (or productions) without any specified (or implied) reference value, and with each estimate (or production) made without regard to the judgments made for previous stimuli [52–59]. Although there has been some discussion regarding this approach [e.g. 60–62], the convincing preponderance of evidence reveals that it is valid, reliable and efficient, and that AMEs and AMPs are readily performed by naive clinical patients as well as laboratory subjects [52–59].

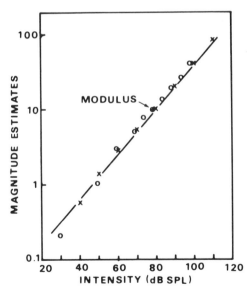

MODULUS≡ REFERENCE STIMULUS.

Figure 7.10 Magnitude estimation of loudness with a modulus (circles) and without a modulus (crosses) as a function of intensity. (Data from Stevens [51].)

Subject bias causes magnitude estimation and production to yield somewhat different results, especially at high and low stimulus levels. Specifically, subjects tend not to assign extreme values in magnitude estimation, or to make extreme level adjustments in magnitude production. These bias effects are in opposite directions, so that the "real" function lies somewhat between the ones obtained from magnitude estimations and productions. This is illustrated in Fig. 7.11 by the divergence of the magnitude estimation (ME) and magnitude production (MP) functions. The unbiased function may be obtained by a calculating the geometric mean of the magnitude estimations and productions along the intensity axis or the loudness axis [29,30]. This result is shown by the curve labeled PMB (for psychological magnitude balance) in Fig. 7.11.

Cross-Modality Matching

A scaling approach related to magnitude estimation and production is called cross-modality matching [44,59,63–65]. In this technique, the subject is asked to express the perceived magnitude for one sense in terms of another sensory modality. For example, loudness might be expressed in terms of line length. A very useful variation of this approach recently

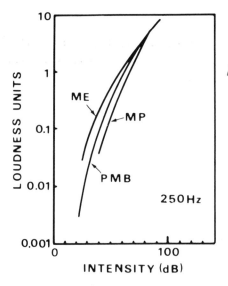

ME : MAGNITUDE ESTIMATION
MP : MAGNITUDE PRODUCTION
PMB : PSYCHOLOGICAL MAGNITUDE
                    BALANCE.

Figure 7.11   Bias effects in magnitude estimation (ME) and magnitude production (MP) are minimized by geometrical averaging in the method of psychological magnitude balance (PMB). (Adapted from Hellman and Zwislocki [54], with permission of *J. Acoust. Soc. Am.*)

developed by Hellman and Meiselman [59]. In this method, the slope of the power function for loudness is derived from that for line length combined with the cross modality match between loudness and line length.

REFERENCES *2/2/94 PRESENTATION*
— KIM

1. D. E. Robinson and C. S. Watson, Psychophysical methods in modern psychoacoustics, in *Foundations of Modern Auditory Theory* (J. V. Tobias, ed.), Vol. 2, Academic Press, New York, 1973, pp. 99–131.
2. R. Carhart and J. Jerger, Preferred method for clinical determination of pure-tone thresholds, *J. Speech Hearing Dis. 24*, 330–345 (1959).
3. G. B. Wetherill and H. Levitt, Sequential estimation of points on a psychometric function, *Br. J. Math. Stat. Psych. 18*, 1–10 (1965).
4. H. Levitt, Transformed up–down methods in psychoacoustics, *J. Acoust. Soc. Amer. 49*, 467–477 (1971).
5. D. L. Bode and R. Carhart, Measurements of articulation functions using adaptive test procedures, *IEEE Trans. Audiol. Electroacoust. AU-21*, 196–201 (1973).
6. H. Levitt, Adaptive testing in audiology, *Scand. Audiol. Suppl. 6*, 241–291 (1978).
7. G. Bekesy, *Experiments in Hearing*, McGraw-Hill, New York, 1960.
8. W. J. Dixon and A. M. Mood, A method for obtaining and analyzing sensitivity data, *J. Amer. Stat. Ass. 43*, 109–126 (1948).
9. G. B. Wetherill, Sequential estimation of quantal responses, *J. Roy. Stat. Soc. 25*, 1–48 (1963).
10. M. M. Taylor and C. D. Creelman, PEST: Efficient estimates on probability functions, *J. Acoust. Soc. Amer. 41*, 782–787 (1967).
11. M. M. Taylor, S. M. Forbes, and C. D. Creelman, PEST reduces bias in forced choice psychophysics, *J. Acoust. Soc. Am. 74*, 1367–1374 (1983).
12. R. A. Campbell, Detection of a noise signal of varying duration, *J. Acoust. Soc. Amer. 35*, 1732–1737 (1962).
13. R. A. Campbell and S. A. Counter, Temporal energy integration and periodicity pitch, *J. Acoust. Soc. Amer. 45*, 691–693 (1969).
14. C. D. Creelman and M. M. Taylor, Some pitfalls in adaptive testing: Comments on "Temporal integration and periodicity pitch." *J. Acoust. Soc. Amer. 46*, 1581–1582 (1969).
15. H. Levitt and L. R. Rabiner, Use of a sequential strategy in intelligibility testing, *J. Acoust. Soc. Amer. 42*, 609–612 (1967).
16. W. Jesteadt, An adaptive procedure for subjective judgments, *Percept. Psychophys. 28*, 85–88 (1980).
17. D. L. Bode and R. Carhart, Stability and accuracy of adaptive tests of speech discrimination, *J. Acoust. Soc. Amer. 56*, 963–970 (1974).
18. R. Plomp and A. M. Mimpen, Speech-reception threshold for sentences as a function of age and noise, *J. Acoust. Soc. Am. 66*, 1333–1342 (1979).

19. A. J. Duquesnoy, Effect of a single interfering noise or speech sound upon the binaural sentence intelligibility of aged persons, *J. Acoust. Soc. Am. 74*, 739–743. (1983).

20. J. R. Dubno, D. D. Dirks, and D. E. Morgan, Effects of age and mild hearing loss on speech recognition in noise, *J. Acoust. Soc. Am. 76*, 87–96 (1984).

21. S. A. Gelfand, L. Ross, and S. Miller, Sentence reception in noise from one versus two sources: Effects of aging and hearing loss, *J. Acoust. Soc. Am. 83*, 248–256 (1988).

22. H. Levitt, Testing for sequential dependencies, *J. Acoust. Soc. Amer. 43*, 65–69 (1968).

23. H. Levitt and M. Treisman, Control charts for sequential testing, *Psychometrika 34*, 509–518 (1969).

24. H. Levitt and D. E. Bock, Sequential programmer for psychophysical testing, *J. Acoust. Soc. Amer. 42*, 911–913 (1967).

25. J. M. Findlay, Estimates on probability functions: A more virulent PEST, *Percept. Psychophys. 23*, 181–185 (1978).

26. J. L. Hall, Maximum-likelihood sequential procedure for estimation of psychometric functions, *J. Acoust. Soc. Am. 44*, 370 (1968).

27. J. L. Hall, PEST: Note on the reduction of variance of threshold estimates, *J. Acoust. Soc. Am. 55*, 1090–1091 (1974).

28. J. L. Hall, Hybrid adaptive procedure for estimation of psychometric functions, *J. Acoust. Soc. Am. 69*, 1763–1769 (1981).

29. J. L. Hall, A procedure for detecting variability of psychophysical thresholds, *J. Acoust. Soc. Am. 73*, 663–669 (1983).

30. A. Pentland, Maximum likelihood estimation: The best PEST, *Percept. Psychophys. 28*, 377–379 (1980).

31. A. B. Watson, and D. P. Pelli, QUEST: A Bayesian adaptive psychometric method, *Percept. Psychophys. 33*, 113–120 (1983).

32. P. L. Emmerson, Observations on a maximum likelihood method of sequential threshold estimation and a simplified approximation, *Percept. Psychophys. 36*, 199–203 (1984).

33. W. A. Simpson, The step method: A new adaptive psychophysical procedure, *Percept. Psychophys. 45*, 572–576 (1989).

34. W. A. Simpson, The method of constant stimuli is efficient, *Percept. Psychophys. 44*, 433–436 (1988).

35. B. R. Shelton, M. C. Picardi, and D. M. Green, Comparison of three adaptive psychophysical procedures, *J. Acoust. Soc. Am. 71*, 1527–1532 (1983).

36. B. R. Shelton and I. Scarrow, Two-alternative versus three-alternative procedures for threshold estimation, *Percept. Psychophys. 35*, 385–392 (1984).

37. A. Hesse, Comparison of several psychophysical procedures with respect to threshold estimates, reproducibility, and efficiency, *Acoustica 59*, 263–266 (1986).

38. L. Marshall and W. Jesteadt, Comparison of pure-tone audibility thresholds obtained with audiological and two-interval forced-choice procedures, *J. Speech Hear. Res. 29*, 82–91 (1986).

39. R. Madigan and D. Williams, Maximum-likelihood procedures in two-alternative forced-choice: evaluation and recommendations, *Percept. Psychophys. 42,* 240–249 (1987).

40. B. Kollmeier, R. H. Gilkey, and U. K. Sieben, Adaptive staircase techniques in psychoacoustics: A comparison of human data and a mathematical model, *J. Acoust. Soc. Am. 83,* 1852–1862 (1988).

41. S. S. Stevens, Mathematics, measurement, and psychophysics, in *Handbook of Experimental Psychology* (S. S. Stevens, ed.), Wiley, New York, 1951.

42. S. S. Stevens, Problems and methods in psychophysics, *Psych. Bull. 55,* 177–196 (1958).

43. S. S. Stevens, The psychophysics of sensory function, in *Sensory Communication* (W. A. Rosenblith, ed.), MIT Press, Cambridge, Mass., 1961.

44. S. S. Stevens, *Psychophysics,* Wiley, New York, 1975.

45. C. H. Coomb, Theory and methods of measurement, in *Research Methods in the Behaviorial Sciences* (L. Festinger and D. Katz, eds.), Holt, Rinehart, and Winston, New York, 1953, pp. 471–535.

46. R. P. Abelson and J. W. Tukey. Efficient conversion of non-metric information into metric information, in *The Quantitative Analysis of Social Problems* (E. R. Tufte, ed.), Addison Wesley, Reading, Massachusetts, 1959, pp. 407–417.

47. S. S. Stevens, Ratio scales, partition scales and confusion scales, in *Psychological Scaling: Theory and Applications* (H. Gulliksen and S. Messick, eds.), Wiley, New York, 1960.

48. S. S. Stevens, A scale for the measurement of a psychological magnitude: Loudness, *Psych. Rev. 43,* 405–416 (1936).

49. S. S. Stevens, J. Volkmann, and E. B. Newman, A scale for the measurement of the psychological magnitude pitch, *J. Acoust Soc. Amer. 8,* 185–190 (1937).

50. S. S. Stevens and J. Volkmann, The relation of pitch to frequency: A revised scale, *Amer. J. Psych. 53,* 329–353 (1940).

51. S. S. Stevens, The direct estimation of sensory magnitudes—loudness, *Amer. J. Psych. 69,* 1–25 (1956).

52. R. P. Hellman, and J. J. Zwislocki, Some factors affecting the estimation of loudness, *J. Acoust. Soc. Am. 33,* 687–694 (1961).

53. R. P. Hellman and J. Zwislocki, Monaural loudness function of a 1,000-cps tone and interaural summation, *J. Acoust. Soc. Amer. 35,* 856–865 (1963).

54. R. P. Hellman and J. Zwislocki, Loudness summation at low sound frequencies, *J. Acoust. Soc. Amer. 43,* 60–63 (1968).

55. R. P. Hellman, Growth of loudness at 1000 and 3000 Hz, *J. Acoust. Soc. Am. 60,* 672–679 (1976).

56. J. J. Zwislocki and D. A. Goodman, Absolute scaling of sensory magnitudes: A validation, *Percept. Psychophys. 28,* 28–38 (1980).

57. R. P. Hellman, Stability of individual loudness functions obtained by magnitude estimation and production, *Percept. Psychophys. 29,* 63–78 (1981).

58. J. J. Zwislocki, Group and individual relations between sensation magnitudes and their numerical estimates, *Percept. Psychophys. 33,* 460–468 (1983a).

59. R. P. Hellman and C. H. Meiselman, Prediction of individual loudness exponents from cross-modality matching, *J. Speech Hear. Res. 31*, 605–615 (1988).
60. B. A. Mellers, Evidence against "absolute" scaling, *Percept. Psychophys. 33*, 523–526 (1983a).
61. B. A. Mellers, Reply to Zwislocki's views on "absolute" scaling, *Percept. Psychophys. 34*, 405–408 (1983b).
62. J. J. Zwislocki, Absolute and other scales: The question of validity views on "absolute" scaling, *Percept. Psychophys. 33*, 593–594 (1983b).
63. S. S. Stevens and M. Guirao, Subjective scaling of length and area and the matching of length to loudness and brightness, *J. Exp. Psychol. 66*, 177–186 (1963).
64. J. C. Stevens and L. M. Marks, Cross-modality matching of brightness and loudness, *Proc. Nat. Acad. Sci. 54*, 407–411 (1965).
65. J. C. Stevens and L. M. Marks, Cross-modality matching functions generated by magnitude estimation, *Precept. Psychophys. 27*, 379–389 (1980).

8
Theory of Signal Detection

The previous chapter addressed itself to classical and modern psycho-physical methods and the direct rating of sensory magnitudes, with respect to hearing. It left essentially unresolved, however, the problem of how to effectively separate sensitivity from response proclivity. In this chapter, we shall approach this problem from the standpoint of the theory of signal detection.

FACTORS AFFECTING RESPONSES

The theory of signal detection [1–3] provides the best approach to separating the effects of sensitivity from those of response bias. We might think of the theory of signal detection (TSD) as asking "what led to a 'yes' (or 'no') decision?" as opposed to "what did the subject hear (or not hear)?"

Suppose a subject is asked to say "yes" when he hears a tone during a test trial and "no" when a tone is not heard. A large number of trials are used for each of several stimulus levels, and half of those at each level are "catch trials" during which signals are not actually presented. There are thus four possible outcomes for each test trial. Two of these are correct:

The signal is present and the subject says "yes" (a hit).
The signal is absent and the subject says "no" (a correct rejection).

The other two alternatives are wrong:

The signal is present but the subject says "no" (a miss).
The signal is absent but the subject says "yes" (a false alarm).

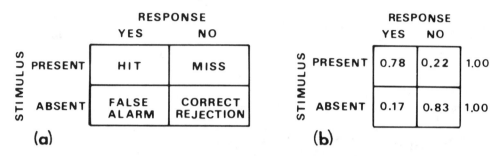

Figure 8.1   (a) Stimulus-response table showing the four possible outcomes for any given trial. Correct responses may be "hits" or "correct rejections," whereas errors may also be of two types, "misses" or "false alarms." (b) Hypothetical results (in proportions) for 100 trials actually containing stimuli and 100 catch trials under a particular test condition.

A convenient way to show these possible outcomes is in the form of a stimulus-response matrix (Fig. 8.1).

The stimulus-response table is generally used to summarize the results of all trials at a particular test level; there would thus be such a table for each stimulus level used in an experiment. For example, Fig. 8.1b shows the results of 100 trials containing a signal and 100 catch trials. The subject responded to 78 of the signal trials (so that the probability of a hit was 0.78), did not respond to 22 signals (the probability of a miss is 0.22), said "yes" for 17 out of 100 catch trials (the probability of a false alarm is 0.17), and said "no" for the remaining absent-stimulus trials (the probability of a correct rejection is 0.83). One is tempted to say that the percent correct at this stimulus level is 78% (the hit rate), but the fact that the subject also responded 17 times when there was no stimulus present tells us that even the 78% correct includes some degree of chance success or guessing. One way to account for this error is to use the proportion of false alarms as an estimate of the overall guessing rate, and to correct the hit rate accordingly. The traditional formula to correct the hit rate for chance success is

$$p(hit)_{corrected} = \frac{p(hit) - p(false\ alarm)}{1 - p(false\ alarm)}$$

In other words, the probability p of a hit corrected for chance success is obtained by dividing the difference between the hit rate and the false alarm rate by one* minus the false alarm rate. Thus, for this example

---

*Recall that the total probability of all catch trials is 1.0, so that $1 - p$ (false alarm) is the same as the probability of a correct rejection.

$$p(hit)_{corrected} = \frac{0.78 - 0.17}{1.0 - 0.17} = \frac{0.61}{0.83} = 0.735$$

The original 78% correct thus falls to 73.5% when we account for the proportion of the "yes" responses due to chance.

Correcting for chance success is surely an improvement over approaches that do not account for guessing, but it still does not really separate the effects of auditory factors (sensitivity) and nonauditory factors. In essence, this process highlights the importance of nonauditory factors in determining the response, because the very fact that the subject said "yes" to catch trials and "no" to stimulus trials indicates that his *decision* to respond was affected by more than just sensitivity to the stimulus. The TSD is concerned with the factors that enter into this decision.

Let us, at least for the moment, drop the assumption that there is some clear-cut threshold that separates audibility from inaudibility, and replace it with the following assumptions of TSD. First, assume that there is always some degree of noise present. This may be noise in the environment, instrumentation noise, or noise due to the subject's moving around and fidgeting. Even if all of these noises were miraculously removed, there would still remain the subject's unavoidable physiological noises (heartbeat, pulse, breathing, blood rushing through vessels, stomach gurgles, etc.). Indeed, the noise is itself often presented as part of the experiments. For example, the task may be to detect a tone in the presence of a noise. Since there is always noise, which is by nature random, we also assume that the stimulation of the auditory system varies continuously. Finally, we shall assume that all of the stimulation occurs (or is at least measurable) along a single continuum. In other words, the subject must decide whether the stimulation in the auditory system (e.g. energy) is due to noise alone (N) or to signal-plus-noise (SN). This process may be represented by distributions of a "decision axis" like the one in Fig. 8.2. Here the abscissa may be conceived of as representing the energy contained in the noise and in the noise plus signal. The x-axis may also be conceived of as representing the magnitude of sensory activation resulting from such stimulation. The ordinate denotes the probability of an event occurring. Hence, the N distribution shows the probability of occurrence of a noise alone as a function of x; and the SN curve shows the chances of a noise-plus-signal as a function of x. The convention is to use the term "probability density" (as opposed to "probability") for the y-axis in order to reflect the fact that values of x change continuously rather than in discrete steps. The subject's response is a decision between "yes" ("I hear the signal as well as the noise") and "no" ("I hear the noise alone").

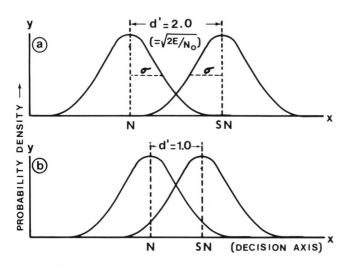

Figure 8.2   Separation between the noise alone (N) and signal-plus-noise (SN) distributions determines the value of d'.

The N and SN distributions in Fig. 8.2 show the probability functions of noise alone (N) and signal-plus-noise (SN). We might think of these curves as showing the chances (or likelihood) of there being respectively a noise alone or a signal-plus-noise during a particular test trial. Obviously, there must always be more energy in SN than in N, due to the presence of the signal. The separation between the N and SN curves thus becomes a measure of sensitivity. This is an unbiased measure because the separation between the two curves is not affected by the subject's criteria for responding (biases). The separation is determined solely by the energy in the signals and the sensitivity of the auditory system. This separation is measured in terms of a parameter d'. The value of d' is equal to the difference between the means ($\bar{X}$) of the N and SN distributions divided by their standard deviation σ*

---

*It is assumed that SN and N are normally distributed with equal variances. Since σ is the square root of the variance, and the variances of SN and N are assumed to be equal, then only one value of σ need be shown. The value of d' is equal to the square root of twice the energy in the signal (2E) divided by the noise power (N_0) in a band that is one cycle wide [5], or: $d' = (2E / N_0)^{1/2}$. Tables of d' are available in the literature [6]. However, since the standard deviation of SN is actually larger than that of N in some cases, a corrected value of d' may be a more valid measure [7].

Theory of Signal Detection 317

$$? \quad d' = \frac{\bar{X}_{SN} - \bar{X}_N}{\sigma}$$

Comparing Figs. 8.2a and b, we see that the greater the separation between N and SN distributions, the larger the value of d'. This value does not change even when different experimental methods are used [4].

How, then does a subject decide whether to say "yes" or "no" for a given separation between the N and SN curves? Consider the N and SN distributions in Fig. 8.3. A vertical line has been drawn through the overlapping N and SN distribution in each frame of this figure. This line represents the subject's *criterion* for responding. Whenever the energy is greater than that corresponding to the criterion the subject will say "yes." This occurs to the right of the criterion along the x-axis. On the other hand, the subject will say "no" if the energy is less than (to the left of) the criterion value. The value (or placement) of this criterion depends on several factors which we will examine next.

The first factor affecting the criterion may be expressed by the question "what is the probability that there is a noise alone compared to the probability that there is a signal-plus-noise for a given value of x?" For any point along the decision axis, this question is the same as comparing the height of the N curve with the height of the SN curve (Fig. 8.3). Otherwise stated, this value is the ratio of the likelihoods that the observation is from the N versus SN distributions for the two overlapping curves at any value of x. The ratio of these two probabilities is called beta (β). The value of the criterion is affected by the amount of overlap

$$\beta = \frac{|N|_{x=a}}{|SN|_{x=a}}$$

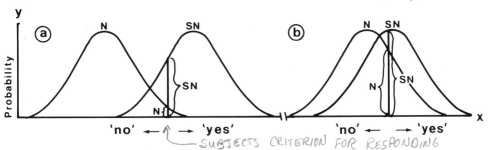

Figure 8.3   Criterion points (shown by vertical lines) for two degrees of overlapping of the N and SN distributions. The probabilities corresponding to the SN and N distributions at the criterion point are highlighted by brackets. Values of x below (to the left of) the criterion result in "no" decisions and those greater than (to the right of) the criterion yield "yes" decisions.

between the N and SN distributions, and by what the subject knows about the relative chances of a signal actually being presented.

Comparison of Figs. 8.3a and 8.3b shows how overlapping of the N and SN functions affects this ratio. At any point, the heights of the two curves becomes close as the separation between them decreases from that in Fig. 8.3a to that in Fig. 8.3b. An "ideal observer" (which is) actually a mathematical concept rather than a real subject) would place the criterion point at the ratio which minimizes the chances of error; that is, at the point at which misses and false alarms are minimized. However, the placement of the criterion point will also be adjusted somewhat by what the subject knows about the chances of occurrence of a noise alone versus a signal-plus noise. Let us now address ourselves to this factor.

Up to this point, it has been assumed that N and SN will be presented on a fifty-fifty basis. However, if the subject knows that a signal will actually be presented one-third of the time, then he will of course adjust his criterion β accordingly. In other words, he will adopt a stricter criterion. Alternatively, if the subject knows that a signal will occur more often than the noise alone, then he will relax his criterion for responding, adjusting for the greater chances of the signal actually being presented. An "ideal observer" always knows these probabilities; a real subject is often, but not always, told what they are.

The last factor that we will discuss which affects the final value of the criterion β has to do with how much a correct response is worth and how much a wrong response will cost. We are therefore concerned with the chance of an error associated with a particular criterion for responding. These chances are shown in Fig. 8.4. The subject will say "no" whenever the actual presentation falls to the left of the criterion, and will say "yes" when the presentation is to the right of the criterion. As a result of the fact that the N and SN distributions are overlapping, it turns out that there will be both "yes" and "no" decisions for a certain proportion of *both* signal and no-signal presentation. With the criterion placed as shown in the figure, most of the "yes" decisions will be in response to actual SN presentations; i.e., the subject will say "yes" when there actually was a signal present. Recall that such a correct identification of the presence of the signal is called a "hit." On the other hand, a certain percentage of the N trials will fall to the right of the criterion, so that the subject will say "yes" even though there was actually no signal presented. This incorrect decision that a signal was present even though it really was not there is a "false alarm." A stimulus-response table similar to the one in Fig. 8.1a is shown next to the N and SN distributions in Fig.

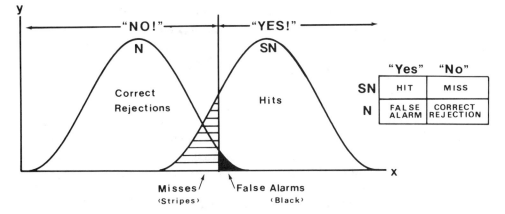

Figure 8.4   The four possible outcomes of a "yes" or "no" response based upon a given criterion value (vertical line). The corresponding stimulus-response table is shown to the right.

8.4 to illustrate how the two curves and the criterion relate to the possible outcomes of an experiment.

Now, suppose that a subject is told that it is imperative that he never miss a signal. He would thus move the criterion point toward the left to increase the hit rate; however, this shift would also have the effect of increasing the number of false alarms. The result would occur because moving the criterion toward the left increases the proportions of *both* the N and SN curves that fall inside of the "yes" region. On the other hand, suppose that the subject is advised that a false alarm is the worst possible error. Under such circumstances, the criterion point would be shifted toward the right, minimizing false alarms. Of course, this shift would also increase the number of misses, because a larger portion of the SN curve would now be in the "no" region.

Instead of telling the subject that one or another type of response is more (or less) important, the subject might be given a nickel for each correct response, lose three cents for a false alarm, etc. This, too, would cause the subject to adjust the criterion point so as to maximize the payoff associated with his responses. In effect, then, a set of values are attached to the responses so that each correct response has a *value* and each erroneous response has a *cost*.

An optimum criterion point (optimum β) is based upon the probabilities of noise alone (p_N) and of signal-plus-noise (p_{SN}), combined with the payoff resulting from the costs and values of each response. The payoff

$\beta \equiv$ OPTIMUM CRITERION POINT

$P_N \equiv$ PROBABILITY OF NOISE ALONE

$P_{SN} \equiv$ PROBABILITY OF SIGNAL-PLUS-NOISE

$V_H \equiv$ VALUES OF HITS
$V_{CR} \equiv$ VALUES OF CORRECT REJECTIONS
$C_M \equiv$ COSTS OF MISSES
$C_{FA} \equiv$ COSTS OF FALSE ALARMS

is the net result of the values of hits (V_H) and correct rejections (V_{CR}) and of the costs of misses (C_M) and false alarms (C_{FA}). In other words

$$\text{optimum } \beta = \left(\frac{p_N}{p_{SN}} \right) \left(\frac{V_{CR} - C_{FA}}{V_H - C_M} \right)$$

The decision criterion is an attempt to maximize the payoff associated with the task. However, the subject in the real world is either not aware of all factors, or not able to use them as efficiently as the mathematically ideal observer. Therefore, the actual performance observed in an experiment generally falls short of what would have resulted had the subject been an ideal observer.

In summary, two types of information are obtained from the subject's responses in a TSD paradigm. One of these, d', is a measure of sensitivity which is determined strictly by the separation between the N and SN distributions and by the ability of the auditory system to make use of this separation. The other measure is the subject's criterion for responding, which does not affect the actual measure of sensitivity.

How can we show all of this information at the same time in a meaningful manner? Consider the effects of several different response criteria for the same value of d'. These criteria may be obtained by changing the directions given to the subject, or by changing the payoff scheme. Another way would be to have the subject rank the degree of certainty with which he makes each yes/no decision (see the discussion of TSD methods, below, for the rationale of this approach).

For a given amount of sensitivity (i.e., a given value of d'), different criteria will result in different proportions of hits and false alarms. This result is shown for two arbitrarily selected values of d' in Fig. 8.5. We may plot the proportions of hits versus false alarms for each criterion point, as in the center of Fig. 8.5. Such a graph is called a receiver-operating characteristic (ROC) curve. Notice that the ROC curve allows both the effects of sensitivity and response criterion to be illustrated at the same time. Sensitivity is shown by the distance of the ROC curve from the diagonal (at which d' = 0), or by the area under the ROC curve. On the other hand, the response criterion is indicated by the particular point along the ROC curve. Specifically, points a, b, and c in the figure (where d' = 2) differ in terms of sensitivity from points d, e, and f (for which d' = 1). However, even though points a, b, and c are the same in terms of sensitivity (d' = 2), they differ from each other in terms of response criteria. (A similar relationship exists among points d, e and f, where d' = 1.)

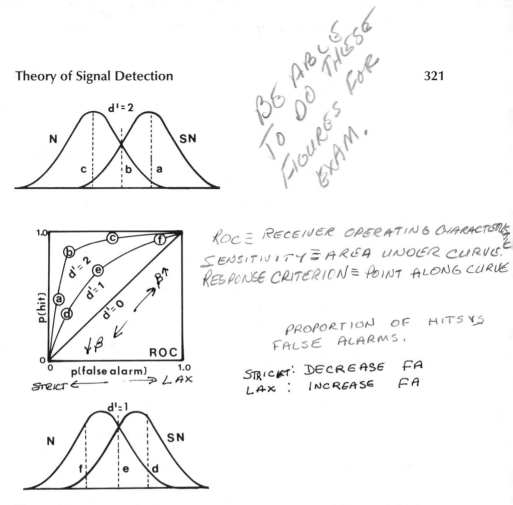

Handwritten annotations:

BE ABLE TO DO THESE FIGURES FOR EXAM.

ROC ≡ RECEIVER OPERATING CHARACTERISTIC
SENSITIVITY ≡ AREA UNDER CURVE.
RESPONSE CRITERION ≡ POINT ALONG CURVE

PROPORTION OF HITS VS FALSE ALARMS.

STRICT: DECREASE FA
LAX : INCREASE FA

Figure 8.5 Relationship between ROC curves (center) and the N and SN distributions for two values of d' (d' = 2, upper curves; d' = 1, lower curves) and various response criteria (letters a,b,c; d,e,f). Sensitivity is shown by the distance of the ROC curve from the diagonal (center). Different response criteria correspond to various points along the ROC curve (indicated by the letters).

PSYCHOPHYSICAL METHODS IN TSD

Yes/No Methods

This discussion of the theory of signal detection has dealt primarily with the yes/no method. To recapitulate: The subject is presented with a large number of trials for each stimulus level, and a large proportion of these are actually catch trials. For each trial the subject says "yes" when a signal is detected and "no" when a signal is not detected. Fundamentally, then, the yes/no method in TSD is somewhat akin to the classical method of constant stimuli, although there are obvious differences in the number of trials, the large proportion of catch trials, and the manner of data analysis.

As in the classical methods, the TSD experiment is easily modified for use in a study of differential sensitivity. In this case, two signals are presented in a trial and the subject's task is to say "yes" ("they are different") or "no" ("they are not different").

The yes/no method is actually a subcategory of a larger class of experiments in which each trial contains one of two alternative signals. In this general case, the subject's task is to indicate which of two possible signals was present during the trial. For example, in the differential sensitivity experiment mentioned in the last paragraph, the decisions "same" versus "different"; or else the subject might be asked to decide between two alternative speech sounds (e.g. /p/ and /b/) while some parameter is varied. In this light the yes/no method might be thought of as a single-interval forced-choice experiment. In other words, the subject is presented with a stimulus interval during each trial, and is required to choose between signal-plus-noise (one of the alternatives) and noise alone (the other alternative).

Two- (and Multiple-) Interval Forced-Choice Methods

Just as the subject may be asked to choose between two alternatives in a single-interval trial, he might also be asked to decide *which* of two successive intervals contained a signal. In this case, the trial consists of two intervals, A and B, which are presented one after the other. One of the intervals (SN) contains the signal and the other (N) does not. The subject must indicate whether the signal as presented in interval A or in interval B.

In multiple-interval forced-choice experiments, several (e.g. four) intervals are included in each trial, among which the subject must choose the one that contained the signal.

Confidence Rating Methods

Recall that various points along the same ROC curve represent different response criteria with the same sensitivity d'. We might think of the response criterion as a reflection of how much confidence a subject has in his decision. In other words, a strict criterion means that the subject must have a great deal of confidence in his decision that the signal is present before he is willing to say "yes." In this case the criterion value β is pushed toward the right along the decision axis. Alternatively, a lax criterion means that the subject does not require as much confidence in his "yes" decision, which moves the criterion point toward the left.

We might apply this relationship between the confidence in the decision and the criterion point by asking the subject to rate how much confidence he has in each of his responses. For example, the subject might be instructed to rate a "yes" response as "five" when he is absolutely positive that there was a signal, and "four" when he thinks there was a signal. A rating of "three" would mean "I'm not sure whether there was a signal or no signal." "Two" would indicate that there probably was no signal present, and a rating of "one" would suggest that the subject is positive that a signal was not presented. This procedure is the same as adopting a series of criterion points located successively from right to left along the decision axis. Thus, the use of confidence ratings enables the experimenter to obtain several points along the ROC curve simultaneously. This approach results in data which are comparable to those obtained by the previously discussed direct methods [8].

IMPLICATIONS OF TSD

The theory of signal detection has importance in psychoacoustics because its application allows the experimenter to ferret out the effects of sensitivity and response criterion. Furthermore, TSD lends itself to experimental confirmation, and can be used to test theories and their underlying assumptions. A key application of TSD has been the testing of the classical concept of threshold as an absolute boundary separating sensation from no sensation. It is implicit in this discussion that such a concept of a clear-cut threshold is not supported by TSD. However, the more general concept of threshold remains unresolved. Threshold theory is beyond the scope of this text. The student is therefore referred to the very informative discussions in papers by Swets [9] and Krantz [10].

REFERENCES

1. J. A. Swets, Ed., *Signal Detection and Recognition by Human Observers*, Wiley, New York, 1964.
2. D. M. Green and J. A. Swets, *Signal Detection Theory and Psychophysics*, Krieger, New York, 1974.
3. J. P. Egan, *Signal Detection Theory and ROC Analysis*, Academic Press, New York, 1975.
4. J. A. Swets, Indices of signal detectability obtained with various psychophysical procedures, *J. Acoust. Soc. Amer. 31*, 511–513 (1959).
5. J. A. Swets, W. P. Tanner, Jr., and T. G. Birdsall, Decision processes in perception, *Psych. Rev. 68*, 301–340 (1961).

6. P. B. Elliot, Tables of d′, in *Signal Detection and Recognition by Human Observers* (J. A. Swets, ed.), Wiley, New York, 1964, pp. 651–684.

7. L. H. Theodore, A neglected parameter: Some comments on "A table for calculation of d′ and β," *Psych. Bull. 78,* 260–261 (1972).

8. J. P. Egan, A. I. Schulman, and G. Z. Greenberg, Operating characteristics determined by binary decisions and by ratings, *J. Acoust. Soc. Amer. 31,* 768–773 (1959).

9. J. A. Swets, Is there a sensory threshold? *Science 134,* 168–177 (1961).

10. D. H. Krantz, Threshold theories of signal detection, *Psych, Rev. 76,* 308–324 (1969).

9

Auditory Sensitivity

The ear's extremely wide range of sensitivity is one of the most striking aspects of audition. The preceding chapters emphasized that hearing measurements are affected by psychophysical methods and other non-auditory factors; nevertheless, a reliable picture of auditory sensitivity has been provided by research over the years. Briefly, the ear is sensitive to a range of intensities from about 0 dB SPL (which is an amplitude of vibration of about the size of a hydrogen molecule) to roughly 140 dB (at which pain and damage to the auditory mechanism ensue). This dynamic range of the approximately 140 dB corresponds to a pressure ratio of $10^7:1$. In other words, the most intense sound pressure that is bearable is on the order of 10 million times as great as the softest one that is perceivable under optimum listening conditions. In terms of frequency, humans can hear tones as low as 2 Hz (although roughly 20 Hz is required for a perception of "tonality") and as high as about 20,000 Hz. Even the most avid hi-fi/stereo enthusiast must be impressed by the range over which the ear is responsive. Furthermore, the auditory system is capable of resolving remarkably small temporal differences.

The frequency and intensity sensitivities of the ear interact, affecting each other to a greater or lesser degree. In addition, when the duration of a sound is less than about half of a second, it affects both frequency and intensity sensitivity. Longer durations may be thought of as being infinitely long as far as auditory sensitivity is concerned.

Finally, the ear is able to discriminate small differences in a wide range of stimuli, i.e., it has remarkable differential sensitivity—the ability to detect very small differences between similar sounds. This ability applies to all three parameters: intensity, frequency, and time.

So much for sweeping generalizations. Let us now look at the details.

ABSOLUTE SENSITIVITY

Minimum Audible Levels

The problem of absolute sensitivity is essentially one of describing how much sound intensity is necessary for a typical, normally hearing person to just detect the presence of a stimulus. We must realize at the outset that these values are actually measures of central tendencies (means, medians, and/or modes) which describe a group of ostensibly normal subjects. In addition, it is essential to know how and where the minimum audible sound intensity is measured.

Two fundamental methods have been used to measure the intensity of a minimum audible stimulus [1]. The first involves testing a subject's thresholds through earphones, and then actually monitoring the sound pressures in the ear canal (between the earphone and eardrum) that correspond to these thresholds. This procedure yields a measure of minimum audible *pressure* (MAP). The alternative approach is to seat the subject in a sound field and test his thresholds for sounds presented through a loudspeaker. The subject then leaves the sound field and the threshold intensity is measured with a microphone placed where his head had been. This method measures the minimum audible *field* (MAF). It is important to dichotomize between the MAP and MAF methods, because they result in different threshold values. This discrepancy has been one of the most elusive problems in psychoacoustics.

Ostensibly, MAP refers to the sound pressure at the eardrum. This quantity is monitored by placing a probe tube in the subject's ear canal. The probe tube passes through the earphone enclosure and leads to a microphone, which measures the sound pressure at the tip of the probe tube. Since it is difficult to place the probe right at the drum (as well as potentially painful and dangerous), the probe is generally located somewhere in the ear canal, as close to the drum as is practicable.

Minimum audible pressures are often stated in terms of the sound pressure generated by an earphone in a standardized 6 cc metal cavity (coupler), which approximates the volume under an earphone on the subject's ear. Such coupler pressures form the reference levels used in audiometric standards (see below). Coupler-referred MAP values are more appropriately called MAPC to distinguish them from the probe tube MAP data obtained from actual ear canals [2].

Sivian and White [1] reviewed the minimum audibility data available as of 1933, and reported the results of their own classic MAP and MAF experiments. Their work was essentially confirmed by Dadson and King [3] and by Robinson and Dadson [4], whose data are shown in the lower portion of Fig. 9.1. These curves show monaural MAP and binaural MAF (from a loudspeaker located directly in front of the subject, i.e., at 0° azimuth) as a function of frequency. Monaural MAP values extending to very low frequencies are also shown. The MAP values for frequencies between 10,000 and 18,000 Hz are shown in the figure on an expanded frequency scale. As these MAP and MAF curves clearly show, human hearing is most sensitive between about 2000 and 5000 Hz, and reasonably good sensitivity is maintained in the 100 Hz–10 kHz range. Absolute sensitivity becomes poorer above and below these frequencies.

While the general relationship between auditory sensitivity and frequency is well established, one should be aware that more recent experi-

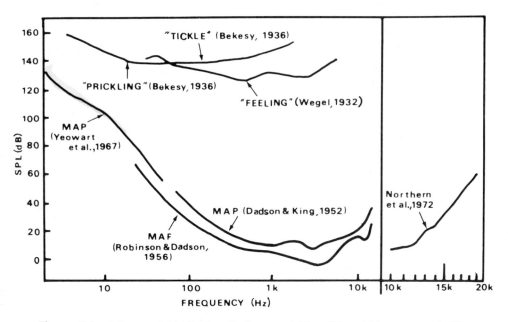

Figure 9.1 Monaural MAP after Dadson and King [3] and Yeowart et al. [5]. High frequency MAP after Northern et al. [6] is shown on the expanded scale to the right for clarity. Upper limits of "usable" hearing after Bekesy [7] and Wegel [8].

ments have provided detailed estimates of absolute sensitivity in the lower and upper frequency ranges. For example, one should refer to Berger [9] for a detailed analysis of hearing sensitivity in the low frequency range (50–1000 Hz), and to Schechter et al. [10] for a detailed analysis of thresholds for the high frequencies (8000–20,000 Hz).

An intriguing phenomenon, demonstrated in Fig. 9.1, is that the MAF curve falls consistently below the MAP curve. In other words, a lower intensity is needed to reach threshold in a sound field (MAF) than under earphones (MAP). This fact was first demonstrated by Sivian and White [1]; and the discrepancy of 6–10 dB is called the "missing 6dB" [11]. Sivian and White proposed that the MAP/MAF discrepancy might be due to physiological noises picked up by the ear when it is covered by an earphone. These physiological noises would partially mask (see Chap. 10) the signal presented by the earphone, so that more sound pressure would be needed to achieve MAP than for the unmasked MAF. While this explanation accounts for part of the missing 6 dB problem, it falls short of accounting for the whole difference.

Several more recent studies have formed the basis for resolving the MAP/MAF difference [2,12–18]. This explanation has been presented in a cohesive manner by Killion [2]. To begin with, recall from Chap. 3 that diffraction and ear canal resonance enhance the pressure of a free field signal reaching the eardrum [19]. Thus, a corrected version of the international standard reference MAF curve* [20] may be converted to eardrum pressure by applying Shaw's [19] free field/eardrum pressure data. Since binaural thresholds are somewhat better than monaural ones (see Chap. 13), a correction is also made to account for the advantage of binaural MAF over monaural MAP. By accounting for differences between real-ear (MAP) and coupler (MAPC) values, the effects of impedance changes and ear canal distortion due to the placement of the earphone, and the effects of physiological noises, the MAP/MAF discrepancy is essentially resolved.

Threshold Microstructure

The MAP and MAF curves in Fig. 9.1 are drawn as smooth curves. It is commonly (and generally implicitly) assumed that an individual's threshold curve is similarly represented by a smooth line. The ubiquitous nature of this assumption is revealed by the fact that both clinicians and researchers make most of their threshold measurements at frequencies that are an

---

*The correction accounts for an apparent error in the low-frequency MAF levels [2].

octave apart, and very rarely sample at intervals that are less than a half-octave wide. However, a number of studies have shown that this may not be the case [21–25]. Instead, a rippled or jagged configuration is often obtained when thresholds are sampled at numerous frequencies that are measured at very close intervals. Moreover, these patterns are highly repeatable. These irregularities in the threshold microstructure are associated with (particularly spontaneous) otoacoustic emissions, and it is believed that they reflect active processes in the cochlea [24–28]. Discussions of active cochlear processes and otoacoustic emissions may be found in Chap. 4.

Upper Limits of Hearing *IS IT A FUNCTION OF FREQUENCY?*

Just as we may conceive of the minimum audibility (MAP and MAF) curves as the lower limit of hearing sensitivity, the upper limits of hearing may be thought of as the sound pressure levels (SPLs) which result in discomfort. These levels are also referred to as the threshold of feeling, tickle, touch, tolerance, or pain. In general, these sensations occur at SPLs of about 120 dB or more, depending upon the laboratory and how the sensation is defined (discomfort, pain, etc.). However, this is not to imply that a pain threshold of about 140 dB SPL must be reached in order to define a subject's tolerance for intense sounds. Uncomfortable loudness has been associated with SPLs of more than 100 dB [29–31]; and Silverman et al. [32] reported discomfort to occur at about 120 dB SPL.

Standard Zero Reference Levels

One might now ask what constitutes a reasonable conception of normal hearing sensitivity for the population as a whole. That is, how much SPL does the average person who is apparently free of pathology need to detect a particular sound? The answer permits standardization of audiometric instruments so that we may quantify hearing loss relative to "what most people can hear."

Prior to 1964 several countries had their own standards for normal hearing and audiometer calibration based upon locally obtained data. For example, the 1954 British Standard [33] was based upon one group of studies [3,34], whereas the 1951 American Standard [35] reflected other findings [36,37]. Unfortunately, these standards differed by about 10 dB; and the American Standard was actually too lax at 250 and 500 Hz, and too strict at 4000 Hz [38]. This situation was rectified in 1964 with the issuance of Recommendation R389 by the International Organization for Standardization (ISO) [39]. This standard is generally referred to as ISO-

1964. It was based upon a round-robin of loudness-balance and threshold experiments involving American, British, French, Russian, and West German laboratories, and as a result equivalent reference SPLs were obtained for the earphones used by each country [40].

Table 9.1 shows these SPLs for the Western Electric (WE) 705A earphones used in the ISO study. These reference levels were subsequently incorporated into the American National Standards Institute (ANSI) S3.6-1969 *American National Standard Specifications for Audiometers* [41]. Also shown in Table 9.1 are the equivalent zero reference levels for the Telephonics TDH-39 earphone [41], which is more commonly used in clinical audiometers. These are MAPC values since they represent the equivalent SPLs, measured in a 6 cc coupler, that correspond to normal threshold levels. Reference values are also available for receivers which are inserted into the ear canal, such as the Etymotic Research ER-3A insert earphones [42].

Hearing Level

Because each of the SPLs in Table 9.1 corresponds to minimum audibility, we may think of them as all representing the same *hearing level.* Thus, each zero reference SPL may also be referred to as 0 dB hearing level (0 dB HL) for its respective frequency. For example, the zero reference level for a 1000 Hz tone (TDH-39 earphones) is 7 dB SPL, so that 0 dB HL corresponds to 7 dB SPL at 1000 Hz. At 250 Hz, more sound pressure is required to reach the normal zero reference threshold level,

Table 9.1 Standard Reference Levels for 0 dB HL for WE 705A and TDH-39 Earphones

	Reference level (dB SPL)	
Frequency (Hz)	Western Electric WE 705A	Telephonics TDH-39
125	45.5	45
250	24.5	25.5
500	11	11.5
1000	6.5	7
1500	6.5	6.5
2000	8.5	9
3000	7.5	10
4000	9	9.5
6000	8	15.5
8000	9.5	13

so that 0 dB HL equals 25.5 dB SPL at this frequency. The relationship between SPL and HL is exemplified in Fig. 9.2. Figure 9.2a shows the minimum audible zero reference threshold values in dB SPL as a function of frequency. As in Fig. 9.1, intensity increases upward on the y-axis. Figure 9.2b shows the same information in dB HL. Notice that the minimum audible value (0 dB HL) all lie along a straight line in terms of hearing level. In other words, the HL scale calls each zero reference SPL value "0 dB HL," so that thresholds can be measured in comparison to a straight line rather than a curved one.

The graph in Fig. 9.2b is the conventional audiogram used in clinical audiology. (Actually, the term "audiogram" may legitimately be used to describe any graph of auditory sensitivity as a function of frequency.) By convention, increasing intensity (which indicates a hearing loss) is read downward on the y-axis when thresholds are plotted in dB HL.

Now, suppose that we measure the thresholds of a person whose cochlea has been partially damaged by excessive noise exposure. This kind of trauma often appears as a hearing loss in the higher frequencies. The triangles in Fig. 9.2 show the impaired threshold in terms of both SPL and HL. The difference in dB between the impaired thresholds and the reference values (circles) is the amount of hearing loss at that frequency. For example, our hypothetical patient has a threshold of 5 dB HL at 1000 Hz. This means that he requires 5 dB HL to just detect the tone, as opposed to only 0 dB HL for a normal person. In SPL, this

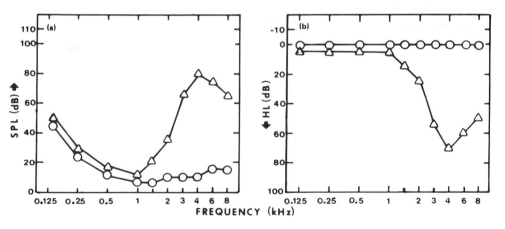

Figure 9.2 Audiograms showing normal hearing (circles) and a hearing loss in the high frequencies (triangles), expressed in (a) dB SPL and (b) dB HL. Note that intensity is shown downward on the clinical audiogram in dB HL.

corresponds to a threshold of 12 dB (i.e., the 7 dB SPL zero reference level for 0 dB HL plus the 5 dB hearing loss. Had the threshold been 40 dB HL, the corresponding value would have been 47 dB SPL. Similarly, the 70 dB HL threshold at 4000 Hz is equivalent to 79.5 dB SPL (70 dB over the 9.5 dB SPL zero reference level). As one might expect, audiometers are calibrated to dB HL values by measuring the output of the earphone in SPL and then converting to HL by subtracting the zero reference in Table 9.1.

Effects of Duration

Thus far we have been considering tones lasting for about a second or more. From the standpoint of audition, such durations may be viewed as infinite. Auditory sensitivity is altered, however, for durations much shorter than a second. Extremely short durations, on the order of 10 msec or less, result in transients that spread energy across the frequency range. These transients will confound the result of an experiment if they are audible [43,44], so that special care is needed in the design and interpretation of studies using short durations.

The perception of tonality appears to change in a somewhat orderly manner as the duration of a very short tone burst is increased [45,46]. A click is heard at the shortest durations, then a click with tonal qualities (click pitch) at slightly longer durations. For frequencies below about 1000 Hz, a tonal pitch is perceived when the duration of the tone burst is long enough for the subject to hear several cycles (periods) of the tone. Thus, the duration threshold for tonality decreases from about 60 msec at 50 Hz to approximately 15 msec at 500 Hz. Above 1000 Hz, the threshold for tonality is essentially constant, and is on the order of about 10 msec.

Absolute sensitivity decreases when the duration of a stimulus becomes much shorter than a second; and the nature of this phenomenon reveals an interesting property of the auditory system. Although the exact results of individual experiments differ, two observations are routinely encountered [47–52]. First, for durations up to roughly 200–300 msec, a tenfold (decade) change in duration can offset an intensity change on the order of about 10 dB. In other words, reducing the duration of a tone burst at threshold from 200 msec to 20 msec (a decade reduction) reduces sensitivity to the degree that the intensity must be increased by 10 dB to reattain threshold. Alternatively, the threshold intensity decreases by about 10 dB when the duration of a tone burst is increased from 20 msec to 200 msec. Second, durations longer than about ⅓ sec are treated by the ear as though they are infinitely long. That is, increasing or decreasing durations which are longer than approximately 300 msec does not change the threshold level. These observations are shown in idealized form in Fig. 9.3a.

The phenomenon under discussion is called temporal integration (or summation). It demonstrates that the ear operates as an energy detector which samples the amount of energy present within a certain time frame (or window). A certain amount of energy is needed within this time window for the threshold to be attached. This energy may be obtained by using a higher intensity for less time or a lower intensity for more time. The ear integrates energy over time *within* an integration time frame of roughly 200 msec. This interval might also be viewed as a period during which energy may be stored, and can be measured as a

[handwritten margin notes:] EAR IS ENERGY DETECTOR

[handwritten margin notes:] ≈ 200 msec

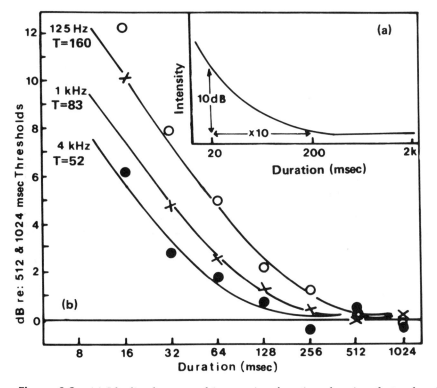

Figure 9.3 (a) Idealized temporal integration function showing that a decade change in duration is offset by an intensity change of about 10 dB up to 200–300 msec. Threshold remains essentially constant at longer durations. (b) Effect of frequency on temporal integration. (Adapted from Watson and Gengel [52], with Permission of *J. Acoust. Soc. Amer.*)

time constant τ [48]. Energy available for longer periods of time is not integrated with the energy inside the time window. This additional energy thus does not contribute to the detection of the sound, so that the threshold does not change durations longer than 200 msec. Photographers might think of this situation as analogous to the interaction of f-stop (intensity) and shutter speed (duration) in summating the light energy for a certain film speed (integration time): The lens opening and shutter speed may be traded against one another as long as the same amount of light is concentrated upon the film.

Figure 9.3b shows the effect of frequency upon temporal integration at threshold. Thresholds for shorter durations are shown relative to the threshold levels obtained for 512 msec, which are represented by the horizontal line. Notice that although temporal integration occurs for all frequencies shown, the functions become flatter (i.e., the time constant τ for integration becomes shorter) as frequency increases from 250 to 4000 Hz.

Temporal integration is observed at higher levels as well as at absolute threshold. Temporal summation of loudness is discussed in Chap. 11, and Chap. 3 covers this topic with respect to the acoustic reflex.

DIFFERENTIAL SENSITIVITY

Having examined the lower and upper bounds of hearing, we may now ask what is the smallest perceivable difference between two sounds. This quantity is called either the difference limen (DL) or the just noticeable difference (jnd); these terms will be used interchangeably in this text. The DL is the smallest perceivable difference in dB between two intensities (ΔI) or the smallest perceivable change in Hz between two frequencies (Δf). We may think of the jnd in two ways. One is as the absolute difference between two sounds, and the other is as the relative difference between them. The latter is obtained by dividing the absolute DL by the value of the starting level. Thus, if the starting level I is 1000 units and the DL ΔI is 50 units, then the relative DL $\Delta I/I$ is 50/1000 = 0.05. This ratio, $\Delta I/I$, is called the Weber fraction.

A point about absolute versus relative DLs should be clarified before proceeding. The frequency DL Δf is an absolute difference in Hz, as opposed to the relative frequency DL obtained by dividing Δf by the starting frequency f. Suppose it is necessary to change a 1000 Hz tone (f) by a 3.6 Hz Δf in order for a particular subject to just detect the frequency difference. His absolute frequency DL is thus 3.6 Hz, whereas his relative DL is 0.0036. The situation is different, however, for the intensity DL, because we measure ΔI in dB. Since decibels are actually ratios, ΔI in dB is really a relative value. (This is why ΔI and I were expressed as "units" in the above example.) For continuity, we shall discuss differential sensitivity for intensity in terms of the Weber fraction $\Delta I/I$*

An important concept in psychophysics is Weber's law, which states that the value of $\Delta I/I$ (the Weber fraction) is a constant (k) regardless of the stimulus level, or

$$\frac{\Delta I}{I} = k$$

A classic illustration of this law is the number of candles one must add to a number of candles which are already lit in order to perceive a difference in the amount of light [53]. If 10 candles are lit, then only one more will produce a jnd of light (DL = 1). However, if there are originally 100 candles then 10 must be added to result in a perceptible difference; and to notice an increase in the light provided by 1000 candles, 100 must be added! Thus, the absolute value of the DL increases from 1 to 100, whereas the Weber fraction k has remained constant at 0.1 (since $\frac{1}{10} = \frac{10}{100} = \frac{100}{1000} = 0.1$), illustrating Weber's law.

Intensity Discrimination

In 1928, Riesz [54] reported on the differential sensitivity for intensity over a wide range of frequencies (35 Hz to 10 kHz) and sensation levels (0–100 dB). Riesz also overcame a major problem of previous experiments [55]: The abrupt switching on and off of the stimuli in these experiments had been marked by audible transient noises. These noises occur because abrupt switching causes energy to spread to other frequencies than the one being tested, and as a result it is unclear whether the subject is responding to the stimulus or to the audible transient. Riesz avoided this problem by using beating tones. When two tones of slightly different frequencies (e.g. 1000 and 1003 Hz) are presented simultaneously, the resulting tone will fluctuate in intensity (beat) at a rate equal to the difference in frequency between the two original tones. Thus, combining a 1000 Hz tone with a 1003 Hz tone results in three beats per second (beat frequency of 3 Hz). This method, which is essentially the same as amplitude modulation, produces no switching transients. Riesz found that DLs were optimized when the modulation rate was 3 beats/sec.

---

*Both $\Delta I/I$ and ΔI in dB are commonly encountered in the literature. They are related by the formula ΔI in dB = $10 \log(1 + \Delta I/I)$. Thus, for $\Delta I/I = 1.0$, ΔI in dB is $10 \log(I + 1) = 10 \log 2$, or 3 dB. When $\Delta I/I$ is 0.5, $\Delta I = 10 \log(1 + 0.5) = 1.76$ dB.

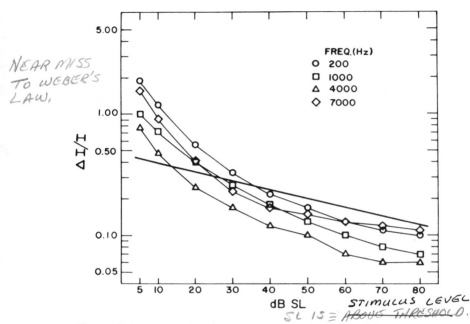

NEAR MISS
TO WEBER'S
LAW,

Figure 9.4 The Weber fraction $\Delta I/I$ as a function of SL. Riesz's [54] data are shown by the curves with symbols; the straight line shows the results of Jesteadt et al. (From Jesteadt, Wier, and Green [56], with permission of *J. Acoust. Soc. Amer.*)

Riesz's subjects adjusted the amplitude of one of the two beating tones until the beats became minimally audible. The intensity difference between the two tones was then taken as the measure of the DL. Figure 9.4 shows the results ($\Delta I/I$ as a function of sensation level) for several frequencies. Weber's law predicts that the data should fall along a horizontal line, indicating that $\Delta I/I$ remains constant at all stimulus levels (SLs). Contrary to Weber's law, Riesz found that $\Delta I/I$ decreased with increasing intensity, especially at low SLs. The curves became flatter at moderate and high SLs (with the Weber fraction approximating 0.3), but did not quite achieve the constant value of $\Delta I/I$ dictated by Weber's law. This discrepancy has come to be known as the "near miss" to Weber's law, and has been corroborated by numerous subsequent studies [e.g., 56–63].* Several examples are illustrated in Fig. 9.5. Although the nature

---

*A "severe departure" from Weber's law has been reported to occur under special conditions [64–66]. It involves a large increase in the size of the Weber fraction at SPLs of approximately 55–65 dB for very brief (under 50 msec.) high-

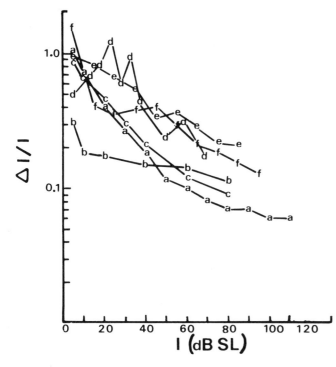

Figure 9.5   The Weber fraction as a function of SL (for 1000 Hz) from several studies: (a) Riesz [54]; (b) and (c) Harris [69]; (d) McGill and Goldberg [57]; (e) Campbell and Lasky [70]; (f) Luce and Green [71]. (Adapted from Luce and Green [71], with permission of *J. Acoust. Soc. Amer.*)

of models to explain the near miss to Weber's law go beyond our scope, several have been proposed. By way of example, one approach involves the spread of the excitation pattern (see Chaps. 4, 5, 10) to a larger number of channels as the signal level increases [67]. Current discussions of these models are provided by Florentine et al., [61], Viemeister and Brown [62], and Green [68].

Riesz [54], using the amplitude modulation method, also reported that the Weber fraction is frequency dependent: He found that $\Delta I/I$ be-

---

frequency signals (over 4000 Hz) that are presented under the gated (versus continuous) pedestal condition; and under similar conditions when the task involves the detection of a signal a band-reject masker (see Chap. 10), expressed as the signal-to-noise ratio. One should refer to Carlyon and Moore [64–66] for the details and implications of this phenomenon.

came smaller as frequency increased from 35 Hz up to about 1000 Hz. The Weber fraction remained more or less constant for the frequencies above this, at least for SLs above 20 dB. This result has not been confirmed by subsequent studies [e.g., 56, 69, 73, 74]. In 1977, Jesteadt et al. [56] reported on an extensive study of the intensity DL using pulsed pure tones. They demonstrated that $\Delta I/I$ does not change with frequency, so that a single straight line may be used to show $\Delta I/I$ as a function of sensation level. This result is shown by the straight line in Fig. 9.4. Jesteadt et al. also demonstrated that the function relating $\Delta I/I$ to SL holds even for sensation levels as low as 5 dB. In contrast, a recent study by Florentine et al. [61] involving a very wide frequency range from 0.25–12 kHz did find a frequency dependency for intensity DLs. They pointed out that the discrepancy is probably due to the much wider range of frequencies used in their study. This is likely because their data did not show a clear frequency effect for the frequencies that were similar to those used by Jesteadt et al.

Rabinowitz et al. [72] combined and summarized the results for differential sensitivity at 1000 Hz. Their results are shown in Fig. 9.6 in

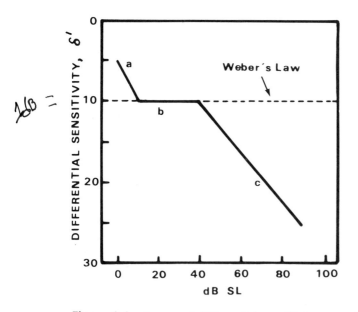

Figure 9.6 Averaged differential sensitivity normalized at 40 dB SL; see text. (δ' is related to the DL for intensity as follows: $\delta'(I) = 10/10 \log(1 + \Delta I/I)$, when 10 log ($\Delta I/I$) produces a d' of 1.0). (Modified after Rabinowitz et al. [72].)

adapted form. Note that Weber's law holds for SLs between 10 and 40 dB (segment b in Fig. 9.6), although differential sensitivity changes with sensation level above and below this range (segments a and c). The horizontal dashed line is the function predicted by Weber's law. Viemeister and Bacon [62] similarly suggested that the function relating the Weber fraction [measured as 10 log ($\Delta I/I$)] to SL (for gated pulsed tones) can be approximated by a horizontal line segment between 20–50 dB SL and a sloping one for higher levels.

Some of the inconsistencies existing in the intensity DL data may be due to the use of alternative methods of presenting the stimuli. Recall here that the DL experiment basically asks whether the subject can hear a difference (which is equal to ΔI) between a baseline signal presented at level I and a more intense signal presented at I + ΔI. We might call the baseline signal the pedestal. There are two general ways to present the increment. The first approach involves leaving the pedestal on all the time and to add ΔI on top of it at various times. This is the continuous pedestal method, and is shown schematically in the lower section of Fig. 9.7, from a recent experiment by Turner, et al. [63]. Alternatively, the pedestal alone (I) may be presented for some period of time, and then be turned off; followed after a brief interval by the presentation of the pedestal together with the increment on top of it (I + ΔI). This strategy is called the gated pedestal method, and is shown in the upper part of the figure. As Turner, et al. have pointed out, the continuous pedestal method is analogous to the types of listening conditions used in early DL papers [e.g., 54,75,76], while the pulsed-tone methods used by Jesteadt et al. and other more recent studies [e.g., 56,61–63,67] involve the gated pedestal technique.

Quite a few studies have directly or indirectly compared intensity DLs using the continuous and gated pedestal methods [e.g., 62,63,65, 77–79]. The general finding has been that smaller intensity DLs are produced by the continuous pedestal method than by the gated pedestal approach. Representative mean results from the study by Turner, et al. are shown in Fig. 9.8 for stimuli presented at three frequencies.

The reason(s) for the gated-continuous difference is not clearly established. Turner et al. have suggested that it might involve a short-term memory effect, and that (citing data by Gescheider et al.) it is probably not a specifically auditory phenomenon because similar findings are also found for touch.

In summary, differential sensitivity for intensity ($\Delta I/I$) becomes more acute with increasing sensation level in a manner which is a near miss to the constant predicted by Weber's law. It difficult to state in a definitive manner whether the Weber fraction for intensity is constant across the

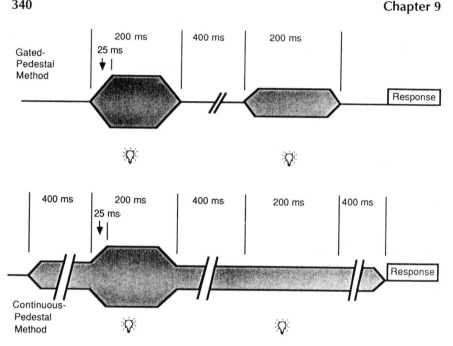

Figure 9.7 The upper diagram shows the gated pedestal method and the lower diagram shows the continuous pedestal method (see text). The level of the pedestal corresponds to I and the level of the pedestal plus increment to $I + \Delta I$. The light bulbs represent warning lights which indicate the listening intervals to the subjects. (From Turner, et al. [63], with permission of *J. Acoust. Soc. Am.*)

audible frequency range. However, it appears safe to say that it is reasonably constant for the middle frequencies.

Frequency Discrimination

The early work [55] on differential frequency sensitivity, like that on intensity discrimination was plagued by transient noise problems associated with the presentation of the stimuli. Shower and Biddulph [80] circumvented this problem by using frequency-modulated (FM) tones as the stimuli. In other words, the test tone was varied continuously in frequency at a rate of twice per second. The subject's task was to detect the presence of a modulated tone as opposed to a steady tone. The DL was taken as the smallest difference in frequency that produced a perceptible modulation of the original tone. Since Shower and Biddulph's classic study included a very wide range of frequencies (62–11,700 Hz) and sensation levels (5–80 dB), it has remained the most widely cited study

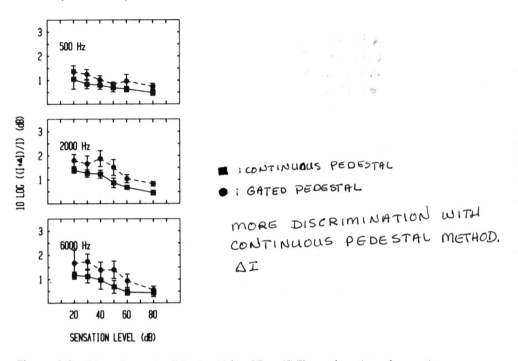

Figure 9.8   Mean intensity DLs (as 10 log [(I + ΔI)/I] as a function of sensation level at three frequencies for the continuous (squares/solid lines) versus gated (circles/dashed lines) pedestal methods. (From Turner, et al. [63], with permission of *J. Acoust. Soc. Am.*)

of differential frequency sensitivity for many years. However, subsequent studies using pulsed tones have generally resulted in better (smaller) DLs at low frequencies and poorer (larger) DLs at higher frequencies than were found with the FM tones [81–88]. We shall return to this point below. The most likely reason for the discrepancy is that frequency modulation results in a stimulus with a complex spectrum, so that we really cannot be sure what serves as the basis for the subject's responses.

Wier et al. [86] recently reported an extensive frequency-discrimination study using pulsed pure tones from 200 to 8000 Hz at sensation levels between 5 and 80 dB. They took the DL to be the smallest frequency difference Δf that the subject could detect 71% of the time. Figure 9.9 shows some of their results at four SLs. The important observations are that the frequency DL Δf becomes larger as frequency increases, and that Δf becomes smaller as sensation level increases. The best (smallest)

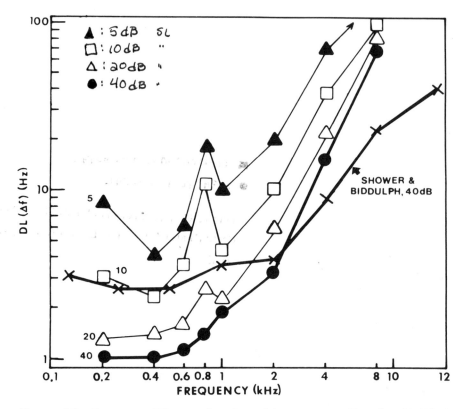

Figure 9.9 Frequency DL as a function of frequency at SLs of 5 dB (filled triangles, 10 dB (open squares), 20 dB (open triangles), and 40 dB (filled circles); based on data of Wier et al. [86]. Shower and Biddulph's [80] data at 40 dB SL (X's) are shown for comparison.

values of Δf—on the order of 1 Hz—occur for low frequencies presented at about 40 dB SL or more. The DL increases substantially above about 1000 Hz, so that Δf at 40 dB SL is roughly 16 Hz at 4000 Hz and 68 Hz by 8000 Hz. The figure also shows that Δf is not simply a monotonic function of frequency; it does not *always* get larger as frequency increases. We see a departure from a monotonically rising function between 200 and 400 Hz, and there are rather dramatic peaks in the curves in the vicinity of 800 Hz. Unfortunately, the origin of these peaks is unclear. We also find that sensation level is relatively more important at low frequencies than at high ones, where the curves tend to converge.

Figure 9.9 also shows the data obtained by Shower and Biddulph for FM tones at 40 dB SL (X's). Comparison of this curve with the one obtained by Wier et al. at the same SL (filled circles) demonstrates that Δf is larger for FM tones at low frequencies, smaller for FM tones at high frequencies, and about the same for the two kinds of stimuli at around 2 kHz. Other studies using pulsed tones at various frequencies and sensation levels are in essential agreement with the findings of Wier et al. [81–85,87,88]. (Nordmark's data [84] are in agreement with those of Wier et al. when the latter are corrected for differences in experimental methodology [89]). Nelson et al. [88] recently replicated the Wier et al. study using a somewhat different methodology. On the basis of their data, they developed a general equation to predict frequency discrimination given the frequency and level of the stimulus. This approach also predicted the Weir et al data extremely well, and was also able to successfully estimate earlier frequency DL data by Harris [81].

Differential sensitivity is shown as the Weber fraction $\Delta f/f$ in Fig. 9.10. Again, the data obtained by Wier et al. are shown along with Shower and Biddulph's data at 40 dB SL for comparison. Notice that $\Delta f/f$

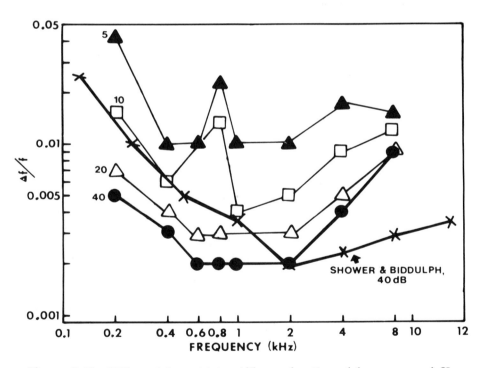

Figure 9.10 Differential sensitivity $\Delta f/f$ as a function of frequency and SL. Symbols same as in Fig. 9.9

improves (becomes smaller) as SL increases, so that the Weber fraction approximates 0.002 for the mid-frequencies at 40 dB SL. The value of $\Delta f/f$ is relatively constant for moderate sensation levels between about 600 and 2000 Hz, but becomes larger at higher and lower frequencies. In summary, then, $\Delta f/f$ is a somewhat complex function of both frequency and intensity, unlike $\Delta I/I$ (Fig. 9.4), which appears to depend upon SL alone [56].

Temporal Discrimination

There are several interesting aspects of temporal discrimination which we shall touch upon. The importance of being able to make fine temporal discriminations should become obvious when one realizes that speech is made up of signals that change rapidly over time. We will briefly look at several general aspects of the temporal realm. The first deals with temporal resolution, the second with the nature of successiveness and temporal order, and the last is the difference limen for duration.

Temporal resolution refers to the shortest period of time over which the ear can discriminate two signals. One way to measure this period is by asking a subject to discriminate between signals that are exactly the same except for a phase difference. Green [90–92] has referred to this quantity as temporal auditory acuity or minimum integration time. The latter phrase suggests that the ear's most sensitive temporal discriminations also provide an estimate of the shortest time period within which the ear can integrate energy. We could think of this time period as the "low end" of the scale for temporal integration, as discussed earlier in the chapter.

Experiments on temporal auditory acuity have been done using a variety of stimuli and approaches [e.g., 90–98]; however, the preponderance of recent studies have used the gap detection technique [97–106]; which was introduced in 1964 by Plomp [107]. The strategy of the gap detection experiment is actually quite straightforward. Moreover, it provides a lucid picture of the temporal resolution concept itself. Suppose we have a continuous burst of noise lasting 500 msec. We could "chop out" a short segment in the center of the noise lasting, say, 30 msec. We now have a (leading) noise burst lasting 285 msec, followed by a 30 msec silent period, followed by a (trailing) 285 msec noise burst. Hence, we have a *gap* lasting 30 msec surrounded in time by leading and trailing noise bursts. The subject is asked whether he hears the gap, hence, the paradigm is called gap detection. The duration of the gap is varied according to some psychophysical method (see Chaps. 7 and 8) in order to find the shortest detectable gap between the two noise bursts, which is called the gap detection threshold (GDT). Thus, the GDT reflects the shortest time interval we can resolve, and it is taken as a measure of temporal resolution.

The essential finding of GDT experiments is that auditory temporal resolution is on the order of 2–3 msec. Such GDTs are obtained when the noise signal contains the higher frequencies and when these are presented at levels which are adequately audible. That the ear can make temporal discriminations as small as about 2 msec is a consistent finding for the various approaches which have been used to study temporal auditory acuity. Detailed discussions of gap detection parameters and models of temporal resolution are available for the more advanced student in numerous recent papers [e.g., 96,97,102,104,105].

The nature of the listener's task is extremely important in measuring temporal discrimination; different values are obtained when different methods are employed. Suppose, for example, that a subject is presented with two signals ("high" and "low") in rapid succession. The subject will be able to detect a difference as small as 2 msec between the onsets of the two signals if we ask him to tell whether there was one signal or two successive ones. On the other hand, he will require on the order of 20 msec in order to say which one came first. The former results in the two signals if we ask him to tell whether there was one signal or two successive ones. On the other hand, he will require on the order of 20 msec in order to be able to say which one came first. The former result may be viewed as an estimate of auditory successiveness (versus simultaneity), while the latter is a measure of perceived temporal order [108,109]. Highly trained subjects can identify a rapid sequence of three tone bursts for durations as small as 2–7 msec [110]. Divenyi and Hirsh [110] pointed out that auditory discrimination performance is substantially affected by at least four factors: (1) the number of stimuli in the sequence of items to be discriminated, (2) how the sequences are presented (separate presentations or continuously), (3) the kind of task which the subject must perform, and (4) the amount of training the subject has had.

We have seen that ΔI depends upon intensity and that Δf is affected by both intensity and frequency. Differential sensitivity for the duration of a signal has also been investigated, although not as extensively as the other two parameters. The general finding that the DL for duration (ΔT) becomes smaller as the overall duration decreases [111–114]. Abel [112] studied ΔT for durations between 0.16 and 960 msec, using various bandwidths of noise from 200 to 300 Hz wide and also 1000 Hz tone bursts. She presented subjects with two intervals, one containing a standard stimulus duration T and the other containing a slightly longer

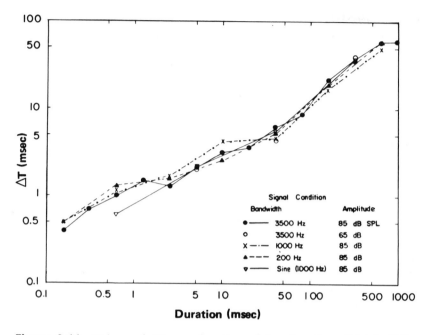

Figure 9.11   Values of ΔT as a function of duration from 0.16 to 960 msec. (From Abel [112], with permission of *J. Acoust. Soc. Am.*)

duration T + ΔT. The subject listened to the two intervals (which were presented randomly), and indicated the one with the longer-duration signal. The smallest time difference correctly detected 75% of the time was taken as the DL for duration ΔT. As Fig. 9.11 shows, ΔT decreases from about 50 msec at durations of 960 msec to on the order of 0.5 for durations of less than 0.5 msec. Differential sensitivity in terms of the Weber fraction ΔT/T is not a constant, but changes with duration so that ΔT/T is about 1.0 at 0.5–1 msec, roughly 0.3 at 10 msec, and approximately 0.1 from 50 to 500 msec. The results were essentially independent of bandwidth and intensity. More recent observations by Sinnott et al. [113] and Dooley and Moore [114] are in essential agreement with these findings.

REFERENCES

1. L. J. Sivian and S. D. White, On minimal audible sound fields, *J. Acoust. Soc. Amer. 4*, 288–321 (1933).
2. M. C. Killion, Revised estimate of minimum audible pressure: Where is the "missing 6 dB"? *J. Acoust. Soc. Amer. 63*, 1501–1508 (1978).

3.   R. S. Dadson and J. H. King, A determination of the normal threshold of hearing and its relation to the standardization of audiometers, *J. Laryng. Otol. 46*, 366–378 (1978).

4.   D. W. Robinson and R. S. Dadson, A re-determination of the equal loudness relations for pure tones, *Brit. J. Appl. Phys. 7*, 166–181 (1956).

5.   N. S. Yoewart, M. Bryan, and W. Tempest, The monaural MAP threshold of hearing at frequencies from 1.5 to 100 c/s, *J. Sound Vib. 6*, 335–342 (1967).

6.   J. L. Northern, M. P. Downs, W. Rudmose, A. Glorig, and J. Fletcher, Recommended high-frequency audiometric threshold levels (8000–18000 Hz), *J. Acoust. Soc. Amer. 52*, 585–595 (1972).

7.   G. Bekesy, *Experiments in Hearing*, McGraw-Hill, New York, 1960.

8.   R. L. Wegel, Physical data and physiology and excitation of the auditery nerve, *Ann. Otol. 41*, 740–779 (1932).

9.   H. Berger, Re-examination of the low-frequency (50–1000 Hz) normal threshold of hearing in free and diffuse sound fields, *J. Acoust. Soc. Am. 70*, 1635–1645 (1981).

10.   M. A. Schechter, S. A. Fausti, B. Z. Rappaport, and R. H. Frey, Age categorization of high-frequency auditory threshold data, *J. Acoust. Soc. Am. 79*, 767–771 (1986).

11.   W. A. Munson and F. M. Wiener, In search of the missing 6 dB, *J. Acoust. Soc. Amer. 24*, 498–501 (1952).

12.   W. Rudmose, On the lack of agreement between earphone pressures and loudspeaker pressures for loudness balances at low frequencies, J. Acoust. Soc. Amer. 35, S1906 (1963).

13.   E. Villchur, Free-field calibration of earphones, *J. Accoust. Soc. Amer. 46*, 1527–1534 (1969).

14.   E. Villchur, Audiometer-earphone mounting to improve intersubject and cushion-fit reliability, *J. Acoust. Soc. Amer. 48*, 1387–1396 (1970).

15.   E. Villchur, Comparison between objective and threshold-shift methods of measuring real-ear attenuation of external sound by earphones, *J. Acoust. Soc. Amer. 51*, 663–664 (1972).

16.   D. W. Morgan and D. D. Dirks, Loudness discomfort level under earphone and in the free field: The effect of calibration, *J. Acoust. Soc. Amer. 56*, 172–178 (1974).

17.   R. W. Stream and D. D. Dirks, Effects of loudspeaker on difference between earphone and free-field thresholds (MAP and MAF), *J. Speech Hearing Res. 17*, 549–568 (1974).

18.   W. Rudmose, The case of the missing 6 dB, *J. Acoust. Soc. Am. 71*, 650–659 (1982).

19.   E. A. G. Shaw, Transformation of sound pressure level from the free field to the eardrum in the horizontal plane, *J. Acoust. Soc. Amer. 56*, 1848–1861 (1974).

20.   International Organization for Standards, R226-1961, Normal equal-loudness contours for pure tones and normal threshold of hearing under free-field listening conditions, 1961.

21.   E. Elliot, A ripple effect in the audiogram, *Nature 181*, 1076 (1958).

22. G. van den Brink, Experiments on binaural diplacusis and tone perception, in *Frequency Analysis and Periodicity Detection in Hearing* (R. Plomp and G. F. Smoorenburg, eds.), Sitjhoff, The Netherlands, 1970, pp. 64–67.

23. M. F. Cohen, Detection threshold microstructure and its effect on temporal integration data, *J. Acoust. Soc. Am. 71*, 405–409 (1982).

24. G. R. Long, The microstructure of quiet and masked thresholds, *Hearing Res. 15*, 73–87 (1984).

25. G. R. Long and A. Tubis, Modification of spontaneous and evoked otoacoustic emissions and associated psychoacoustic microstructure by aspirin consumption, *J. Acoust. Soc. Am. 84*, 1343–1353 (1988).

26. J. P. Wilson, Evidence for a cochlear origin for acoustic re-emissions, threshold fine-structure and tonal tinnitus, *Hearing Res. 2*, 233–252 (1980).

27. E. Schloth, Relation between spectral composition of spontaneous otoacoustic emissions and fine-structure of thresholds in quiet, *Acoustica 53*, 250–256 (1983).

28. E. Zwicker and E. Schloth, Interrelation of different oto-acoustic emissions, *J. Acoust. Soc. Am. 75*, 1148–1154 (1983).

29. J. D. Hood, Observations upon the relationship of loudness discomfort level and auditory fatigue to sound-pressure-level and sensation level, *J. Accoust. Soc. Amer. 44*, 959–964 (1968).

30. J. D. Hood and J. P. Poole, Tolerable limit of loudness: Its clinical and physiological significance, *J. Acoust. Soc. Amer. 40*, 47–53 (1966).

31. J. D. Hood and J. P. Poole, Investigations on hearing upon the upper physiological limit of normal hearing, *Intl. Aud. 9*, 250–255 (1970).

32. S. R. Silverman, C. E. Harrison, and H. S. Lane, Tolerance for pure tones and speech in normal and hard-of-hearing ears, OSRD Rept. 6303, Central Institute for the Deaf, Missouri (1946).

33. British Standards Institute, Standard 2497, The normal threshold of hearing for pure tones by earphone listening, 1954.

34. L. J. Wheeler and E. D. D. Dickson, The determination of the threshold of hearing, *J. Laryng. Otol. 46*, 379–395 (1952).

35. American Standards Association, ASA-Z24.5-1951, Specifications for audiometers for general diagnostic purposes, 1951.

36. U.S. Public Health Service, National Health Survey: Preliminary Reports, *Hearing Study Series Bulletins 1–7*, 1935–1936.

37. J. C. Steinberg, H. C. Montgomery, and M. B. Gardner, Results of the World's Fair hearing tests, *J. Acoust. Soc. Amer. 12*, 291–301 (1940).

38. H. Davis and F. W. Krantz, The international standard reference zero for pure-tone audiometers and its relation to the evaluation of impairment of hearing, *J. Speech Hearing Res. 7*, 7–16 (1964).

39. International Organization for Standards, Recommendation R389, Standard reference zero for the calibration of pure-tone audiometers, 1964.

40. P. G. Weissler, International standard reference for audiometers. *J. Acoust. Soc. Amer. 44*, 264–275 (1968).

41. American National Standards Institute, ANSI-S3.6-1969(R1973), American national standard specifications for audiometers, 1969, 1973.

42. L. A. Wilber, B. Kruger, and M. C. Killion, Reference thresholds for the ER-3A insert earphone, *J. Acoust. Soc. Am. 83*, 669–676 (1988).
43. H. N. Wright, Audibility of switching transients, *J. Acoust. Soc. Amer. 32*, 138 (1960).
44. H. N. Wright, An artifact in the measurement of temporal summation at the threshold of hearing, *J. Speech hearing Dis. 32*, 354–359 (1967).
45. W. Bürck, P. Kotowski, and H. Lichte, Die Lautstärke von Knacken. Geräuchen und Tönen, *Elek. Nachr.-Tech. 12*, 278–288 (1935).
46. J. M. Doughty and W. R. Garner, Pitch characteristics of short tones. 1. Two kinds of pitch threshold, *J. Exp. Psych. 37*, 351–365 (1947).
47. J. W. Hughes, The threshold of audition for short periods of stimulation, *Proc. Roy. Soc. B133*, 486–490 (1946).
48. R. Plomp and M. A. Bouman, Relation between hearing threshold and duration for pure tones, *J. Acoust. Soc. Amer. 31*, 749–758 (1959).
49. J. Zwislocki, Theory of auditory summation, *J. Acoust. Soc. Amer. 32*, 1046–1060 (1960).
50. A. M. Small, J. F. Brandt, and P. G. Cox, Loudness as a function of signal duration, *J. Acoust. Soc. Amer. 34*, 513–514 (1962).
51. R. S. Campbell and S. A. Counter, Temporal integration and periodicity pitch, *J. Acoust. Soc. Amer. 45*, 691–693 (1969).
52. C. S. Watson and R. W. Gengel, Signal duration and signal frequency in relation to auditory sensitivity, *J. Acoust. Soc. Amer. 46*, 989–997 (1969).
53. I. J. Hirsh, *The Measurement of Hearing*, McGraw-Hill, New York, 1952.
54. R. R. Riesz, Differential intensity sensitivity of the ear for pure tones, *Physiol. Rev. 31*, 867–875 (1928).
55. V. O. Knudsen, The sensibility of the ear to small differences in intensity and frequency, *Physiol. Rev. 21*, 84–103 (1923).
56. W. Jesteadt, C. C. Wier, and D. M. Green, Intensity discrimination as a function of frequency and sensation level, *J. Acoust. Soc. Amer. 61*, 169–177 (1977).
57. W. J. McGill and J. P. Goldberg, Pure-tone intensity discrimination as energy detection, *J. Acoust. Soc. Amer. 44*, 576–581 (1968).
58. W. J. McGill and J. P. Goldberg, A study of the near-miss involving Weber's law and pure tone intensity discrimination, *Percept. Psychophys. 4*, 105–109 (1968).
59. N. F. Viemeister, Intensity discrimination of pulsed sinusoids: The effects of filtered noise, *J. Acoust. Soc. Amer. 51*, 1265–1269 (1972).
60. B. C. J. Moore and D. H. Raab, Pure-tone intensity discrimination: Some experiments relating to the "near-miss" to Weber's law, *J. Acoust. Soc. Amer. 55*, 1049–1054 (1974).
61. M. Florentine, S. Buus, and C. R. Mason, Level discrimination as a function of level for tones from 0.25 to 16 kHz, *J. Acoust. Soc. Am. 81*, 1528–1541 (1987).
62. N. F. Viemeister and S. P. Brown, Intensity discrimination, and magnitude estimation for 1-kHz tones, *J. Acoust. Soc. Am. 84*, 172–178 (1988).
63. C. W. Turner, J. J. Zwislocki, P. R. Filion, Intensity discrimination deter-

mined with two paradigms in normal and hearing-impaired subjects, *J. Acoust. Soc. Am. 86*, 109–115 (1989).

64. R. P. Carlyon and B. C. J. Moore, Intensity discrimination: A "severe departure" from Weber's law, *J. Acoust. Soc. Am. 76*, 1369–1376 (1984).

65. R. P. Carlyon and B. C. J. Moore, Continuous versus gated pedestals and the "severe departure" from Weber's law, *J. Acoust. Soc. Am. 79*, 453–460 (1986).

66. R. P. Carlyon and B. C. J. Moore, Detection of tones in noise and the "severe departure" from Weber's law, *J. Acoust. Soc. Am. 79*, 461–464 (1986).

67. M. Florentine and S. Buus, An excitation-pattern model for intensity discrimination, *J. Acoust. Soc. Am. 70*, 1646–1654 (1981).

68. D. M. Green, *Profile Analysis: Auditory Intensity Discrimination*, Oxford University Press, New York, 1988.

69. J. D. Harris, Loudness Discrimination, *J. Speech Hearing Dis.*, Mono. Suppl. 11 (1963).

70. R. A. Campbell and E. Z. Lasky, Masker level and sinusoidal signal detection, *J. Acoust. Soc. Amer. 42*, 972–976 (1967).

71. R. D. Luce and D. M. Green, Neural coding and physiological discrimination data, *J. Acoust. Soc. Amer. 56*, 1554–1564 (1974).

72. W. M. Rabinowitz, J. S. Lim, L. D. Braida, and N. I. Durlach, Intensity perception: VI. Summary of recent data on deviations from Weber's law for 1000-Hz tone pulses, *J. Acoust. Soc Amer. 59*, 1506–1509 (1976).

73. P. N. Schacknow and D. H. Raab, Intensity discrimination of tone bursts and the form of the Weber function, *Percept. Psychophys. 14*, 449–450 (1973).

74. M. J. Penner, B. Leshowitz, E. Cudahy, and G. Richard, Intensity discrimination for pulsed sinusoids of various frequencies, *Percept. Psychophys. 15*, 568–570 (1974).

75. E. Lüscher and J. Zwislocki, A simple method for indirect monaural determination of the recruitment phenomena (Difference limen in intensity in different types of deafness), *Acta Otol. Suppl. 78*, 156–168 (1949).

76. J. Jerger, A difference limen recruitment test and its diagnostic significance, *Laryngoscope 62*, 1316–1332 (1952).

77. R. A. Campbell and E. Z. Lasky, Masker level and sinusoidal detection, *J. Acoust. Soc. Am. 42*, 972–976 (1967).

78. D. M. Green, Masking with continuous and pulsed tones, *J. Acoust. Soc. Am. 46*, 939–946 (1969).

79. D. M. Green, J. Nachmias, J. K. Kearny, and L. A. Jeffress, Intensity discrimination with gated and continuous sinusoids, *J. Acoust. Soc. Am. 66*, 1051–1056 (1979).

80. E. G. Shower and R. Biddulph, Differential pitch sensitivity of the ear, *J. Acoust. Soc. Amer. 3*, 275–287 (1931).

81. J. D. Harris, Pitch discrimination, *J. Acoust Soc. Amer. 24*, 750–755 (1952).

82. W. A. Rosenblith and K. N. Stevens, On the DL for frequency, *J. Acoust. Soc. Amer. 25*, 980–985 (1953).

83. G. B. Henning, Frequency discrimination in noise, *J. Acoust. Soc. Amer. 41*, 774–777 (1967).

84. J. O. Nordmark, Mechanisms of frequency discrimination, *J. Acoust. Soc. Amer. 44*, 1533–1540 (1968).
85. B. C. J. Moore, Frequency difference limens for short duration tones, *J. Acoust. Soc. Amer. 54*, 610–619 (1973).
86. C. C. Wier, W. Jesteadt, and D. M. Green, Frequency discrimination as a function of frequency and sensation level, *J. Acoust. Soc. Amer. 61*, 178–184 (1977).
87. W. Jesteadt and C. C. Wier, Comparison of monaural and binaural discrimination of intensity and frequency, *J. Acoust. Soc. Amer. 61*, 1599–1603 (1977).
88. D. A. Nelson, M. E. Stanton, and R. L. Freyman, A general equation describing frequency discrimination as a function of frequency and sensation level, *J. Acoust. Soc. Am. 73*, 2117–2123 (1983).
89. C. C. Wier, W. Jesteadt, and D. M. Green, A comparison of method-of-adjustment and forced-choice procedures in frequency discrimination, *Percept. Psychophys. 19*, 75–79 (1976).
90. D. M. Green, Temporal auditory acuity, *Psych. Rev. 78*, 540–551 (1971).
91. D. M. Green, Temporal integration time, in *Basic Mechanisms in Hearing* (A. R. Møller, ed.), Academic Press, New York, 1973, pp. 829–846.
92. D. M. Green, Temporal acuity as a function of frequency, *J. Acoust. Soc. Amer. 54*, 373–379 (1973).
93. D. A. Ronken, Monaural detection of a phase difference between clicks, *J. Acoust. Soc. Amer. 47*, 1091–1099 (1970).
94. J. Patterson and D. M. Green, Discrimination of transient signals having identical energy spectra, *J. Acoust. Soc. Amer. 48*, 894–905 (1970).
95. N. F. Viemeister, Temporal modulation transfer functions based upon modulation thresholds, *J. Acoust. Soc. Am. 66*, 1364–1380 (1979).
96. D. M. Green, Temporal factors in psychoacoustics, in *Time Resolution in Auditory Systems* (A. Michelsen, ed.), Springer, New York, 1985, pp. 122–140.
97. T. G. Forest and D. M. Green, Detection of partially filled gaps in noise and the temporal modulation transfer function, *J. Acoust. Soc. Am. 82*, 1933–1943 (1987).
98. C. Formby and K. Muir, Modulation and gap detection for broadband and filtered noise signals, *J. Acoust. Soc. Am. 84*, 545–550 (1988).
99. M. J. Penner, Persistence and integration: Two consequences of a sliding integrator, *Percept. Psychophys. 18*, 114–120 (1975).
100. M. J. Penner Detection of temporal gaps in noise as a measure of the decay of auditory sensation *J. Acoust. Soc. Am. 61*, 552–557 (1977).
101. P. J. Fitzgibbons and F. L. Whightman, Gap detection in normal and hearing-impaired listeners, *J. Acoust. Soc. Am. 72*, 761–765 (1982).
102. P. J. Fitzgibbons, Temporal gap detection in noise as a function of frequency, bandwidth and level, *J. Acoust. Soc. Am. 74*, 67–72 (1983).
103. P. J. Fitzgibbons, Temporal gap resolution in masked normal ears as a function of masker level, *J. Acoust. Soc. Am. 76*, 67–70 (1984).
104. M. J. Shailer and B. C. J. Moore, Gap detection as a function of frequency, bandwidth, and level, *J. Acoust. Soc. Am. 74*, 467–473 (1983).

105. S. Buus and M. Florentine, Gap detection in normal and impaired listeners: The effect of level and frequency, in *Time Resolution in Auditory Systems* (A. Michelsen, ed.), Springer, Berlin, 1985, pp. 159–179.

106. P. J. Fitzgibbons and S. Gordon-Salant, Temporal gap resolution in listeners with high-frequency sensorineural hearing loss, *J. Acoust. Soc. Am. 81*, 133–137 (1987).

107. R. Plomp, Rate of decay auditory sensation, *J. Acoust. Soc. Am. 36*, 277–282 (1964).

108. I. J. Hirsh, Auditory perception of temporal order, *J. Acoust. Soc. Amer. 31*, 759–767 (1959).

109. I. J. Hirsch and C. E. Sherrick, Jr., Perceived order in different sense modalities, *J. Exp. Psych. 62*, 423–432 (1961).

110. P. L. Divenyi and I. J. Hirsh, Identification of temporal order in three-tone sequences, *J. Acoust. Soc. Amer. 56*, 144–151 (1974).

111. A. M. Small, Jr. and R. A. Campbell, Temporal differential sensitivity for auditory stimuli, *Amer. J. Psych. 75*, 401–410 (1962).

112. S. M. Abel, Duration discrimination of noise and tone bursts, *J. Acoust. Soc. Amer. 51*, 1219–1223 (1972).

113. J. M. Sinnott, M. J. Owren, and M. R. Petersen, Auditory duration discrimination in Old World monkeys (*Macaca, Cercopithecus*) and humans, *J. Acoust. Soc. Am. 82*, 465–470 (1987).

114. G. J. Dooley, and B. C. J. Moore, Duration discrimination of steady and gliding tones: A new method for estimating sensitivity to rate of change, *J. Acoust. Soc. Am. 84*, 1332–1337 (1988).

10
Masking

The previous chapter dealt with auditory sensitivity. This one is concerned with masking, or how sensitivity for one sound is affected by the presence of another sound; and also with psychoacoustic phenomena which are for one reason or another typically associated with masking.

Suppose that the threshold for a sound A is found to be 40 dB SPL. A second sound B is then presented and the threshold of A is measured again, but this time in the presence of sound B. We now find that sound A must be presented at, say, 52 dB in order to be detected. In other words, sound A has a threshold of 40 dB when measured in quiet, but of 52 dB when determined in the presence of sound B. This increase in the threshold of one sound in the presence of another is called masking [1]. Our definition of masking may be expanded to include the reduction in loudness that can occur when a second sound is presented, a process referred to as partial masking [2,3].

We may use the word "masking" to denote either the threshold shift per se or the amount (in dB) by which the threshold is raised. Thus, sound A has been *masked* by sound B; and the amount of *masking* due to the presence of B is equal to 52 dB − 40 dB, or 12 dB. In this case, 40 dB is the *unmasked threshold* and 52 dB is the *masked threshold*, and 12 dB is the *amount of masking*. We may also say that since B causes 12 dB of masking to occur for A, the *effective level* of B is 12 dB. Finally, we may adopt the convention of calling around B the *masker*, and sound A the *maskee*, test signal, or probe signal. As will become obvious, masking not only tells us about how one sound affects another, but also provides insight into the frequency-resolving power of the ear. This is the case because the masking pattern to a large extent reflects the excitation pattern along the basilar membrane. In Chap. 13 we shall see how masking is modified under certain conditions of binaural hearing.

The basic masking experiment is really quite straightforward. First, the unmasked threshold of the test stimulus is determined and recorded. This unmasked threshold becomes the baseline. Next, the masker is presented to the subject at a fixed level. The test stimulus is then presented to the subject and its level is adjusted (by whatever psychoacoustic method is being used) until its threshold is determined in the presence of the masker. This level is the masked threshold. As just described, the amount of masking is simply the difference in decibels between this masked threshold and the previously determined unmasked (baseline) threshold. This procedure may then be repeated for all parameters of the test stimulus and masker. An alternative procedure is to present the test stimulus at a fixed level and then to vary the masker level until the stimulus is just audible (or just marked).

MONAURAL MASKING

The masking produced by a particular sound is largely dependent upon its intensity and spectrum. Let us begin with pure tones, which have the narrowest spectra. As early as 1894, Mayer [4] had reported that, while low-frequency tones effectively mask higher frequencies, higher frequencies are not good maskers of lower frequencies. Masking, then, is not necessarily a symmetric phenomenon. This spread of masking to frequencies higher than that of the masker has been repeatedly demonstrated for tonal maskers [5–8]. We must therefore focus our attention not only upon the amount of masking, but also upon the frequencies at which masking occurs.

Figure 10.1 shows a series of masking patterns (sometimes called masking audiograms) obtained by Ehmer [6]. Each panel shows the amount of masking produced by a given pure tone masker presented at different intensities. In other words, each curve shows as a function of maskee frequency the masked thresholds of the maskee which are produced by a given masker presented at a given intensity. Masker frequency is indicated in each frame and masker level is shown near each curve. Several observations may be made from these masking patterns. First, the strongest masking occurs in the immediate vicinity of the masker frequency; the amount of masking tapers with distance from this "center" frequency. Second, masking increases as the intensity of the masker is raised.

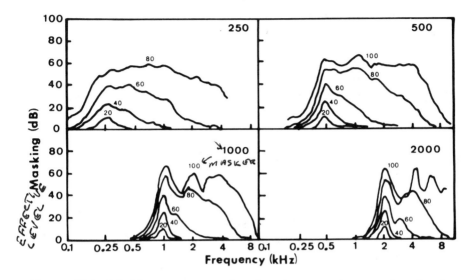

Figure 10.1 Masking patterns produced various pure tone maskers (masker frequency indicated in each frame). Numbers on curves indicate masker level. (Adapted from Ehmer [6], with permission of *J. Acoust. Soc. Amer.*)

The third observation deals with how the masking pattern depends upon the intensity and frequency of the masker. Concentrate for the moment upon the masking pattern produced by the 1000 Hz masker. Note that the masking is quite symmetric around the masker frequency for relatively low masker levels (20 and 40 dB). However, the masking patterns become asymmetrically wider with increasing masker intensity, with the greatest masking occurring for tones higher than the masker frequency, but with very little masking at lower frequencies. Thus, as masker intensity is raised, there is considerable spread of masking upward in frequency but minimal downward spread. Note too that there are peaks in some of the masking patterns corresponding roughly to the harmonics of the masker frequency. Actually, however, these peaks are probably not due to aural harmonics (see Chap. 12) because they do not correspond precisely to multiples of the masker [6,7]. Small [7] found that these peaks occurred when the masker frequency was about 0.85 times the test tone frequency.

Finally, notice that the masking patterns are very wide for low-frequency maskers, and are considerably more restricted for high-frequency maskers. In other words, high-frequency maskers are only effective over a relatively narrow frequency range in the vicinity of the masker frequency, but low frequencies tend to be effective maskers over a very wide range of frequencies.

These masking patterns reflect the activity along the basilar membrane. Recall from Chap. 4 that the traveling wave envelope has a gradually increasing amplitude along its basal (high-frequency) slope, reaches a peak, and then decays rapidly with a steep apical (low-frequency) slope. It is thus expected that higher (more basal) frequencies would be most affected by the displacement pattern caused by lower-frequency stimuli. In addition, the high-frequency traveling wave peaks and "decays away" fairly close to the basal turn, so that its masking effect would be more restricted. Lower frequencies, on the other hand, produce basilar membrane displacements along most of the partition. In addition, the excitation pattern become wider as the signal level increases.

Although a great deal of information about masking has been derived from studies using tonal maskers, difficulties become readily apparent when both the masker and test stimulus are tones. Two major problems are due to the effects of beats and combination tones.

Beats are audible fluctuations that occur when a subject is presented with two tones differing in frequency by only a few cycles per second (e.g., 1000 and 1003 Hz) at the same time. Consequently, when the masker and test tones are very close in frequency, one cannot be sure whether the subject has responded to the beats or to the test tone. These audible beats can result in notches at the peaks of the masking patterns when the masker and maskee are close in frequency [5]. The situation is further complicated because combination tones are also produced when two tones are presented together. Combination tones are produced at frequencies equal to numerical combinations of the two original tones (f1 and f2), such as f2–f1 or 2f1–f2. Beats and combination tones are covered in Chap. 12. Beats may be partially (though not totally) eliminated by replacing the tonal maskers with narrow bands of noise centered around given frequencies; however, the elimination of combination tones requires more sophisticated manipulations [9]. The results of narrow-band noise masking experiments have essentially confirmed the masking patterns generated in the tonal masking studies [10–12].

We have seen that upward spread of masking is the rule as masker level is increased. However, a very interesting phenomenon appears when the stimulus level is quite high, for example, at spectrum levels* of

MASKER OR MASKEE

*"Spectrum level" refers to the power in a one-cycle-wide band. In other words, spectrum level is level per cycle. It may be computed by subtracting 10 times the log of the bandwidth from the overall power in the band. Thus: $dB_{spectrum\ level} = dB_{overall} - 10\log(bandwidth)$. If bandwidth is 10 kHz and overall power is 95 dB, then the spectrum level is $95 - 10\log 10{,}000$, or $95 - 40 = 55$ dB.

about 60 to 80 dB. Bilger and Hirsch [13] found that threshold shifts (masking) also occurred at *low* frequencies when higher-frequency noise bands (maskers) were presented at intense levels. This is called "remote masking" because the threshold shifts occur at frequencies below and remote from the masker. In general, the amount of remote masking increases when the bandwidth of the masking noise is widened or its spectrum level is raised [14]. We might expect that remote masking is the result of the low-frequency effect of the acoustic reflex (see Chap. 3) since it occurs as higher masker levels. However, remote masking has been reported to occur even in the absence of the acoustic reflex [15]. Thus, although there is support for some contribution of the reflex to remote masking [16], remote masking is most likely due primarily to envelope detection of distortion products generated within the cochlea at high masker intensities [17–19]. (See Chap. 4 for a discussion of cochlear distortion.)

It is apparent from Fig. 10.1 that masking increases as the level of the masker is raised. We may now ask how the amount of masking relates to the intensity of the masker. In other words, how much of a threshold shift results when the masker level is raised by a given amount? This question was addressed in the classical studies of Fletcher [20] and Hawkins and Stevens [21]. Since the essential findings of the two studies agreed, let us concentrate upon the data reported by Hawkins and Stevens in 1950. They measured the threshold shifts for pure tones (and for speech) produced by various levels of a white noise masker. (It should be pointed out that although "white" noise connotes equal energy at all frequencies, the actual spectrum reaching the subject is shaped by the frequency response of the earphone or loudspeaker used to present the signal. Therefore, the exact masking patterns produced by a white noise depend upon the transducer employed, as well as on bandwidth effects that will be discussed in the next section.)

Figure 10.2 shows Hawkins and Stevens' data as masked threshold contours. These curves show the masked thresholds produced at each frequency by a white noise presented at various spectrum levels. The curves have been idealized in that the actual results were modified to reflect the masking produced by a true white noise. The actual data were a bit more irregular, with peaks in the curves at around 7 kHz, reflecting the effects of the earphone used. The bottom contour is simply the unmasked threshold curve. The essential fidning is that these curves are parallel and spaced at approximately 10 dB intervals, which is also the interval between the masker levels. This result suggests that a 10 dB increase in masker level produces a 10 dB increase in masked threshold; a point which will become clearer soon.

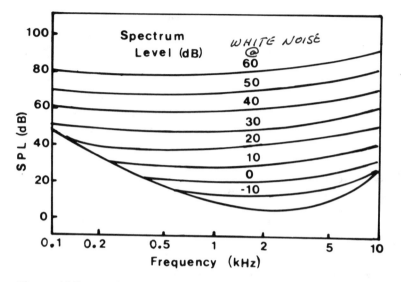

Figure 10.2   Masking contours showing masking as a function of frequency for various spectrum levels of an idealized white noise. Bottom curve is threshold in quiet. (Adapted from Hawkins and Stevens [21], with permission of *J. Acoust. Soc. Amer.*)

The actual amount of masking may be obtained by subtracting the unmasked threshold (in quiet) from the masked threshold. For example, the amount of masking produced at 1000 Hz by a white noise with a spectrum level of 40 dB is found by subtracting the 1000 Hz threshold in quiet (about 7 dB SPL) from that in the presence of the 40 dB noise spectrum level (roughly 58 dB). Thus, the amount of masking is 58 − 7 = 51 dB in this example. Furthermore, since the masked thresholds are curved rather than flat, the white noise is not equally effective at all frequencies. We might therefore express the masking noise in terms of its effective level at each frequency. We may now show the amount of masking as a function of the effective level of the masking noise (Fig. 10.3). As Fig. 10.3 shows, once the masker attains an effective level, the amount of masking is a linear function of masker level. That is, a 10 dB increase in masker level results in a corresponding 10 dB increase in the masked threshold of the test signal. Hawkins and Stevens demonstrated that this linear relationship between masking and masker level is independent of frequency (as shown in the figure), and that it applies to speech stimuli as well as to pure tones.

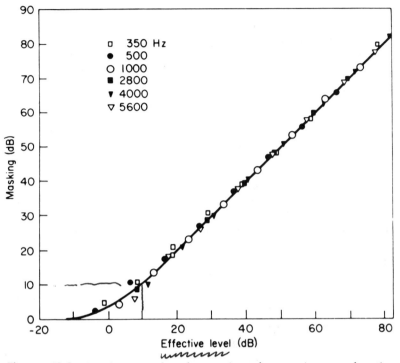

Figure 10.3 Masking produced at various frequencies as a function of the effective level of the masker. (Adapted from Hawkins and Stevens [21], with permission of *J. Acoust. Soc. Amer.*)

FREQUENCY SELECTIVITY

Filters are used in our daily lives to select among various things which may be tangible or intangible. We have all seen change sorters. Even though mixed change is dropped into the same hole, dimes end up in one section, quarters in another, etc. The discrete and large size differences among coins makes this straightforward. However, a selection process must work within the limits of the filters. A clear albeit distasteful example of this point relates to the inevitable grading process in college courses. Grading represents a filtering process: The input to a bank of filters is a continuum from 70–100%, and the output is an "A" or a "B" or a "C." The "B" filter goes from 80–89% Thus, it can select between 78 and 81%, or 89 and 90%; but it cannot differentiate between 83 and 85% Otherwise stated, values that fall within the range of the same filter cannot be differentiated, whereas values the fall across the border of two filters can be isolated from one another. The same issue of selectivity applies to hearing. The ear's ability to analyze a sound so that we can separate one frequency from the other also implies a filtering capability, which we call frequency selectivity. Our ability to analyze the components of a sound depends on the width of our auditory filters.

What does all of this have to do with masking? As we shall see, masking and related experiments reveal the frequency selectivity of the ear and provide insight into the nature of the underlying auditory filter.

Since a tone may be masked by another tone or by a narrow band of noise as well as by white noise, it is reasonable to ask how much of the white noise actually contributes to the masking of a tone. Otherwise stated, does the entire bandwidth of the white noise contribute to the masking of a given tone, or is there a certain limited ("critical") band-width around the tone that alone results in masking? Fletcher [22] at-tacked this problem by finding for tones and masked thresholds pro-duced by various bandwidths of noise centered around the test tones. He held the spectrum level constant, and found that the masked thresh-old of a tone increased as the bandwidth of the masking noise was widened. However, once the noise band reached a certain critical band-width, further widening of the band did not result in any more masking of the tone. Thus, Fletcher demonstrated that only a certain critical band-width within the white noise actually contributes to the masking of a tone at the center of the band, a finding which has been repeatedly confirmed [23–27].

This finding is easily understood if we think of the critical band-width as a filter. More and more of the energy in the white noise will be made available by the filter as the filter's bandwidth is widened. On the other hand, energy present in the white noise that lies above and below the upper and lower cutoff frequencies of the filter is "wasted" from the standpoint of the filter (Fig. 10.4). Now, if this filter defines the critical bandwidth that contributes to the masking of a tone at the center of the band, then it is easy to see how only that portion of the noise that is inside the filter will be useful in masking the tone. Adding to the noise band beyond the limits of this filter (the areas labeled "b" in Fig. 10.4) will not add any more masking, although it will cause the noise to sound louder (see Chap. 11).

Fletcher [22] hypothesized that the signal power (S) would be equal to the noise power (N_0) located within the critical bandwidth (CB) when the tone was at its masked threshold: $S = CB \cdot N_0$. Thus, the critical band would be equal to the ratio of the signal power to the noise power; or CB $= S/N_0$. In decibels, this corresponds to $dB_S - dB_{N_0}$. Hawkins and Ste-vens [21] found that the masked threshold of a 1000 Hz tone was approxi-

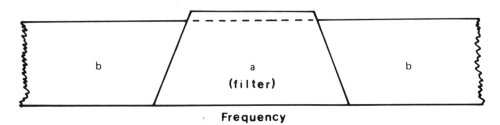

Figure 10.4 Energy within the filter (a) contributes to the masking of the tone at the center, whereas energy outside of the filter (b) does not contribute to the masking (see text).

mately 58 dB in the presence of a white noise whose spectrum level was 40 dB. The resulting estimate of the critical band is therefore 58 dB − 40 dB = 18 dB, which corresponds to a bandwidth of 63. 1 Hz. This estimate of the critical band is shown by the X in Fig. 10.5. Notice that this indirect estimate of the critical bandwidth based upon the power ratio of signal to noise is actually quite a bit narrower than the other more direct estimates of the critical band shown in the figure. For this reason, the indirect estimate based upon Fletcher's formula are referred to as *critical ratios*, as opposed to the *critical bands* obtained by other, direct means. Good correspondence to the critical band is obtained when the critical ratio is multiplied by a factor of 2.5 [28]. This correspondence is demonstrated by the open circles in Fig. 10.5, which are the values of the critical ratios multiplied by 2.5 (based upon Hawkins and Stevens' [21] data).*

---

*Bilger [31] proposed that the listener performs an intensity discrimination between the noise power in the critical band and the combined power of the noise plus signal at the masked threshold; as a result the critical ratio is equated to the familiar Weber fraction (Chap. 9):

$$\frac{S}{CB \cdot N} = \frac{\Delta I}{I}$$

This equation is solved for critical bandwidth by multiplying S/N by the reciprocal of the Weber fraction

$$CB = \frac{S}{N} \cdot \frac{I}{\Delta I}$$

Since the critical ratio is multiplied by 2.5 to obtain the critical band, this leads to a Weber fraction of $\frac{1}{2.5} = 0.4$, or a difference limen of 1.46 dB, a value that is in reasonable agreement with intensity DL data.

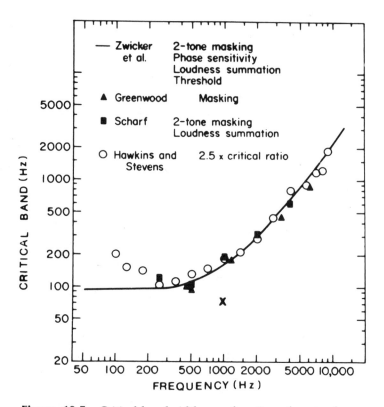

Figure 10.5 Critical bandwidth as a function of center frequency for various studies. The X is the critical ratio estimate of Hawkins and Stevens [21] for a 1000 Hz tone. [Adapted from Scharf [29], Critical bands, in *Foundations of Modern Auditory Theory* (J. V. Tobias, ed.), Vol. 1, ©1970, Academic Press.]

Note that there is good agreement with Greenwood's [12] masking data, as well aa with the critical bands directly derived from loudness studies (see Chap. 11).

Figure 10.5 indicates that the critical band becomes wider as the center frequency increases. Scharf [29] has provided a table of critical bandwidth estimates based upon the available data. Examples are a critical bandwidth of 100 Hz for a center frequency of 250 Hz, a 160 Hz band for 1000 Hz, and a 700 Hz band for 4000 Hz. Similar data and formulas for calculation of the critical bandwidth and critical band rate have been provided by Zwicker and Terhardt [30]. Actually, one should be careful not to conceive of a series of discrete critical bands laid as it were end to end, but rather of a bandwidth around any particular frequency that defines the phenomenon we have discussed with respect to that frequency. (One should remember in this context Scharf's [29, p. 159] elegant definition: "the critical band is that bandwidth at which subjective responses rather abruptly change.") We should thus think of critical bandwidths as overlapping filters rather than as discrete, contiguous filters.

It would appear that the original concept [22] of the critical bandwidth as defining an internal auditory filter is fundamentally correct. Its location is more than likely peripheral, with critical bandwidths probably corresponding to 1–2 mm distances along the human cochlear partition [29]. Thus, the critical band presents itself as a fundamental concept in the frequency-analysis capability of the cochlea, the physiological aspects of which are discussed in Chap. 4. Detailed reviews of the critical band concept may be found in the work of Scharf [29] and Bilger [31]. ←ref. mat.

The idea of the internal filter originally embodied in the critical band concept, particularly in its conceptualization as a rectangular filter around the center frequency [22], has been modified and updated by numerous studies [32–42]. Figure 10.6 shows the shapes of the auditory filter over a wide range of intensities, as derived in a recent paper by Moore and Glasberg [42]. (The curves were based on raw data from young, normal hearing subjects from variety of studies.*) The figure reveals that the filter becomes increasingly more asymmetric with increasing level. The major aspect of this asymmetry is that the slope of the low-frequency (left-hand) branch of the filter decreases with increasing level. This widening of the left-hand branch of the filter that corresponds to the phenomenon of upward spread of masking we saw earlier in this chapter. The reason is that the left-hand branch of this filter determines the high-frequency aspect of the excitation pattern.[†]

With an idea of the shape of the auditory filter, we may ask how it is related to frequency and to the critical band (cf. Fig. 10.5). To do this, we need to summarize the nature of the filters in some valid and convenient way. This can be done by using what is called the equivalent rectangular

---

*The auditory filter tends to widen with age [9]. (Also see Patterson et al. [37] for other findings, and Gelfand and Silman [43] for a general discussion of factors relating to aging and hearing impairment.)

[†]Our interest in the latter point is the agreement between the auditory filter and the spread of masking effect. The details of why the low-frequency branch of the filter determines the high-frequency aspect of the excitation pattern is beyond the current scope. See Moore and Glasberg [42] for the underpinnings and formulas, including a FORTRAN program for calculation of excitation patterns.

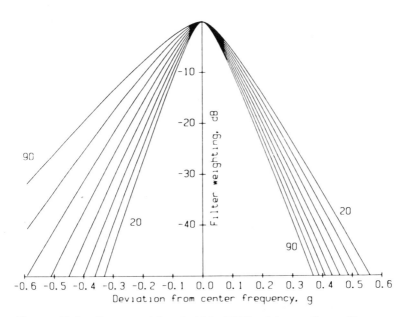

Figure 10.6 Shape and bandwidth (ERB) of the auditory filter expressed in terms increasing level in 10 dB steps from 20 to 90 dB SPL/ERB. (Note the opposite directions in which the left- and right-hand slope change is level increases from 20 to 90 dB. The left-hand slope shown on these filters determine the high frequency aspect of the excitation pattern.) (From Moore and Glasberg [42], with permission of *Hearing Research.*)

bandwidth (ERB) of the filter. An ERB is simply the rectangular filter that passes the same amount of power as would pass through the filter we are trying to specify. Thus, if a white noise is directed to the inputs of a filter of any given configuration and also through its ERB, then the power at their outputs (passed through them) would be the same. Using this approach, Moore and Glasberg [44] have shown how the auditory filter changes with frequency. Figure 10.7 shows the ERB of the auditory filter as a function of its center frequency. Here we see that the width of the auditory filter widens as frequency increases, and also that this relationship is quite consistent across several studies. Also shown in the figure is an equivalent line based upon the classical critical band. (The latter was derived using a formula by Zwicker and Terhardt [30].) Observe that the more recent measurements of auditory filter width are slightly narrower but generally parallel with the older ones based upon classical critical band data. The parallel relationship breaks down below about 500 Hz, where unlike the earlier critical band data, the newer

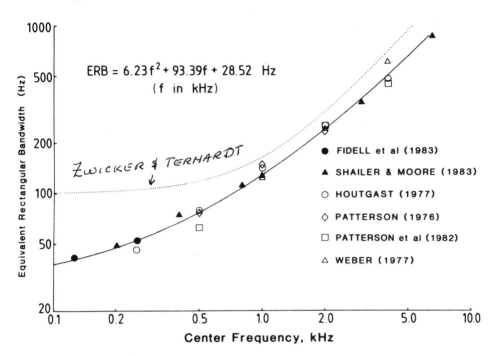

Figure 10.7 The solid line shows the width of the auditory filter (in terms of ERB) as a function of center frequency based on the data of various studies. The dotted line summarizes the same relationship for classical critical band data. (From Moore and Glasberg [44], with permission of *J. Acoust. Soc. Am.*)

observations suggest that the auditory filter continues to be a function of frequency.*

We have already seen that beats and combination tones can adversely affect tone-on-tone masking measurements. Now that we have an idea of the auditory filter, we may consider another factor which can confound masking (among other) experiments. This phenomenon is off-frequency listening [9,33]. Recall from the previous discussion the notion of a continuum of overlapping auditory filters. We typically presume that the subject is listening to some tone "through" the auditory filter, which is centered at that test frequency. However, the subject might also "shift" to another auditory filter, which includes the test

---

*One should refer to Patterson and Moore [9], whose extensive discussion of this topic includes arguments addressing the discrepancy below 500 Hz in the light of differences in processing efficiency.)

frequency but is not centered there. The example in Fig. 10.8 shows why
this might happen. The vertical line depicts a tone of some frequency
and the solid bell curve portrays the auditory filter centered around this
tone. The square represents a low-pass noise masker. Look first at Fig.
10.8a. Notice that part of the masker falls within the auditory filter

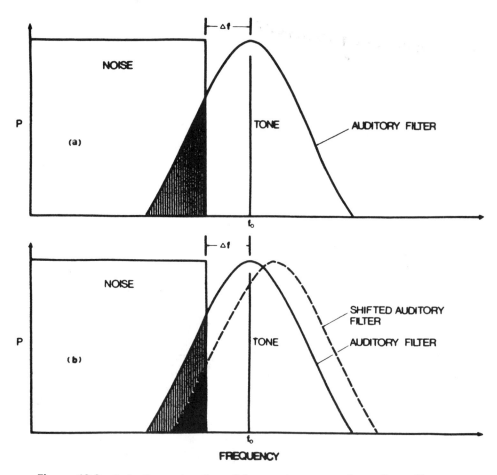

Figure 10.8 In both graphs, the solid curve represents the auditory filter centered at the test tone and the square at the left portrays a lower frequency
masking noise. Off-frequency listening occurs when the subject shifts to another
auditory filter (indicated by the dashed curve in graph *b*) in order to detect the
presence of a test signal. (Adapted from Patterson [33], with permission of *J.
Acoust. Soc. Am.*)

(shaded area). If the tone were presented *without* the noise, then the signal-to-noise (S/N) ratio coming out of this auditory filter would be very high. Hence, the subject would detect the tone. When the *noise is presented* along with the tone, then the portion of the noise falling inside of this auditory filter causes the S/N ratio to be diminished. This, in turn, reduces the chances that the subject will detect the tone.

All of this supposes that the only way to listen to the tone is through the auditory filter centered at that tone's frequency. However, the dashed curve in Fig. 10.8b shows that a sizable proportion of this test tone is also passed by a neighboring auditory filter, which itself is centered at a slightly higher frequency. Moreover, a much smaller part of the masking noise is passed by this neighboring filter. Hence, that the S/N ratio between the test tone and the masking noise is increased when the subject listens "through" this shifted auditory filter. Consequently, the likelihood that the tone will be detected is improved due to such off-frequency listening.

An effective approach to minimize the confounding effects of off-frequency listening is to present the signals involved in an experiment (such as the test tone and masker tone) along with additional noise(s) which will mask-out the frequencies above and below the range of interest [45].

So far, we have described masking in terms of the level of the tone (or other signal) which has been masked. Thus, the masking patterns in Figs. 10.1 and 10.2 expressed the amount of masking produced for various test tones as a function of frequency by a given masker (at some fixed level). That is, "30 dB of masking" on one of these graphs means that the masker caused the threshold of the test signal to be increased by 30 dB above its unmasked threshold. If this experiment were done using the Bekesy tracking method (Chap. 7), the "raw" results might look something like the left panel in Fig. 10.9. Here, the lower tracing shows the threshold of the test signal, which is a tone sweeping in frequency from 500–4000 Hz. The upper tracing shows the masked threshold tracing in the presence of a fixed masker (which is a 1000 Hz tone at 60 dB). Subtracting the lower (unmasked) tracing from the upper (masked) threshold tracing would result in a familiar masking pattern similar to those in Fig. 10.1.

Another way to look at masking was initiated by Chistovich [47], Small [7], and Zwicker [48]. This approach essentially asks the question, what levels of the masker are needed to mask the test signal? Now, the test tone (maskee) is kept at a fixed level and frequency, and the level of the *masker* tone is adjusted until it just masks the test tone. This is done at many different frequencies of the masker, resulting in a curve very different from the familiar masking audiogram seen above.

psychoacustic
tuning (PTC)
curve

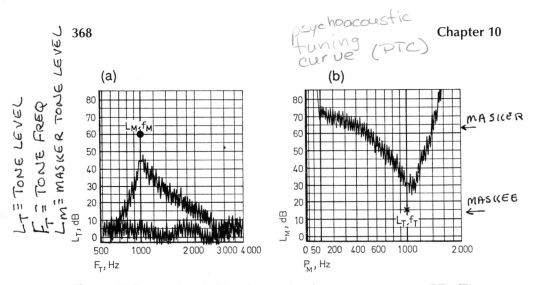

$L_T \equiv$ TONE LEVEL
$F_T \equiv$ TONE FREQ
$L_M \equiv$ MASKER TONE LEVEL

MASKER ←

MASKEE ←

Figure 10.9 (a) Thresholds of sweeping-frequency *test* tones (LT, dB) as a function of frequency (of the test tones, FT, Hz) in quiet (lower tracing) and in the presence of a fixed masker (upper tracing). The filled circle shows the level and frequency of the fixed masker (60 dB, 1000 Hz; LM, FM). (b) These tracings show the levels of sweeping-frequency *masker* tones (LM,dB) needed to just mask the fixed test tone of 1000 Hz at 15 dB (LT,FT). (From Zwicker and Schorn [46], with permission of *Audiology*.)

This approach is easily understood by referring to the right panel of Fig. 10.9. (A careful look at this graph will reveal differences from the left panel not only in the tracing but also in the captions for the x- and y-axes.) The tonal signal (the maskee) is a 1000 Hz tone at 15 dB (indicated by the X). Now it is the *masker* tone which sweeps across the frequency range, and the subject uses the Bekesy tracking method to keep the masker at a level which will just mask the fixed test tone. The resulting diagram shows the level of the masker needed to keep the test tone just-masked as a function of the masker frequency.

It should be immediately apparent to the reader that this tracing bears a striking resemblance to the auditory neuron tuning curves seen in earlier chapters. It is thus called a psychophysical (or psychoacoustic) tuning curve (PTC). Psychophysical tuning curves provide as a very good representation of the ear's frequency selectivity. This occurs based on the notion that we are sampling the output of just one auditory filter when a very low signal is used. As the masker gets closer and closer to the frequency of the test signal, less and less level will be required to mask it, and hence the function of masker level needed to just mask the tone provides a picture of the filter.

However, one must avoid the temptation to think of the PTC as the psychoacoustic analogy of an individual neural tuning curve. It is clear that much more than a single neuron is being sampled, and that PTCs are wider than neural tuning curves. Moreover, the earlier discussions dealing with the implications of beats, combination tones and off-frequency listening in masking are particularly applicable to PTCs. For example, PTCs become wider when off-frequency listening is minimized by the use of notched noise [49]. A notched noise is simply a band-reject noise (see Chap. 1) in which the band being rejected is centered where we are making our measurement. Therefore, the notched noise masks the frequency regions above and below the one of the interest, so that off-frequency listening is reduced.

Figure 10.10 shows two sets of individual PTCs at four test tone frequencies (500–4000) from a more recent experiment. These PTCs were obtained using simultaneous masking (triangles) versus forward masking (squares) were obtained using differing kinds of masking conditions, to be discussed later.

WHAT IS CENTRAL MASKING?

CENTRAL MASKING

The typical arrangement of a masking experiment involves presenting both the masker and the test stimulus to the same ear. Up to now, we have been discussing this ipsilateral type of masking. Another approach is to present the masker to one ear and the test signal to the opposite ear. Raising the intensity of the masker will eventually cause the masker to become audible in the other ear, in which case it will mask the test stimulus (a process known as cross-hearing or contralateralization of the masker). This is actually a case of ipsilateral masking as well, because it is the amount of masker that crosses the head, so to speak, that causes the masking of the signal. However, it has been demonstrated that a masker presented to one ear can cause a threshold shift for a signal at the other ear even when the masker level is too low for it to cross over to the signal ear [50–56]. This contralateral effect of the masker is most likely due to an interaction of the masker and test signal within the central nervous system, probably at the level of the superior olivary complex where bilateral representation is available [40].

Central masking is in some ways similar to, yet in other ways quite different from, the monaural (direct, ipsilateral) masking discussed earlier. In general, the amount of threshold shift produced by central masking is far less than by monaural masking; and more central masking occurs for higher-frequency tones than for low. The amount of masking is greatest at masker onset and decays to a steady-state value within

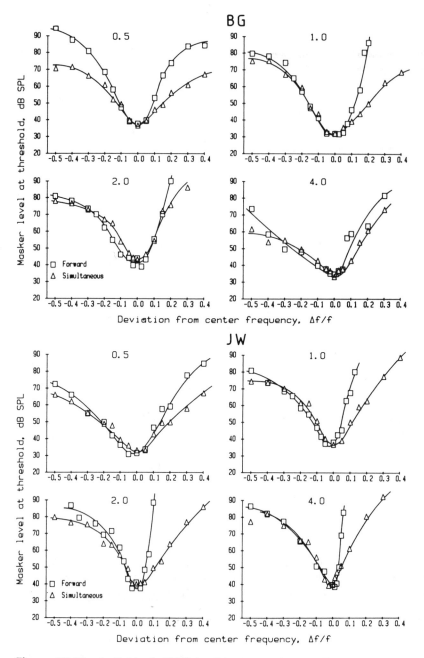

Figure 10.10 Individuals PTCs at 500, 1000, 2000 and 4000 Hz for two listeners. Triangles are simultaneous masking data and squares are forward masking data. Notice that the forward masking PTCs show sharper tuning. (From Moore et al [49], with Permission of *J. Acoust. Soc. Am.*)

about 200 msec. Of particular interest is the frequency dependence of central masking. The greatest amount of central masking occurs when the masker and test tones are close together in frequency. This frequency dependence is shown rather clearly in Fig. 10.11, in which the masker is a 1000 Hz tone presented at a sensation level of 60 dB to the opposite ear. Note that the most masking occurs in a small range of frequencies around the masker frequency. This frequency range is quite close to critical bandwidth (CB). As the figure also shows, more central masking results when the masker and test tones are pulsed on and off together (curve a) rather than when the masker is continuously on and the signal is pulsed in the other ear (curve b). This is a finding common to most central masking experiments, although the amount of masking produced by a given masker level varies among studies and between subjects in the same study. Furthermore, central masking increases as the level of the masker is raised only for the pulsed masker/pulsed signal arrangement, whereas the amount of masking produced by the continuous masker/pulsed signal paradigm remains between about 1 and 2 dB regardless of masker level.

An excellent review of the relationships between the psychophysical and electrophysiological correlates of central masking may be found in

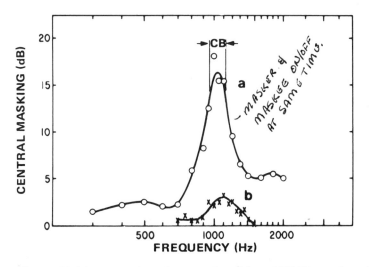

Figure 10.11   Central masking produced by a 1000 Hz tonal masker at 60 dB SL for an individual subject. Curve a is for a masker and maskee pulsed on and off together; curve b is for a continuously on masker and a pulsed signal. (Adapted from Zwislocki et al. [56], with permission of *J. Acoust. Soc. Amer.*)

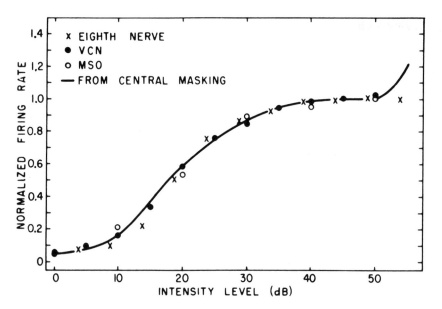

Figure 10.12   Relationship between actually obtained firing rates in the auditory (eighth) nerve, ventral cochlear nucleus (VCN), and medial superior olive (MSO), and rates predicted from central masking data. [From Zwislocki [58], In search of physiological correlates of psychoacoustic characteristics, in *Basic Mechanisms in Hearing* (A. R. Møller, ed.), © 1973 by Academic Press.]

two papers by Zwislocki [57,58]. An example is shown in Fig. 10.12, which demonstrates the firing rates of neurons at various levels of the lower auditory nervous system (see Chaps. 5 and 6), and those predicted on the basis of central masking data. With few exceptions, the agreement shown in the figure of the intensity parameter also holds for frequency and time. Thus, central masking is shown to be related to activity in the lower auditory pathways.

TEMPORAL MASKING

In defining masking as the threshold shift for one sound due to the presence of another sound, we have been considering situations in which the masker and test signal occur simultaneously. Let us now extend our viewpoint to include masking that occurs when the test signal and masker do not overlap in time: temporal masking. This phenomenon may be better understood with reference to the diagrams in Fig. 10.13. In Fig. 10.13a the signal (probe) is presented and terminated,

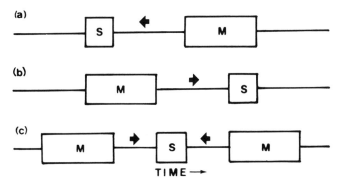

Figure 10.13. Temporal masking paradigms: (a) In backward masking the masker (M) follows the signal (S). (b) In forward masking the masker precedes the signal. (c) Combined forward and backward masking. The heavy arrows show the direction of the masking effect.

and then the masker is presented after a brief time delay following signal offset. Masking occurs in spite of the fact that the signal and masker are not presented together. This arrangement is called backward masking because the masker is preceded by the signal; i.e., the masking effect occurs backward in time (as shown by the arrow in the figure). Forward masking (Fig. 10.13b) is just the opposite. Here, the masker is presented first and then the signal is turned on after an interval following masker offset. As the arrow shows, the masking of the signal now occurs forward in time.

Interest in temporal masking became prevalent with the studies reported by Samoilova [59,60] and Chistovich and Ivanova [61] in the 1950s, although backward and forward masking had been reported upon earlier [62,63]. In the United States, interest began with studies by Pickett [64] and Elliott [65–67]. The basic experiment follows the schemes in Fig. 10.13. The amount of masking of the test signal produced by the following (a) or preceding (b) masker is determined while various parameters of the probe and masker are manipulated. These parameters may be the time interval between probe and masker, masker level, masker duration, etc.

Figure 10.14 shows some results which are typical of temporal masking data. The ordinate is the amount of masking produced by 50-msec noise bursts presented at 70 dB SPL for a test signal of 1000 Hz lasting 10 msec. The abscissa is the time interval between masker and test signal for the backward and forward masking paradigms. Finally, the solid lines show the amount of masking produced when the masker and

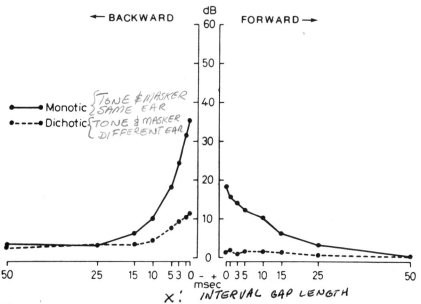

Figure 10.14 Temporal masking in decibels as a function of the interval between signal and masker. (Signal: 10 msec, 1000 Hz tone bursts: masker: 50 msec broad-band noise bursts at 70 dB SPL). (Adapted from Elliott [65], with permission of *J. Acoust. Soc. Amer.*)

probe signal are presented to the same ear (monotically), and the dotted lines reveal the masking that results when the noise goes to one ear and the tone to the other (dichotic masking).

At least three observations may be made from Fig. 10.14. First, backward masking is more effective than forward masking. In other words, more masking occurs when the masker follows the signal by a brief time interval than when the signal follows the masker. Second, more masking occurs when both signal and masker are delivered to the same ear (monotically) than when the probe is presented to one ear and the masker to the other (dichotically). Finally, the closer in time the signal and masker are presented, the more masking results. Conversely, less masking occurs as the time gap between probe and masker widens.

Although Fig. 10.14 shows data for masker-probe separations of up to 50 msec, Elliott [68] has demonstrated significant backward masking for temporal gaps as wide as 100 msec. One would expect to find that temporal masking would increase as the level of the masker is increased. However, the linear increase of masked threshold as a function of masker level seen for simultaneous masking, discussed earlier, is not observed for temporal masking [60,65,69]. That is, increasing the masker level by 10 dB may result in an additional threshold shift on the order of only 3 dB.

Returning to backward masking as a function of the delay between probe and masker, notice in Fig. 10.14 that the amount of masking decreases dramatically as the interval increaes from 0 to 15 msec. For longer delays, the amount of backward masking decreases very little as the interval is lengthened further. The same situation occurs for the forward masking curve, but to a lesser degree. The steep and shallow segments of the monotic temporal masking curves suggest that two different mechanisms might be active [70]. The steeper segments within approximately 15–20 msec of the masker are probably due to over-lapping in time between the traveling wave patterns of the signal and masker; i.e., to a cochlear event. This conclusion is supported by other findings [66,71], as well. It would appear that neural events are responsi-ble for the shallower temporal masking curves at longer delays between the probe and masker. Furthermore, the dichotic temporal masking must rely upon central processing, since the signal and masker are pre-sented to different ears.

The duration of the masker influences the amount of forward mask-ing, but this does not appear to occur for backward masking [68]. That is, more forward masking is produced by a masker 200 msec in duration than by a 25 msec masker. Interestingly, more masking occurs when backward and forward masking are combined than would result if the individual contributions of backward and forward masking were simply added together [72–74]. Such a result is obtained by placing the probe signal between the two maskers, as shown in Fig. 10.13c. Such findings suggest that forward and backward masking may well depend upon different underlying mechanisms.

As we might expect, temporal masking depends upon the frequency relationship between the probe signal and the masker [68,75] just as we have seen to occur for simultaneous masking. In other words, more masking occurs when the signal and masker are close together in fre-quency than when they are far apart.

The underlying mechanisms of temporal masking are not fully re-solved. We have already seen that overlapping in time of the cochlear displacement patterns is a reasonable explanation at very short masker-signal delays. Evidence for the role of central processing in temporal masking has been pointed out in the literature [65,76,77]. Among other factors, forward masking may be due to a persistence of the masker's representation in the auditory neural channel, and/or to a temporary reduction in the absolute sensitivity of the stimulated units resulting from stimulation by the masker. It may be that backward masking occurs because the masker is presented before the signal has been fully processed within the auditory nervous system, thus interfering with the process of its perception. In other words, the occurrence of the masker might be thought of as overriding the in-process processing of the signal.

A large segment of the more recent work involving forward masking has involved psychophysical tuning curves. While this topic is beyond our scope, one should be aware of the most common finding which is that the PTCs generated under forward masking conditions generally show sharper tuning than those described for simultaneous masking conditions [49,78–82]. Examples of this difference are readily seen in Fig. 10.10, above. These discrepancies have often been attributed to possible differences in frequency selectivity, but there is evidence to the contrary [82–85]. There are several informative discussions on this topic to which the interested reader may refer [e.g., 9,81,84,85].

POSTSTIMULATORY FATIGUE

It is not uncommon to experience a period of decreased hearing sensitivity, which lasts for some time, after being exposed to high sound intensities, for example after leaving a discotheque. This temporary shift in auditory threshold may last as long as roughly 16 hours or more, improving gradually. The phenomenon is quite descriptively called post-stimulatory fatigue or temporary threshold shift (TTS).

The nature of the TTS is in clear contrast to the threshold shifts associated with simultaneous masking discused previously in this chapter. Poststimulatory fatigue appears to be a manifestation of temporary changes in the hair cells as a result of exposure to the fatiguing stimulus. As one might expect, excessive and/or long-standing exposures may result in permanent threshold shifts, reflecting pathologic changes or destruction of the hair cells and their associated structures. From the practical standpoint, the amount of TTS produced by exposure to a given fatiguing stimulus has been used as a predictor of individual susceptibility to permanent threshold shifts ("damage risk"). However, this approach is not unchallenged. Since space permits only brief coverage of TTS, the reader is referred to other sources [86–94] for excellent reviews of this topic and related areas.

Except for levels below approximately 80 dB SPL, which do not appear to produce any TTS, the amount of threshold shift increases stimulus intensity is raised [95–97]. Furthermore, it appears that higher-frequency stimuli result in more TTS than do lower frequency fatiguers

[98]. For a given intensity, the amount of TTS will increase with duration [97,99]. In other words, the TTS will become worse as exposure time is increased. Furthermore, the rate at which TTS increases is proportional to the logarithm of the exposure time.

The amount of TTS is smaller for intermittent sounds than for continuous stimulation [99,100]; it appears to be related to the total or average time that the fatiguer is "on" during the course of stimulation [87].

The frequency range over which TTS occurs becomes wider as the stimulus level is raised, and this affect is asymmetric in that the higher frequencies (up to roughly 4000–6000 Hz) are the most severely affected. The TTS reaches a maximum at a higher frequency than the fatiguer frequency, generally about one-half to one octave above [86,87,90–92,94,101]. Physiological work has also revealed that the greatest amount of TTS measured for single auditory neurons occurs when the animal is exposed to high level sounds a half-octave below the neuron's characteristic frequency [102]. The basis of this phenomenon appears to be that the location of the maximum basilar membrane vibration shifts in a basal (higher frequency) direction by an amount equivalent to about a half-octave at high levels of stimulation [103].

The course of recovery from TTS may be measured at various times after the fatiguing tone has been turned off. The course is rather complicated within about 2 min following the offset of the fatiguer [104,105]: It is nonmonotonic, with a "bounce" occurring in the vicinity of the 2 min point. This bounce is a reversal of the recovery, after which the TTS begins to decrease again with time. For longer recovery times, the amount of TTS tends to decrease from the value at the 2 min point (generally called TTS_2) at a rate that is proportional to the logarithm of the time since exposure [106].

REFERENCES

1. American National Standards Institute, Standard S1.1-1960, Acoustical terminology, 1960.
2. M. F. Meyer, Masking: Why restrict it to the threshold level? *J. Acoust.Soc. Amer. 31*, 243 (1959).
3. B. Scharf, Partial masking, *Acoustica 14*, 16–23 (1964).
4. A. M. Mayer, Researches in acoustics, *Philos. Mag. 37*, 259–288 (1894).
5. R. L. Wegel and C. E. Lane, The auditory masking of one pure tone by another and its probable relation to the dynamics of the inner ear, *Physiol. Rev. 23*, 266–285 (1924).
6. R. H. Ehmer, Masking patterns of tones, *J. Acoust Soc. Amer. 31*, 1115–1120 (1959).
7. A. M. Small, Pure tone masking, *J. Acoust. Soc. Amer. 31*, 1619–1625 (1959).

8. A. Finck, Low-frequency pure tone masking, *J. Acoust. Soc. Amer.* 33, 1140–1141 (1961).

9. R. D. Patterson, and B. C. J. Moore, Auditory filters and excitation patterns as representations of frequency resolution, in *Frequency Selectivity in Hearing* (B. C. J. Moore, ed.), Academic Press, London, 1986, pp. 123–177.

10. J. P. Egan and H. W. Hake, On the masking pattern of a simple auditory stimulus, *J. Acoust. Soc. Amer.* 22, 622–630 (1950).

11. R. H. Ehmer, Masking by tones vs. noise bands, *J. Acoust. Soc. Amer.* 31, 1253–1256 (1959).

12. D. D. Greenwood, Auditory masking and the critical band, *J. Acoust. Soc. Amer.* 33, 484–501 (1961).

13. R. C. Bilger and I. J. Hirsh, Masking of tone by bands of noise, *J. Acoust. Soc. Amer.* 28, 623–630 (1956).

14. R. C. Bilger, Intensive determinants of remote masking, *J. Acoust. Soc. Amer.* 30, 817–824 (1958).

15. R. C. Bilger, Remote masking in the absence of intra-aural muscles, *J. Acoust. Soc. Amer.* 39, 103–108 (1966).

16. J. L. Shapely, Reduction in the loudness of a 250-cycle tone in one ear following the introduction of a thermal noise in the opposite ear, *Proc. Iowa Acad. Sci.* 61, 417–422 (1954).

17. W. Spieth, Downward spread of masking, *J. Acoust. Soc. Amer.* 29, 502–505 (1957).

18. B. H. Deatherage, H. Davis, and D. H. Eldredge, Physiological evidence for the masking of low frequencies by high, *J. Acoust. Soc. Amer.* 29, 132–137 (1957).

19. B. H. Deatherage, H. Davis, and D. H. Eldredge, Remote masking in selected frequency regions, *J. Acoust. Soc. Amer.* 29, 512–514 (1957).

20. H. Fletcher, Relation between loudness and masking, *J. Acoust. Soc. Amer.* 9, 1–10 (1937).

21. J. E. Hawkins and S. S. Stevens, The masking of pure tones and of speech by white noise, *J. Acoust. Soc. Amer.* 22, 6–13 (1950).

22. H. Fletcher, Auditory patterns, *J. Acoust. Soc. Amer.* 12, 47–65 (1940).

23. T. H. Schaefer, R. S. Gales, C. A. Shewaker, and P. O. Thompson, The frequency selectivity of the ear as determined by masking experiments, *J. Acoust. Soc. Amer.* 22, 490–497 (1950).

24. P. M. Hamilton, Noise masked thresholds as a function of tonal duration and masking noise band width, *J. Acoust. Soc. Amer.* 29, 506–511 (1957).

25. D. D. Greenwood, Auditory masking and the critical band, *J. Acoust. Soc. Amer.* 33, 484–502 (1961).

26. J. A. Swets, D. M. Green, and W. P. Tanner, On the width of the critical bands, *J. Acoust. Soc. Amer.* 34, 108–113 (1962).

27. C. E. Bos and E. deBoer, Masking and discrimination, *J. Acoust. Soc. Amer.* 39, 708–715 (1966).

28. E. Zwicker, G. Flottrop, and S. S. Stevens, Critical bandwidth in loudness summation, *J. Acoust. Soc. Amer.* 29, 548–557 (1957).

29. B. Scharf, Critical bands, in *Foundations of Modern Auditory Theory* (J. V. Tobias, ed.), Vol. 1, Academic Press, New York, 1970, 157–202.

30. E. Zwicker and E. Terhardt, Analytical expressions of critical-band rate and critical bandwidth as a function of frequency, *J. Acoust. Soc. Am. 68*, 1523–1525 (1980).

31. R. C. Bilger, A revised critical-band hypothesis, in *Hearing and Davis: Essays Honoring Hallowell Davis* (S. K. Hirsh, D. H. Eldredge, eds.) Wash. Univ. Press, St. Louis, 1976, pp. 191–198.

32. R. D. Patterson, Auditory filter shape, *J. Acoust. Soc. Amer. 55*, 802–809 (1974).

33. R. D. Patterson, Auditory filter shapes derived with noise stimuli, *J. Acoust. Soc. Am. 59*, 640–654 (1976).

34. T. Houtgast, Auditory-filter characteristics derived from direct-masking data plus pulsation-threshold data with a rippled-noise masker, *J. Acoust. Soc. Am. 62*, 409–415 (1977).

35. D. L. Weber, Growth of masking and the auditory filter, *J. Acoust. Soc. Am. 62*, 424–429 (1977).

36. B. C. J. Moore and B. R. Glasberg, Auditory filter shapes derived in simultaneous and forward masking, *J. Acoust. Soc. Am. 70*, 1003–1014 (1981).

37. R. D. Patterson, I. Nimmo-Smith, D. L. Webster, and R. Milroy, The deterioration of hearing with age: Frequency selectivity, the critical ratio, the audiogram, and speech threshold, *J. Acoust. Soc. Am. 72*, 1788–1803 (1982).

38. M. J. Shailer and B. C. J. Moore, Gap detection as a function of frequency, bandwidth, and level, *J. Acoust. Soc. Am. 467–473* (1983).

39. S. Fidell, R. Horonjeff, S. Teffeteller, and D. M. Green, Effective masking bandwidths at low frequencies, *J. Acoust. Soc. Am. 73*, 628–638 (1983).

40. B. R. Glasberg, B. C. J. Moore, and I. Nimmo-Smith, Comparison of auditory filter shapes derived with three different maskers, *J. Acoust. Soc. Am. 75*, 536–544 (1984a).

41. B. R. Glasberg, B. C. J. Moore, R. D. Patterson, and I. Nimmo-Smith, Comparison of auditory filter, *J. Acoust. Soc. Am. 76*, 419–427 (1984b).

42. B. C. J. Moore and B. R. Glasberg, Formulae describing frequency selectivity as a function of frequency and level, and their use in calculating excitation patterns, *Hearing Res. 28*, 209–225 (1987).

43. S. A. Gelfand and S. Silman, Future perspectives in hearing and aging: Clinical and research needs, *Seminars in Hearing 6*, 207–219 (1985).

44. B. C. J. Moore and B. R. Glasberg, Suggested formulae for calculating ← auditory-filter bandwidths and excitation patterns, *J. Acoust. Soc. Am. 74*, 750–753 (1983b).

45. B. J. O'Loughlin and B. C. J. Moore, improving psychoacoustic tuning curves, *Hearing Res. 5*, 343–346 (1981).

46. E. Zwicker and K. Schorn, Psychoacoustical tuning curves in audiology, *Audiology 17*, 120–140 (1978).

47. L. A. Chistovich, Frequency characteristics of masking effect, *Biophys. 2*, 708–715 (1957).

48. E. Zwicker, on a psychoacoustical equivalent of tuning curves, in *Facts and Models in Hearing* (E. Zwicker and E. Tehrhardt, eds.), Springer, Berlin, 1974, pp. 95–99.

49. B. C. J. Moore, B. R. Glasberg, and B. Roberts, Refining the measurement of psychophysical tuning curves, *J. Acoust. Soc. Am. 76*, 1057–1066 (1984).

50. R. Chocolle, La sensibilité auditive différentielle d'intensité en présence d'un son contralatéral de même fréquence, *Acoustica 7*, 75–83 (1957).

51. J. G. Ingham, Variations in cross-making with frequency, *J. Exp. Psych. 58*, 199–205 (1959).

52. C. E. Sherrick and P. L. Mangabeira-Albarnaz, Auditory threshold shifts produced by simultaneous pulsed contralateral stimuli, *J. Acoust. Soc. Amer. 33*, 1381–1385 (1961).

53. D. D. Dirks and C. Malmquist, Changes in bone-conduction thresholds produced by masking of the non-test ear, *J. Speech Hearing Res. 7*, 271–287 (1964).

54. D. D. Dirks and J. C. Norris, Shifts in auditory thresholds produced by pulsed and continuous contralateral masking, *J. Acoust. Soc. Amer. 37*, 631–637 (1966).

55. J. Zwislocki, E. N. Damianopoulus, E. Buining, and J. Glantz, Central masking: Some steady-state and transient effects, *Percept. Psychophys 2*, 59–64 (1967).

56. J. Zwislocki, E. Buining, and J. Glantz, Frequency distribution of central masking, *J. Acoust. Soc. Amer. 43*, 1267–1271 (1968).

57. J. Zwislocki, A theory of central masking and its partial validation, *J. Acoust. Soc. Amer. 52*, 644–659 (1972).

58. J. Zwislocki, In search of physiological correlates of psychoacoustic characteristics, in *Basic Mechanisms in Hearing* (A. R. Møller, ed.), Academic Press, New York, 1973, pp. 787–808.

59. I. K. Samoilova, Masking effect of a strong sound stimulus on a previously applied weak one, *Biofizika 1*, 79–97 (1956).

60. I. K. Samoilova, Masking of short tone signals as a function of the time between masked and masking sounds, *Biofizika 4*, 550–558 (1959).

61. L. A. Chistovich and V. A. Ivanova, Mutual masking of short sound pulses, *Biofizika 4*, 170–180 (1959).

62. H. Werner, Studies on contour. I. Qualitative analyses, *Amer. J. Psych. 47*, 40–64 (1935).

63. E. Lüscher and J. Zwislocki, Adaptation of the ear to sound stimuli, *J. Acoust. Soc. Amer. 21*, 135–139 (1949).

64. J. M. Pickett, Backward masking, *J. Acoust. Soc. Amer. 31*, 1613–1615 (1959).

65. L. L. Elliott Backward masking: Monotic and dichotic conditions, *J. Acoust. Soc. Amer. 34*, 1108–1115 (1962).

66. L. L. Elliott, Backward and forward masking of probe tones of different frequencies, *J. Acoust. Soc. Amer. 34*, 1116–1117 (1962).

67. L. L. Elliott, Backward masking: Different durations of the masker stimulus, *J. Acoust. Soc. Amer. 36*, 393 (1964).

68. L. L. Elliott, Development of auditory narrow-band frequency contours, *J. Acoust. Soc. Amer. 42*, 143–153 (1967).

69. H. Babkoff and S. Sutton, Monaural temporal masking of transients, *J. Acoust. Soc. Amer. 44*, 1373–1378 (1968).

70. H. Duifhuis, Consequences of peripheral frequency selectivity for nonsimultaneous masking, *J. Acoust. Soc. Amer. 54*, 1471–1488 (1973).

71. J. H. Patterson, Additivity of forward and backward masking as a function of signal frequency, *J. Acoust. Soc. Amer. 50*, 1123–1125 (1971).

72. I. Pollack, Interaction of forward and backward masking, *J. Aud. Res. 4*, 63–67 (1964).

73. L. L. Elliott, Masking of tones before, during, and after brief silent periods in noise, *J. Acoust. Soc. Amer. 45*, 1277–1279 (1969).

74. R. H. Wilson and R. Carhart, Forward and backward masking: Interactions and additivity, *J. Acoust. Soc. Amer. 49*, 1254–1263 (1971).

75. H. N. Wright, Backward masking for tones in narrow-band noise, *J. Acoust. Soc. Amer. 36*, 2217–2221 (1964).

76. D. H. Raab, Forward and backward masking between acoustic clicks, *J. Acoust. Soc. Amer. 33*, 137–139 (1961).

77. B. H. Deatherage and T. R. Evans, Binaural and masking: Backward, forward and simultaneous effects, *J. Acoust. Soc. Amer. 46*, 362–371 (1969).

78. T. Houtgast, Psychophysical evidence for lateral inhibition in hearing, *J. Acoust. Soc. Am. 51*, 1885–1894 (1972).

79. H. Duifhuis, Cochlear nonlinearity and second filter. Possible mechanisms and implications, *J. Acoust. Soc. Am. 59*, 408–423 (1976).

80. F. L. Wightman, T. McGee, and M. Kramer, Factors influencing frequency selectivity in normal and hearing-impaired listeners, in *Psychophysics and Physiology of Hearing* (E. F. Evans and J. P. Wilson, eds.), Academic Press, London 1977, pp. 295–306.

81. D. L. Weber, Do off-frequency maskers suppress the signal?, *J. Acoust. Soc. Am. 73*, 887–893 (1983).

82. R. A. Lufti, Predicting frequency selectivity in forward masking from simultaneous masking, *J. Acoust. Soc. Am. 76*, 1045–1050 (1984).

83. P. G. Stelmachowicz and W. Jesteadt, Psychophysical tuning curives in normal-hearing listeners: Test reliability and probe level effects, *J. Speech Hear. Res. 27*, 396–402 (1984).

84. W. Jesteadt and S. J. Norton, The role of suppression in psychophysical measures of frequency selectivity, *J. Acoust. Soc. Am. 78*, 365–374 (1985).

85. R. A. Lufti, Interpreting measures of frequency selectivity: Is forward masking special?, *J. Acoust. Soc. Am. 83*, 163–177 (1988).

86. D. N. Elliott and W. Fraser, Fatigue and adaptation, in *Foundations of Modern Auditory Theory* (J. V. Tobias, ed.), Vol. 1, Academic Press, New York, 1970, pp. 115–155.

87. W. D. Ward, Adaptation and fatigue, in *Modern Developments In Audiology* (J. Jerger, ed.), 2nd Ed., Academic Press, New York, 1973, pp. 301–344.

88. K. D. Kryter, Impairment to hearing from exposure to noise, *J. Acoust. Soc.*

Amer. 53, 1211–1234 (1973). [Also: comments by A. Cohen, H. Davis, B. Lempert, and W. D. Ward, and reply by K. D. Kryter, *J. Acoust. Soc. Amer. 53,* 1235–1252 (1973)].

89. D. Henderson, R. P. Hamernick, D. S. Dosanjh, and J. H. Mills, Eds., *Effects of Noise on Hearing,* Raven, New York, 1976).

90. J. D. Miller, Effects of noise on people, *J. Acoust. Soc. Am. 56,* 729–764 (1974).

91. W. Melnick, Auditory effects of noise, in *Occupational Hearing Conservation* (M. H. Miller and C. A. Silverman, eds.), Prentice-Hall, Englewood Cliffs, New Jersey, 1984, pp. 100–132.

92. R. A. Schmiedt, Acustic injury and the physiology of hearing, *J. Acoust. Soc. Am. 76,* 1293–1317 (1984).

93. K. D. Kryter, *The Effects of Noise on Man, Second Edition,* Academic Press, New York, 1985.

94. J. C. Saunders, S. P. Dear, and M. E. Schneider, The anatomical consequences of hearing loss: A review and tutorial, *J. Acoust. Soc. Am. 78,* 833–860 (1985).

95. I. J. Hirsh and R. C. Bilger, Auditory-threshold recovery after exposures to pure tones, *J. Acoust. Soc. Amer. 27,* 1186–1194 (1955).

96. W. D. Ward, A. Glorig, and D. L. Sklar, Temporary threshold shift from octave-band noise: applications to damage-risk criteria, *J. Acoust. Soc. Amer. 31,* 522–528 (1959).

97. J. H. Mills, R. W. Gengel, C. S. Watson, and J. D. Miller, Temporary changes in the auditory system due to exposure to noise for one or two days. *J. Acoust. Soc. Amer. 48,* 524–530 (1970).

98. W. D. Ward, Auditory fatigue and masking, in *Modern Developments in Audiology* (J. Jerger, ed.), Academic Press, New York, 1963, pp. 241–286.

99. W. D. Ward, A. Glorig, and D. L. Sklar, Dependence of temporary threshold shift at 4kc on intensity and time, *J. Acoust. Soc. Amer. 30,* 944–954 (1958).

100. W. D. Ward, A. Glorig, and D. L. Sklar, Temporary threshold shift produced by intermittent exposure to noise, *J. Acoust. Soc. Amer. 31,* 791–794 (1959).

101. W. D. Ward, Damage-risk criteria for line spectra, *J. Acoust. Soc. Amer. 34,* 1610–1619 (1962).

102. A. R. Cody and B. M. Johnstone, Acoustic trauma: single neuron basis for the "half-octave shift," *J. Acoust. Soc. Am. 70,* 707–711 (1981).

103. B. M. Johnstone, R. Patuzzi, and G. K. Yates, Basilar membrane measurements and the traveling wave, *Hearing Res. 22,* 147–153 (1986).

104. I. J. Hirsch and W. D. Ward, Recovery of the auditory threshold after strong acoustic stimulation, *J. Acoust. Soc. Amer. 24,* 131–141 (1952).

105. I. J. Hirsch and R. C. Bilger, Auditory-threshold recovery after exposures to pure tones, *J. Acoust. Soc. Amer. 27,* 1186–1194 (1955).

106. W. D. Ward, A. Glorig, and D. L. Sklar, Relation between recovery from temporary threshold shift and duration of exposure, *J. Acoust. Soc. Amer. 31,* 600–602 (1959).

11

Loudness

The intensity of a sound refers to its physical magnitude, which may be expressed in such terms as its power or pressure. Turning up the "volume" control on a stereo amplifier thus increases the intensity of the music coming out of the loudspeakers. This intensity is easily measured by placing the microphone of a sound-level meter near thee loudspeaker. The perception of intensity is called loudness; generally speaking, low intensities are perceived as "soft" and high intensities as "loud." In other words, intensity is the physical parameter of the stimulus and loudness is the percept associated with that parameter. However, intensity and loudness are not one and the same; and although increasing intensity is generally associated with increasing loudness, there is not a simple one-to-one correspondence between the two. Furthermore, loudness is also affected by factors other than intensity. For example, it is a common experience to find that loudness changes when the "bass" and "treble" controls of a stereo amplifier are adjusted, even though the volume control itself is untouched.*

LOUDNESS LEVEL

We may begin our discussion of loudness by asking whether the same amount of intensity results in the same amount of loudness for tones of

---

*Bass and treble are the relative contributions of the lower and higher frequency ranges, respectively. Thus, raising the bass emphasizes the low frequencies, and raising the treble emphasizes the high.

different frequencies. For example, does a 100 Hz tone at 40 dB SPL have the same loudness as a 1000 Hz tone also presented at 40 dB? The answer is no. However, a more useful question is to ask how much intensity is needed in order for tones of different frequencies to sound equally loud. These values may be appropriately called equal loudness levels.

Although the exact precedures differ, the fundamental approach for determining equal loudness levels is quite simple. One tone is presented at a fixed intensity level, and serves as the reference tone for the experiment. The other tone is then varied in level until its loudness is judged equal to that of the reference tone. (The traditional reference tone has been 1000 Hz; but Stevens [1] more recently suggested the use of 3150 Hz, where threshold sensitivity is most acute.) A third frequency tone may then be balanced with the reference tone; then a fourth, a fifth, and so on. The result is a list of sound pressure levels at various frequencies, all of which sound equal in loudness to the reference tone. We can then draw a curve showing these equally loud intensity levels as a function of frequency. If the experiment is repeated for different reference tone intensities, the result is a series of contours like the ones in Fig. 11.1.

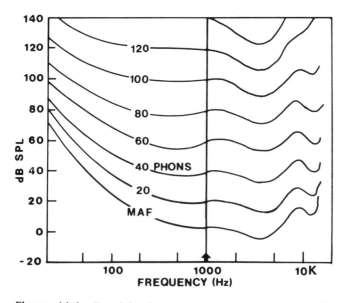

Figure 11.1   Equal loudness contours (phon curves) adapted from Robinson and Dadson [2]. (Permission *British J. Appl. Phys.*, © 1956 by The Institute of Physics.)

The contour labeled "40 phons" shows the intensities needed at each frequency for a tone to sound equal in loudness to a 1000 Hz reference tone presented at 40 dB SPL. Thus, any sound which is equal in loudness to a 1000 Hz tone at 40 dB has a loudness level of 40 phons. A tone which is as loud as a 1000 Hz tone at 50 dB has a loudness level of 50 phons; one that is as loud as a 1000 Hz tone at 80 dB has a loudness level of 80 phons, etc. We may now define the phon as the unit of loudness level. All sounds that are equal in phons have the same loudness level even though their physical magnitudes may be different. Since we are expressing loudness level in phons relative to the level of a 1000 Hz tone, phons and dB SPL are necessarily equal at this frequency.

The earliest equal loudness data were reported by Kingsbury [3] in 1927. However, the first well-accepted phon curves were published in 1933 by Fletcher and Munson [4], and as a result, equal loudness contours have come to be called "Fletcher-Munson curves." Subsequently, extensive equal loudness contours were also published by Churcher and King [5] and by Robinson and Dadson [2]. There are some differences among the curves given by the various studies, although the basic configurations are reasonably similar. Robinson and Dadson's curves appear to be the most accurate, and are the ones shown in Fig. 11.1. Equal loudness contours have also been reported for narrow bands of noise [6].

At low loudness levels the phon curves are quite similar in shape to the minimum audible field (MAF) curve. Thus, more intensity is needed to achieve equal loudness for lower frequencies than for higher ones. However, notice that the phon curves tend to flatten for higher loudness levels, indicating that the lower frequencies grow in loudness at a faster rate than the higher frequencies, overcoming, so to speak, their disadvantage at near-threshold levels. This effect can be experienced in a simple, at-home experiment, We begin by playing a record album at a moderate level, with the bass and treble controls set so that the music is as "natural sounding" as possible. If we decrease the volume to a much softer level, the music will also sound as though the bass was decreased, demonstrating the de-emphasis of the low (bass) frequencies at lower loudness levels. If we raise the volume to a quite loud level, then the music will sound as though the bass was turned up as well. This "boomy" sound reflects the faster rate of growth for the lower frequencies with increasing loudness levels.

Since the same sound pressure level (SPL) will be associated with different loudness levels as a function of frequency, it would be convenient to have a frequency weighting network which could be applied to the wide-band sounds encountered in the environment. Such a weighting function would facilitate calculating the loudness of such sounds as highway noise, sonic booms, etc. This has been done to some extent in the construction of electronic weighting networks for sound level meters (see Peterson and Gross [7] for a complete discussion). These networks are rough approximations to various phon curves. For example, the A-weighting network approximates the general shape of the 40 phon curve by de-emphasizing the low frequencies and more efficiently passing the high. The B-weighting network roughly corresponds to the 70-phon loudness level; and the C-weighting network is designed to mimic the essentially flat response of the ear at high loudness levels.

LOUDNESS CALCULATION REFERENCE

More precise calculation methods have been proposed by Stevens [1,8,9], Zwicker [10], and Kryter [11,12]. We will not discuss these methods except to say that the basic approach is to assign weights to various frequency bands in the sound being measured, and then to combine these weights in order to arrive at the predicted loudness of the sound. Stevens [1] combined the results of 25 equal loudness (and "equal noisiness") contours across a wide variety of studies in order to arrive at the representative contours shown in Fig. 11.2, which serve as the basis for Stevens' "Mark VII" loudness calculation procedure [1].

The use of loudness levels represents a significant improvement over such vague concepts as "more intense sounds are louder." However, the phon itself does not provide a direct measure of loudness, per

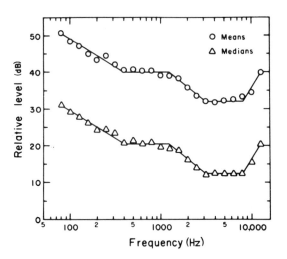

Figure 11.2 Combined equal perceived magnitude (loudness) contours. Circles show mean data across studies and triangles show medians. (From Stevens [1], with permission of *J. Acoust. Soc. Amer.*)

se. We must still seek an answer to the question of how the loudness percept is related to the level of the physical stimulus.

LOUDNESS SCALING

Loudness scales show how the loudness percept is related to the intensity of the sound stimulus. Since we are interested not only in the loudness of a particular sound, but also in how much louder one sound is than another, the relationship between loudness and intensity is best determined with direct ratio scaling techniques (see Chap. 7).* This approach was pioneered by Stevens [15,17–21], whose earliest attempts to define a ratio scale of loudness used the fractionalization method [18]. Stevens later adopted the use of magnitude estimation and magnitude production [20], and subsequent work has almost exclusively employed these techniques alone or in combination [22–28].

The unit of loudness is the sone [18]; one sone is the loudness of a 1000 Hz tone presented at 40 dB SPL. Since SPL in decibels and loudness level in phons are equivalent at 1000 Hz, we may also define one *sone* as the *loudness* corresponding to a *loudness level* of 40 *phons*. We may therefore express loudness in sones as a function of loudness level in phons [13] as well as a function of stimulus intensity. (In this context, recall that Stevens [1] proposed that the reference frequency be moved to about 3150 Hz. This change would lower the reference for one sone to 32 dB SPL at 3150 Hz, as was confirmed by Hellman [28], who measured the loudness functions of 1000 and 3000 Hz tones.) Since loudness level does not vary with frequency (i.e., 40 phons represents the same loudness level at any frequency even though the SPLs are different), we can ignore frequency to at least some extent when assigning loudness in sones to a tone, as long as sones are expressed as a function of phons. As previously mentioned, methods that calculate loudness for complex sounds first weight the frequency bands comprising the complex sound, using what is essentially a phon curve, as in Fig. 11.2. Loudness in sones is then calculated from these weighted bands.

The sone scale is easily understood. Having assigned a value of one sone to the reference sound, we assign a loudness of two sones to the

---

*The intensity difference limen (DL), or just noticeable difference (jnd), has also been proposed as a basis for loudness scaling, as has been the partitioning of the audible intensity range into equal loudness categories. However, the consensus of data supports ratio scaling. See Robinson's [13] review and study, and also Gardner [14] and Stevens [15] for summaries of the controversy; as well as Marks [16] and Stevens [17] for informative treatments within the more general context of psychophysics.

intensity that sounds twice as loud as the reference, 0.5 sones to the level that sounds half as loud, etc. The resulting function appears as shown in Fig. 11.3. Notice that loudness in sones is a straight line when plotted as a function of level on log–log coordinates. This fact is extremely important, because a straight line on a log–log plot indicates a power function. In other words, loudness L may be expressed as a power e of the stimulus level I according to the formula

$$L = kI^e$$

where k is a constant. This is a case of Stevens' law [29], which states that sensation grows as a power of stimulus level. The exponent indi-

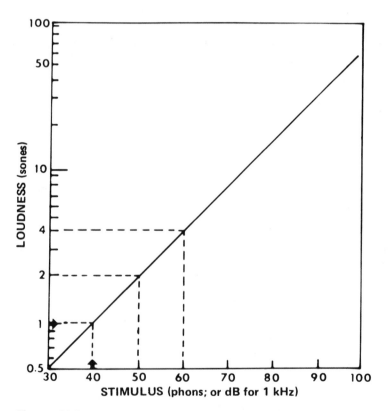

Figure 11.3 Idealized sone scale showing a doubling of loudness for a 10 dB (phon) stimulus increase at and above 30 phons. Actually, at lower stimulus levels, the function curves downward revealing faster growth of loudness near threshold (see text).

cates the rate at which the sensation grows with stimulus magnitude. Thus, an exponent of 1.0 would mean that the magnitude of the sensation increases at the same rate as the stimulus level. Exponents less than 1.0 show that the sensation grows at a slower rate than stimulus level (examples are loudness and brightness); whereas exponents greater than 1.0 indicated that the perceived magnitude grows faster than the physical level (examples are electric shock and heaviness). Conveniently, the exponent also corresponds to the slope of the function. (The constant k depends upon the units used to express the magnitudes.)

The linear relationship (on log–log coordinates) of loudness as a function of phons is shown in Fig. 11.3 for loudness levels as low as 30 phones (or dB at 1000 Hz). Consistent experimental findings have demonstrated that straight-line relationship is not continued at lower sound pressure levels [22,30–32]. Instead, the loudness function begins to curve downward with decreasing stimulus levels as threshold is approached, indicating that loudness grows faster near threshold.

Early studies resulted in a median exponent of 0.6 for loudness as a function of sound pressure level, so that a 10 dB level increase would correspond to a doubling of loudness [19]; and Robinson [13] reported that loudness increased twofold with a change in loudness level of 10 phons. This is essentially equivalent to saying that a doubling of loudness corresponds to a tripling of signal level. However, not all studies have reported this value. For example, Stevens and Guirao [24] reported much faster loudness growth, with exponents averaging 0.77. Stevens' assessment of the data lead him to propose that an exponent of 0.67 more closely typifies the actual relationship, and incorporated this value into his loudness calculation procedure [1]. This slope of two-thirds leads to a doubling of loudness with an increase in sound pressure level of 9 dB. Moreover, it turns out that there is a fair amount of variability in loudness function exponents between subjects; although the individual exponents are very reliable [33–36].

What, then, is the slope of the loudness function? The preponderance of the available data, including much of the most recent experimentation on loudness seems to consistently point to an exponent of 0.6 as the most representative value [31,32,35–38]. One might note that this is also the international standard value of the loudness growth exponent [39]).

CRITICAL BANDS AND LOUDNESS OF COMPLEX SOUNDS

The critical band concept was introduced with respect to masking in the last chapter. As we shall see, loudness also bears in intimate relationship to the critical bandwidth; and loudness experiments provide a direct estimate of the width of the critical band. As Scharf [40] pointed out, it is convenient to think of the critical band as the bandwidth where abrupt changes occur. Consider the following experiment with this concept in mind.

Suppose pairs of simultaneous tones are presented to a subject, both tones always at the same fixed level. The first pair of tones presented are very close together in frequency; and the subject compares their loudness to the loudness of a standard tone. The frequency difference between the two tones is then increased, and the resulting loudness is again compared to the standard. We find that the loudness of the two tones stays about the same as long as the tones are separated by less than the critical bandwidth, but that there is a dramatic increase in loudness when the components are more than a critical bandwidth

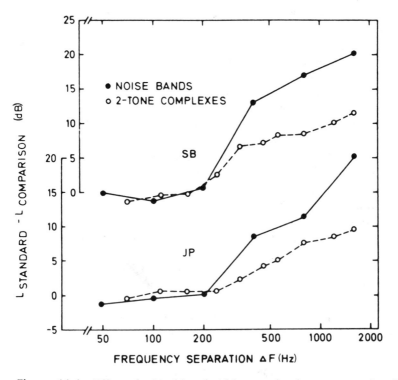

Figure 11.4 Effect of critical bandwidth upon loudness summation for a two-tone complex (open circles) and bands of noise (filled circles) for two subjects (SB and JP). Test level was 65 dB SPL and center frequency was 1000 Hz (see text). (From Florentine et al. [41], with permission of *J. Acoust. Soc. Amer.*)

apart. The open circles in Fig. 11.4 show typical results for two subjects. In this figure the amount of loudness summation is shown as the level difference between the standard and comparison stimuli (ordinate) as a function of bandwidth (abscissa). Notice that the loudness of the two-tone complex stays essentially the same for frequency separations smaller than the critical bandwidth (roughly 200 Hz in this example); whereas loudness increases when the frequency difference is greater than the width of the critical band.

The fact that loudness remains essentially the same for bandwidths (or frequency separations) smaller than the critical band, but increases when the critical band is exceeded, has been demonstrated for two-tone and multitone complexes, and also for bands of noise [41–45]. This loudness summation effect is minimal at near-threshold levels, and the greatest loudness increases occur for moderate signal levels [42,44,45]. As Fig. 11.5 shows, loudness summation becomes greater as

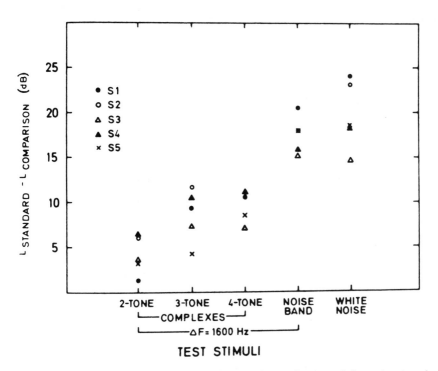

Figure 11.5   Loudness summation for tonal complexes and for noise (symbols show data for individual subjects). (From Florentine et al. [41], with permission of *J. Acoust. Soc. Amer.*)

the number of components of a multitone complex is increased, with the most loudness summation occurring for bands of noise wider than the critical band [41]. This relation is shown in Fig. 11.4, in which the same loudness results from both two-tone complexes (open circles) and noise bands (filled circles) narrower than the critical band, but much greater loudness summation results for the noise when the critical bandwidth is exceeded.

These findings by Florentine et al. [41] are inconsistent with those of Scharf [46], who found that loudness summation was unaffected by the number of components in a tonal complex. Florentine et al. proposed that this difference may have been due to differences in test levels because they found the greatest effect at 65 dB SPL, which was not included in the earlier study by Scharf; or perhaps to the effects of pooling data across subjects in the other study. The small effect associated with the number of components may have been obscured by such differences. In any case, the issue of the effect of the number of components is not clearly resolved [47,48]. The major point, however, that loudness summation occurs when the bandwidth of the signal becomes wider than the critical band, is well established.

TEMPORAL INTEGRATION OF LOUDNESS

Temporal integration (summation) at threshold was discussed in Chap. 10, where we found that sensitivity improves as signal duration increases up to about 200–300 msec, after which thresholds remain essentially constant. Temporal integration was also covered with respect to the acoustic reflex in Chap. 3. A similar phenomenon is also observed for loudness [49–56]. Increasing the duration of a very brief signal at a given level above threshold will, within the same general time frame as in the cases previously discussed, cause it to sound louder.

There are two basic techniques that may be used to study the temporal integration of loudness. One method is similar to that used in establishing phon curves. The subject is presented with a reference sound at a given intensity and is asked to adjust the level of a second sound until it is equal in loudness with the first one [49–51,56]. In such cases, one of the sounds is "infinitely" long (i.e., long enough so that we may be sure that temporal integration is maximal, say 1 sec), and the other is a brief tone burst (of a duration such as 10 msec, 20 msec, 50 msec, etc.). Either stimulus may be used as the reference while the other is adjusted, and the result is an equal loudness contour as a function of signal duration. The alternate method involves direct magnitude scaling [52,53,55] from which equal loudness curves can be derived.

Figure 11.6 shows representative curves for the temporal integration of loudness. These curves are based upon the findings of Richards [56]. In his experiment, test tones of various durations were balanced in loudness to a 500 msec reference tone presented at either 20, 50, or 80 dB SPL. The ordinate shows the test tone levels (in dB SPL) needed to achieve equal loudness with the reference tone. This quantity is plotted as a function of test tone duration on the abscissa. Notice that loudness increases (less intensity is needed to achieve a loudness balance with the reference tone) as test tone duration increases. This increase in loudness is greater for increases in duration up to about 80 msec, and then tends to slow down. In other words, increases in duration from 10 msec to about 80 msec has a steeper loudness summation slope than increases in duration above 80 msec. However, Richards did find that there was still some degree of additional loudness integration at longer durations.

These data are basically typical of most findings on temporal integration of loudness. That is, there is an increase of loudness as duration is increased up to some "critical duration;" and loudness growth essentially stops (or slows down appreciably) with added duration. On the

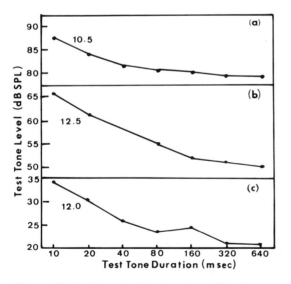

Figure 11.6 Temporal integration of loudness at 1000 Hz based upon loudness balances to a 500 msec tone at (a) 20 dB SPL, and (b) 50 dB SPL and (c) 80 dB SPL. Slopes of the steeper portions (dB per decade duration change) are shown near each curve. (Based upon data by Richards [56].)

other hand, the critical duration is quite variable among studies, and has generally been reported to decrease as a function of sensation level [49,50], though not in every study [53]. In addition, the rate at which loudness has been found to increase with duration varies among studies. McFadden [55] found large differences also among individual subjects. Richards [56] fitted the steeper portions of the temporal integration functions with straight lines, and found that their slopes were on the order of 10–12 dB per decade change in duration. The mean values are shown on the figure, and agree well with other studes [50,53]. One might note at this point that the results of loudness integration experiments have been shown to be affected by the methodology used and the precise nature of the instructions given to the patients, and also by confusions on the part of subjects between loudness and duration of the signal [57].

LOUDNESS ADAPTATION

Loudness adaptation refers to the apparent decrease in the loudness of a signal that is continuously presented at a fixed level for a resonably long period of time. In other words, the signal appears to become softer as time goes on even though the intensity is the same. Hood's [58] classic experiment demonstrates this phenomenon rather clearly. A 1000 Hz tone is presented to the subject's right ear at 80 dB. This adapting stimulus remains on continuously. At the start, a second 1000 Hz tone is presented to the left ear, and the subject adjusts the level of this second (comparison) tone to be equally loud to the adapting tone in the right ear (part a in Fig. 11.7). Thus, the level of the comparison tone is used as an indicator of the loudness of the adapting tone in the opposite ear. This first measurement represents the loudness prior to adaptation (the pre-adaptation balance).

The comparison tone is then turned off while the adapting tone continues to be applied to the right ear (adaptation period b in Fig. 11.7). After several minutes of adaptation, the comparison signal is reapplied to the opposite ear, and the subject readjusts it to be equally loud with the 80 dB adapting tone. This time, however, the comparison tone is adjusted by the subject to only 50 dB in order to achieve a loudness balance with the adaptor (segment c in Fig. 11.7), indicating that the loudness of the adapting tone has decreased by an amount comparable to a 30 dB drop in signal level. Thus, there has been 30 dB of adaptation due to the continuous presentation of the tone to the right ear. Since the loudness decrease occurs during stimulation, the phenomenon is also called *per*stimulatory adaptation. This phenomenon contrasts, of course,

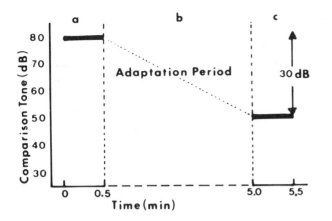

Figure 11.7 Loudness adaptation as shown by the level of the comparison stimulus. (Modified from Hood [58].)

with the TTS described in the previous chapter, which constitutes *post*stimulatory fatigue.

The method just described for the measurement of adaptation may be considered a simultaneous homophonic loudness balance. In other words, the subject must perform a loudness balance between two tones of the same frequency that are presented, one to each ear, at the same time. Other studies employing this approach [59–61] have reported similar findings.

An problem inherent in these early studies of loudness adaptation was their use of simultaneously presented adapting and comparison tones of the same frequency. Although the presumed task was a loudness balance between the ears, the experiments were confounded by the perception of a fused image due to the interaction of the identical stimuli at the two ears. As we shall see in Chap. 13, the relative intensities at the two ears will determine whether the fused image is perceived centralized within the skull or lateralized toward one side or the other. It is therefore reasonable to question whether the loudness adaptation observed in such studies is confounded by interactions between the ears such as lateralization.

One way around the problem is to use a comparison tone having a different frequency than the adapting tone. This procedure would reduce the lateralization phenomenon because the stimuli would be different at the ears. In 1955, Egan [59] found no significant difference in the amount of loudness adaptation caused by this heterophonic method and the homophonic approach described above. Subsquently, however,

Egan and Thwing [62] reported that loudness balances involving lateralization cues did in fact result in greater adaptation than techniques that kept the effects of lateralization to a minimum.

Other studies have shown that loudness adaptation is reduced or absent when binaural interactions (lateralization cues) are minimized [63–68]. This may be accomplished by using adapting and comparison tones of different frequencies (heterophonic loudness balances), or by a variety of other means. For example, Stokinger and colleagues [66,67] reduced or obliterated loudness adaptation by shortening the duration of the comparison tone and by delaying the onset of the comparison tone

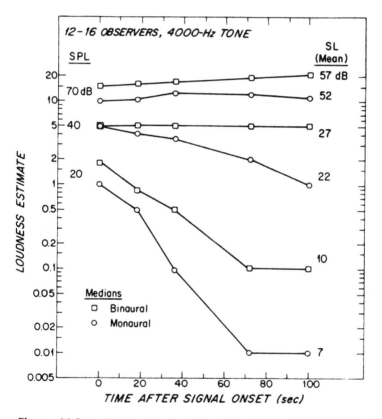

Figure 11.8 Adaptation (medians) for a 4000 Hz tone measured by successive magnitude estimations as a function of the duration of the tone. The parameter is sensation level, or the number of decibels above the subjects' thresholds. See text. [From Scharf [70], Loudness adaptation, in *Hearing Research and Theory, Vol. 2* (J. V. Tobias and E. D. Schubert, eds.), Vol. 1, (C) 1983 by Academic Press.]

after the adapting tone was removed. Both of these approaches had the effects of reducing or removing the interaction of the two tones between the ears. Moreover, it has been demonstrated that the presentation of an intermittent tone to one ear induces adaptation of a continuous tone in the other ear [69,70]. Thus, it appears that lateralization methods foster misleading impressions about loudness adaptation effects, especially with regard to monaural adaptation [70].

What, then, do we know about loudness adaptation based upon experimentation which directly assesses the phenomenon? Scharf [70] has provided a cohesive report of a large number of loudness adaptation experiments using, for the most part, magnitude estimations of loudness that were obtained at various times during the stimulus. Several of his findings may be summarized for our purposes as follows: First, there appears to be a noticeable amount of variability among people in terms of how much adaptation they experience. Second, the loudness of a pure tone adapts when it is presented to a subject at levels up to approximately 30 dB sensation level (SL, i.e., 30 dB above his threshold). This relationship is shown in Fig. 11.8, although one might note that adaptation continues beyond the value of 70 seconds shown in the figure [70]. Third, there is more adaptation for higher frequency tones than for lower frequencies tones or for noises. Fourth, adaptation appears to be the same whether the tones are presented to one ear or to both ears. In the latter case, the amount of adaptation that is measured seems to be primarily determined by the ear with less adaptation. For example, if the right ear adapts in 90 sec and the left ear in 105 sec, then the binaurally presented tone would be expected to adapt in 105 sec. Here, of course, we are assuming that both ears are receiving similar continuous tones. Clearly, these points represent only a brief sampling of Scharf's extensive findings and theoretical arguments. The student should consult his paper for greater elucidation as well as for an excellent coverage of the overall topic.

REFERENCES

1. S. S. Stevens, Perceived level of noise by Mark VII and decibels (E), *J. Acoust. Soc. Amer. 51*, 575–601 (1972).
2. D. W. Robinson and R. S. Dadson, A redetermination of the equal loudness relations for pure tones, *Brit. J. Appl. Phys. 7*, 166–181 (1956).
3. B. A. Kingsbury, A direct comparison of the loudness of pure tones, *Phys. Rev. 29*, 588–600 (1927).
4. H. Fletcher and W. A. Munson, Loudness, its definition, measurement, and calculation, *J. Acoust. Soc. Amer. 5*, 82–105 (1933).
5. B. G. Churcher and A. J. King, The performance of noise meters in terms of the primary standard, *J. Inst. Elec. Eng. 81*, 57–90 (1937).

6. I. Pollack, The loudness of bands of noise, *J. Acoust. Soc. Amer. 24*, 533–538 (1952).

7. A. P. G. Peterson and E. E. Gross, *Handbook of Noise Measurement*, 7th Ed., General Radio, Concord, Massachusetts, 1972.

8. S. S. Stevens, Calculation of the loudness of complex noise, *J. Acoust. Soc. Amer. 28*, 807–832 (1956).

9. S. S. Stevens, Procedure for calculating loudness: Mark VI, *J. Acoust. Soc. Amer. 33*, 1577–1585 (1961).

10. E. Zwicker, Uber psychologische and methodische Grundlagen der Lautheit, *Acoustica 1*, 237–258 (1958).

11. K. D. Kryter, Concepts of perceived noisiness, their implementation and application, *J. Acoust. Soc. Amer. 43*, 344–361 (1968).

12. K. D. Kryter, *The Effects of Noise on Man*, 2nd Ed., Academic Press, New York, 1970.

13. D. W. Robinson, The subjective loudness scale, *Acoustica 7*, 217–233 (1957).

14. W. R. Gardner, Advantages of the discriminability criteria for a loudness scale, *J. Acoust. Soc. Amer. 30*, 1005–1012 (1958).

15. S. S. Stevens, On the validity of the loudness scale, *J. Acoust. Soc. Amer. 31*, 995–1003 (1959).

16. L. E. Marks, *Sensory Processes: The New Psychophysics*, Academic Press, New York, 1974.

17. S. S. Stevens, In *Psychophysics: Introduction to Its Perceptual, Neural and Social Prospects* (G. Stevens, ed.), Wiley, New York, 1975.

18. S. S. Stevens, A scale for the measurement of a psychological magnitude: Loudness, *Psych. Rev. 43*, 405–416 (1936).

19. S. S. Stevens, The measurement of loudness, *J. Acoust. Soc. Amer. 27*, 815–829 (1955).

20. S. S. Stevens, The direct estimation of sensory magnitudes—loudness, *Amer. J. Psychol. 69*, 1–25 (1956).

21. S. S. Stevens, Concerning the form of the loudness function, *J. Acoust. Soc. Amer. 29*, 603–606 (1957).

22. R. P. Hellman and J. Zwislocki, Monaural loudness function at 1000 cps and interaural summation, *J. Acoust. Soc. Amer. 35*, 856–865 (1963).

23. R. P. Hellman and J. Zwislocki, Loudness function of a 1000-cps tone in the presence of a masking noise, *J. Acoust. Soc. Amer. 36*, 1618–1627 (1964).

24. J. C. Stevens and M. Guirao, Individual loudness functions, *J. Acoust. Soc. Amer. 36*, 2210–2213 (1964).

25. S. S. Stevens and H. Greenbaum, Regression effect in psychophysical judgment, *Percept. Psychophysiol. 1*, 439–446 (1966).

26. R. P. Hellman and J. Zwislocki, Loudness determination at low sound frequencies, *J. Acoust. Soc. Amer. 43*, 60–64 (1968).

27. R. R. Rowley and G. A. Studebaker, Monaural loudness-intensity relationships for a 1000-Hz tone, *J. Acoust. Soc. Amer. 45*, 1186–1192 (1969).

28. R. P. Hellman, Growth of loudness at 1000 and 3000 Hz, *J. Acoust. Soc. Amer. 60*, 672–679 (1976).

29. S. S. Stevens, On the psychophysical law, *Psych. Rev. 54*, 153–181 (1957).
30. R. P. Hellman and J. J. Zwislocki, Some factors affecting the estimation of loudness, *J. Acoust. Soc. Am. 33*, 687–694 (1961).
31. B. Scharf, Loudness, in *Handbook of Perception, Vol. IV, Hearing* (E. C. Carterette and M. P. Friedman, eds.), Academic Press, New York, 1978, pp. 187–242.
32. G. Canevet, R. Hellman, and B. Scharf, Group estimation of loudness in sound fields, *Acoustica*, 277–282, (1986).
33. A. W. Logue, Individual differences in magnitude estimation of loudness, *Percept. Psychophys. 19*, 279–280 (1976).
34. J. K. Walsh and C. P. Browman, Intraindividual consistency on a cross-modality matching task. *Percept. Psychophys. 23*, 210–214 (1978).
35. R. P. Hellman, Stability of individual loudness functions obtained by magnitude estimation and production, *Percept. Psychophys. 29*, 63–70 (1981).
36. R. P. Hellman and C. H. Meiselman, Prediction of individual loudness exponents from cross-modality matching, *J. Speech Hear. Res. 31*, 605–615 (1988).
37. L. Marks, On scales of sensation: Prolegomena to any future psychophysics that will be able to come forth as science, *Percept. Psychophys. 16*, 358–376 (1974b).
38. R. P. Hellman, Growth of loudness at 1000 and 3000 Hz, *J. Acoust. Soc. Am. 60*, 672–679 (1976).
39. International Standards Organization, *Expression of the physical and subjective magnitudes of sound*, ISO R-131-1959(E), Geneva, 1959.
40. B. Scharf, Critical bands, in Foundations of Modern Auditory Theory (J. V. Tobias, ed.), Vol. I, New York Academic Press, 1970, pp. 157–202.
41. M. Florentine, S. Buus, and P. Bonding, Loudness of complex sounds as a function of the standard stimulus and the number of components, *J. Acoust. Soc. Amer. 64*, 1036–1040 (1978).
42. E. Zwicker and J. Feldtkeller, Über die Lautstärke von gleichförmigen Geräuschen, *Acoustica 5*, 303–316 (1955).
43. J. Feldtkeller and E. Zwicker, Das Ohr als Nachrichtenempfänger, Hirzel, Stuttgart, 1956.
44. E. Zwicker, G. Flottrop, and S. S. Stevens, Critical bandwidth in loudness summation, *J. Acoust. Soc. Amer. 29*, 548–557 (1957).
45. B. Scharf, Critical bands and the loudness of complex sounds near threshold, *J. Acoust. Soc. Amer. 31*, 365–380 (1959).
46. B. Scharf, Loudness of complex sound as a function of the number of components, *J. Acoust. Soc. Amer. 31*, 783–785 (1959).
47. B. Scharf, Acoustic reflex, loudness summation, and the critical band, *J. Acoust. Soc. Am. 60*, 753–755 (1976).
48. R. Hellman, and B. Scharf, Acoustic reflex and loudness, *The Acoustic Reflex: Basic Principles and Clinical Applications* (S. Silman, ed.), 1984, pp. 469–516.
49. G. A. Miller, The perception of short bursts of noise, *J. Acoust. Soc. Amer. 20*, 160–170 (1948).

50. A. M. Small, J. F. Brandt, and P. G. Cox, Loudness as a function of signal duration, *J. Acoust Soc. Amer. 34*, 513–514 (1962).
51. C. D. Creelman, Detection, discrimination, and the loudness of short tones, *J. Acoust. Soc. Amer. 35*, 1201–1205 (1963).
52. E. Ekman, G. Berglund, and V. Berglund, Loudness as a function of duration of auditory stimulation, *Scand. J. Psych. 7*, 201–208 (1966).
53. J. C. Stevens and J. W. Hall, Brightness and loudness as a function of stimulus duration, *Percept. Psychophysiol. 1*, 319–327 (1966).
54. J. S. Zwislocki, Temporal summation of loudness: An analysis, *J. Acoust. Soc. Amer. 46*, 431–441 (1969).
55. D. McFadden, Duration-intensity reciprocity for equal-loudness, *J. Acoust. Soc. Amer. 57*, 701–704 (1975).
56. A. M. Richards, Loudness perception for short-duration tones in masking noise, *J. Speech Hearing Res. 20*, 684–693 (1977).
57. S. D. G. Stephens, Methodological factors influencing loudness of short duration tones, *J. Sound Vib. 37*, 235–246 (1974).
58. J. D. Hood, Studies on auditory fatigue and adaptation, *Acta Otol.*, Suppl. 92 (1950).
59. J. P. Egan, Perstimulatory fatigue as measured by heterophonic loudness balances, *J. Acoust. Soc. Amer. 27*, 111–120 (1955).
60. H. N. Wright, Measurement of perstimulatory auditory adaptation, *J. Acoust. Soc. Amer. 32*, 1558–1567 (1960).
61. A. M. Small and F. D. Minifie, Effect of matching time on perstimulatory adaptation, *J. Acoust. Soc. Amer. 33*, 1028–1033 (1961).
62. J. P. Egan and E. J. Thwing, Further studies on perstimulatory fatigue, *J. Acoust. Soc. Amer. 27*, 1225–1226 (1955).
63. T. E. Stokinger and G. A. Studebaker, Measurement of perstimulatory loudness adaptation, *J. Acoust. Soc. Amer. 44*, 250–256 (1968).
64. W. D. Fraser, J. W. Petty, and D. N. Elliott, Adaptation: Central or peripheral? *J. Acoust. Soc. Amer. 47*, 1016–1021 (1970).
65. J. W. Petty, W. D. Fraser, and D. N. Elliott, Adaptation and loudness decrement: A reconsideration, *J. Acoust. Soc. Amer. 47*, 1074–1082 (1970).
66. T. E. Stokinger, W. A. Cooper, and W. A. Meissner, Influence of binaural interaction on the measurement of perstimulatory loudness adaptation, *J. Acoust. Soc. Amer. 51*, 602–607 (1972).
67. T. E. Stokinger, W. A. Cooper, W. A. Meissner, and K. O. Jones, Intensity, frequency, and duration effects in the measurement of monaural perstimulatory loudness adaptation, *J. Acoust. Soc. Amer. 51*, 608–616 (1972).
68. D. E. Morgan and D. D. Dirks, Suprathreshold loudness adaptation, *J. Acoust. Soc. Amer. 53*, 1560–1564 (1973).
69. Botte, M.C., G. Canevet, and B. Scharf, Loudness adaptation induced by an intermittent tone, *J. Acoust. Soc. Am. 72*, 727–739 (1982).
70. B. Scharf, Loudness adaptation, in *Hearing Research and Theory, Vol. 2* (J. V. Tobias and E. D. Schubert, eds.), Academic Press, New York, 1983, pp. 1–56.

12

Pitch

In this chapter we will deal with several attributes of sounds, grossly classified as "pitch." Like loudness, the word pitch denotes a perception with which we are all familiar. Yet, in spite of hundreds of years of study, the manner in which pitch is perceived remains enigmatic. For example, the issue of place versus temporal coding of frequency discussed in earlier chapters has been somewhat resolved: we know that both mechanisms are operative. However, the precise interaction of frequency and temporal coding in auditory frequency analysis remains largely unresolved. Furthermore, the perception of pitch, per se, appears to be multifaceted; and it may be that there are various kinds of pitch. Thus, we find that psychoacoustic pitch scales that have been confirmed by the rigors of laboratory replication are often at odds with musical scales that have withstood the tests of time and experience.

In light of these factors, the reader should not be surprised to find his fingers acting as placemarkers to other sections (particularly Chaps. 2, 4–6, 9, and 10) while perusing this chapter. The need to refer back to such phenomena as cochlear and neural coding, distortion, differential sensitivity, and masking should not be viewed as an inconvenience, but rather as exemplary of the pervasiveness of pitch in all aspects of auditory perception: a factor that makes it an exciting area in psychoacoustics.

PITCH SCALES

Started in formal terms, pitch is the psychological correlate of frequency, such that high frequency tones are heard as being "high" in pitch and low frequencies are associated with "low" pitches. We saw in Chap. 9 that not all changes in frequency are perceptible. Instead, a certain amount of frequency change is needed before the difference limen (DL) is reached. In other words, the frequency difference between two tones must be at least equal to the DL before they are heard as being different in pitch. Obviously, pitch and frequency are related, but not in a simple one-to-one manner.

How, then, is pitch related to frequency? This problem was tackled by Stevens et al. [1] using the fractionalization method discussed in Chap. 7. That is, their subjects were presented with a standard tone and were asked to adjust the frequency of a second tone until its pitch was one-half that of the standard. The result was a scale in which pitch is expressed as a function of frequency. This scale was revised by Stevens and Volkmann [2] in 1940. In this study, the subjects were required to adjust the frequencies of five tones within a certain frequency range until they were separated by equal pitch intervals. In other words, their task was to make the distance in pitch between tones A and B equal to that between B and C, which in turn was to be the same as that between C and D, and so on. Stevens and Volkmann also repeated the earlier frac-tionalization experiment, except that they now gave their subjects a 40 Hz tone that was arbitrarily assigned a pitch of zero. (The rationale will become clear momentarily.) Pitch scales have also been developed using the method of magnitude estimation [3,4].

The various methods result in slightly different pitch scales. Keeping this fact in mind, we will examine one scale [2] as an example of the relationship between frequency and pitch.

Figure 12.1 shows the revised pitch scale reported by Stevens and Volkmann [2]. The scale is a good fit to the data they obtained using equal pitch distances and fractionalization. Frequency is shown along the abscissa and pitch on the ordinate. As shown, pitch is expressed in units called *mels* [1,2]. By convention, 1000 mels is the pitch of a 1000 Hz tone presented at 40 phons. This association is shown by the lines la-beled a in the figure. The frequency that sounds twice as high as 1000 mels has a pitch of 2000 mels, while 500 mels is half the pitch of 1000 mels, and so on. Thus, the lines labeled b in the figure indicate that 3000 Hz is 2000 mels. Note that tripling the frequency from 1000 to 3000 Hz only doubles the pitch, from 1000 to 2000 mels. Furthermore, even a cursory look at Fig. 12.1 reveals that the audible frequency range of about 20,000 Hz is focused down to a pitch range of only about 3500 mels. Nevertheless, Stevens and Volkmann demonstrated rather good correspondence between pitch in mels and distance along the basilar membrane, both quantities expressed as a function of frequency. Scharf

PITCH UNIT IS "MELS".

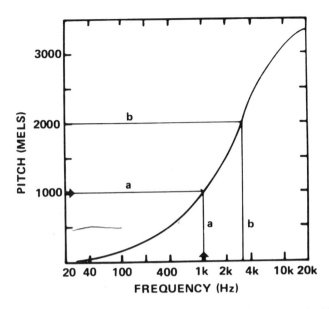

Figure 12.1   The revised pitch (mel) scale (see text). (Adapted from Stevens and Volkmann [2], with permission of *Amer. J. Psychol.*)

[5] pointed out that approximately 150 mels corresponds to the typical critical bandwidth (see Chaps. 10 and 11).

Stevens and Volkmann employed both direct estimates of the pitch remaining below 40 Hz and extrapolations to arrive at 20 Hz as being the lowest perceptible pitch. (The interval between 25 and 40 Hz was equal in pitch to that between 40 and 52 Hz; hence, the assignment of "zero pitch" to 40 Hz in the fractionalization method used in their study.) This estimate is consistent with Bekesy's [6] observation that the lowest frequency yielding a sensation of pitch is approximately 20 Hz.

It is interesting to ask how the psychoacoustic pitch scale (in mels) relates to the musical pitch scales which divide the frequency range into subjective intervals such as octaves (1:2 relationships), fifths (2:3 relationships), etc. For informative reviews of musical perception, see Littler [7] and Ward [8]. A pervasive problem has been that the psychoacoustic and musical pitch scales are often at odds with one another. For example, the musical interval between 100 and 200 Hz corresponds to one octave, as does the interval from 1000 to 2000 Hz. On the other hand, the interval in mels between 100 and 200 Hz is different from the interval between 1000 and 2000 Hz (see Fig. 12.1). Obviously, however, we cannot arbitrarily dismiss one scale in favor of the other simply because they disagree. The evidence for both approaches is firmly defensible. What, then, might be the source of the differences between the psychoacoustic and musical pitch scales?

Insight into this problem was provided by Terhardt [9–12], who suggested a dichotomy between the *spectral pitch* of pure tones and the virtual pitch of tonal complexes. This concept is probably best approached by comparing psychoacoustic and musical consonance. Consonance simply means that when two sounds are presented together they result in a pleasant perception; in contrast, sounds that appear unpleasant together are dissonant. It has been shown [13–15] that consonance for pairs of pure tones depends upon the difference between the two frequencies $(f_2 - f_1)$. If the tones are relatively close in frequency there will be a sensation of "roughness" due to rapid beats between the two tones. (Beats will be discussed later in the chapter. For now, they may be thought of as a waxing and waning in the perception of two simultaneously presented tones that differ slightly in frequency.) This roughness is perceived as being unpleasant or dissonant. If the tones are far enough apart that there is no roughness, then the two tones are consonant. Thus, psychoacoustic consonance relies upon the distance in frequency between two tones. In music, however, consonance is produced by frequency intervals which are small integer ratios (e.g., 1:2, 2:3, 3:4). A complex ratio will be judged dissonant even if there is no sensation of roughness.

Let us return now to the difference between spectral and virtual pitch. While both quantities are of course related to the spectrum of the stimuli, virtual pitch goes beyond the frequency analysis to include the perception of an auditory gestalt calling upon what has been previously learned. We draw upon learned cues in the recognition of virtual pitch in the same way that we use them in Fig. 12.2 to visually synthesize a complete image of the word "hearing" from the incomplete contours. Musical pitch intervals depend upon a knowledge of the intervals between the lowest six to eight harmonics of a complex tone. This knowledge is, in turn, learned in the course of one's ongoing processing of speech. Hence, we might consider the perception of virtual pitch to be a matter of recognizing learned pitch intervals which are familiar to the pitch "processor" in the central auditory nervous system.

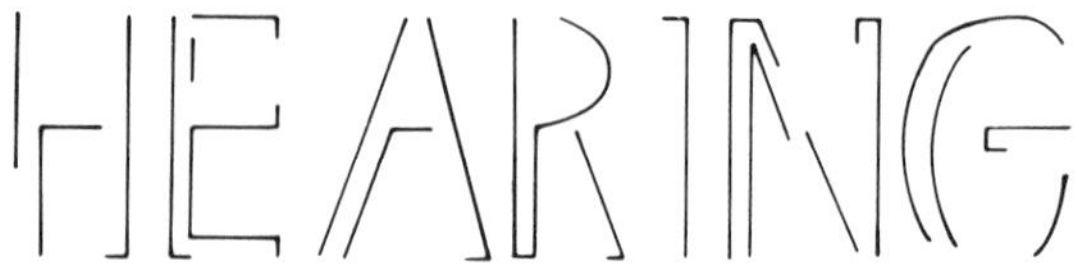

Figure 12.2 Visual analogy for the perception of virtual pitch (see text).

PITCH AND INTENSITY

Is the pitch of a tone changed by varying its intensity? To study this problem, Stevens [16] asked subjects to adjust the intensity of a tone until it had the same pitch as a standard tone of slightly different frequency. The results obtained for one subject who was a "good responder" are summarized in Fig. 12.3. As the figure shows, increasing the intensity of the tone increased its pitch for frequencies 3000 Hz and above, but lowered its pitch for frequencies 1000 Hz and below. The pitch stayed essentially constant as intensity was varied for tones be-

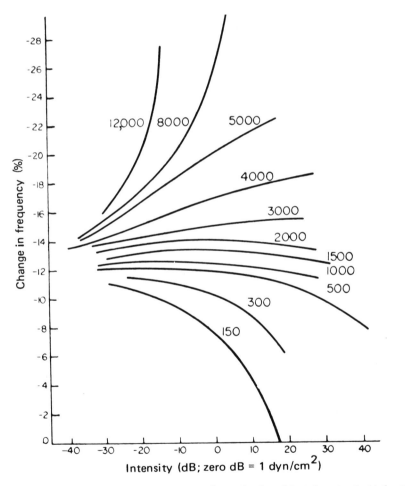

Figure 12.3 Equal pitch contours for a single subject (see text). (Adapted from Stevens [16], with permission of *J. Acoust. Soc. Am.*)

tween 1000 and 3000 Hz. Snow [17] reported that pitch changed substantially as intensity was increased for tones below about 300 Hz, but that there was little or no change between approximately 1000 and 2000 Hz.

Although the data in Fig. 12.3 are frequently cited as representative of how intensity affects pitch, subsequent studies [18–20] have failed to corroborate the large pitch changes associated with intensity increases or the universality of such observations. For example, Ward [19] studied the effect of intensity on pitch at 250 Hz, using five musicians as subjects. He found relatively large pitch changes with increasing intensity for only two subjects, whereas the other three showed essentially no change in pitch between 40 and 90 dB SPL. Furthermore, Cohen [20] found no significant differences in pitch as intensity was increased for low frequencies, and pitch changes of only 2% or less for high frequencies. It thus appears that one set of "representative" curves cannot be used to show how pitch is affected by intensity, and that changes that do occur are rather small.

BEATS, HARMONICS, AND COMBINATION TONES

We have seen in several contexts that a pure tone stimulus will result in a region of maximal displacement along the basilar membrane according to the place principle. Now, suppose that a second tone is added whose frequency f_2 is slightly different from that of the first sinusoid (f_1), as in Fig. 12.4. If the frequency difference between the two tones (f_2-f_1) is

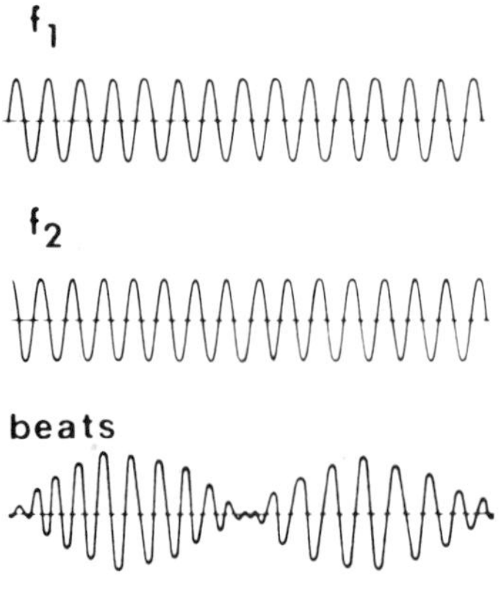

f_1

f_2

beats

Figure 12.4 Tones of slightly different frequency, f1 and f2, result in beats which fluctuate (wax and wane) at a rate equal to the difference between them (f2–f1). See text.

small (say, 3 Hz), then the two resulting excitation patterns along the cochlear partition will overlap considerably, so that the two stimuli will be indistinguishable. However, the small frequency difference between the two tones will cause them to be in phase and out of phase cyclically in a manner that repeats itself at a rate equal to the frequency difference $f_2 - f_1$. Thus, a combination of a 1000 Hz tone and a 1003 Hz tone will be heard as a 1000 Hz tone that waxes and wanes in level (beats) at a rate of three times per second. This perception of aural beats therefore reflects the limited frequency-resolving ability of the ear.

If the two tones are equal in level, then the resulting beats will alternate between maxima that are twice the level of the original tones and minima that are inaudible due to complete out-of-phase cancellation. Such beats are aptly called "best beats." Tones which differ in level result in smaller maxima and incomplete cancellation. As one would expect, the closer are the levels of the two tones, the louder the beats will sound.

As the frequency difference between the two tones widens, the beats become faster. These rapid amplitude fluctuations are perceived as "roughness" rather than as discernible beats, as discussed earlier in the chapter. Further widening of the frequency separation results in the perception of the two original tones, in addition to which a variety of combination tones may be heard. Combination tones, as well as aural harmonics, are the result of nonlinear distortion in the ear.

A simple example demonstrates how nonlinear distortions produce outputs which differ from the inputs. Consider two levers, one rigid and the other springy. The rigid lever represents a linear system. If one moves one arm of this lever up and down sinusoidally (the input) then the opposite arm will also move sinusoidally (the output). On the other hand, the springy lever has a nonlinear response. A sinusoidal input to one arm will cause the other arm to move up and down, but there will also be superimposed overshoots and undershoots in the motion, due to the "bounce" of the springy lever arms. Thus, the responding arm of the lever will move with a variety of superimposed frequencies (distortion products) even though the stimulus is being applied sinusoidally. In other words, the distortion products are those components at the output of the system that were not present at the input.

The simplest auditory distortion products are aural harmonics. As their name implies, these are distortion products which have frequencies that are multiples of the stimulus frequency. For example, a stimulus freqency f_1, when presented at a high enough level, will result in aural harmonics whose frequencies correspond to $2f_1$, $3f_1$, etc. Therefore, a 500 Hz primary tone (f_1) will result in aural harmonics that are multiples of 500 Hz (1000 Hz, 1500 Hz, etc.).

If two primary tones f_1 and f_2 are presented together, nonlinear distortion will result in the production of various combination tones due to the interactions among the primaries and the harmonics of these tones. For convenience, we will call the lower-frequency primary tone f_1 and the higher one f_2. There are several frequently encountered combination tones that we shall touch upon. See Boring [21] and Plomp [22] for interesting historical perspectives, and Goldstein et al. [23] for an excellent review of the compatibility among physiological and psychoacoustic findings on combination tones.

It is necessary to devise methods that enable us to quantify the aspects of combination tones. A rather classical method takes advantage of the phenomenon of aural beats discussed above. Recall that best beats occur when the beating tones are of equal amplitudes. Generally stated, this technique involves the presentation of a "probe" tone at a frequency close enough to the combination tone of interest so that beats will occur between the combination and probe tones. Characteristics of the combination tone are inferred by varying the amplitude of the probe until the subject reports hearing best beats (i.e., maximal amplitude variations). The best beats method, however, has been the subject of serious controversy [24–27], and has been largely replaced by a cancellation technique [28–30]. The cancellation method also employs a probe tone; but in this method, instead of asking the subject to detect best beats, the probe tone is presented at the frequency of the combination tone, and its phase and amplitude are adjusted until the combination tone is cancelled. Cancellation occurs when the probe tone is equal in amplitude and opposite in phase to the combination tone. The characteristics of the combination tone may then be inferred from those of the probe tone that cancels it. A very lucid description of and comparison among all of the major methods has been provided by Zwicker [31].

Techniques such as these have resulted in various observations about the nature of combination tones. We will only mention a few. The simplest combination tones result, of course, from adding or subtracting the two primary tones. The former is the summation tone $f_1 + f_2$. For primaries of 800 Hz (f_1) and 1000 Hz (f_2), the summation tone would be 1800 Hz. We will say little about the summation tone except to point out that it is quite weak and not always audible. On the other hand, the difference tone f_2-f_1 is a significant combination tone which is frequently encountered [22]. For the above-mentioned 800 and 1000 Hz primaries, the difference tone would be 200 Hz. The difference tone is heard only when the primary tones are presented well above threshold. Plomp [22] found, despite wide differences among his subjects, that the primaries had to exceed approximately 50 dB sensation level in order for the difference tone to be detected.

The cubic difference tone $(2f_1-f_2)$ is another significant and frequently encountered combination tone [22]. For our 800 and 1000 Hz primary tones, the resulting cubic difference tone is $2(800) - 1000 = 600$ Hz. The particularly interesting aspect of the cubic difference tone is that it is audible even when the primaries are presented at low sensation levels. For example, Smoorenburg [32] demonstrated that $2f_1-f_2$ is detectable when the primaries are only 15–20 dB above threshold, although he did find variations among subjects.

When the primary tones exceed 1000 Hz, the level of the difference tone f_2-f_1 tends to be rather low (approximately 50 dB below the level of the primaries); in contrast, the difference tone may be as little as 10 dB below the primaries when they are presented below 1000 Hz [28,29, 33,34]. On the other hand, the cubic difference tone $2f_1-f_2$ appears to be limited to frequencies below the lower primary f_1, and its level increases as the ratio f_2/f_1 becomes smaller [29,30,32–34]. Furthermore, the cubic difference tone has been shown to be within approximately 20 dB of the primaries when the frequency ratio of f_2 and f_1 is on the order of 1.2 [32,33]. The student with an interest in this topic should refer as well to the work of Zwicker [31] and Humes [35,36] for insightful reviews and analyses of the nature of combination tones.

An interesting attribute of combination tones is their stimulus-like nature [23]. In other words, the combination tones themselves interact with primary (stimulus) tones as well as with other combination tones to generate beats and higher-order (secondary) combination tones, such as $3f_1-2f_2$ and $4f_1-3f_2$. Goldstein et al. [23] have shown that such secondary combination tones have properties similar to those of combination tones generated by the primaries. Interestingly, Goldstein et al. demonstrated that secondary combination tones generated by the interaction of the cubic difference tone $2f_2-f_2$ and a third primary (stimulus) tone were obliterated when $2f_1-f_2$ was cancelled. This result, of course, supports the concept that combination tones actually exist as distinct entities within the cochlea once they have been generated by nonlinear processes. The exact nature(s) of these distortion process(es) have yet to be unquestionably established.

COMPLEX TONES AND PERIODICITY PITCH

We generally think of the pitch of a sound as being dependent upon the frequencies at which energy is physically present. Thus, high-frequency energy would be associated only with high pitch, as predicted by the place principle. However, we have also seen (Chap. 5) that auditory neurons fire in synchrony with the period of a tone for frequencies up to about 1100 Hz, and that statistically significant phase locking occurs for frequencies as high as approximately 5000 Hz, regardless of the neurons's characteristic frequency. On this basis, we should not be surprised to find that pitch perception may be based upon temporal factors (periodicity) as well as upon the coding of frequency by place (see also Chap. 2).

Pitch perception based upon the periodicity of the stimulus waveform is descriptively called periodicity pitch. For reasons that will become readily apparent, it is also known as residue pitch, low pitch, and repetition pitch, and by other such terms. Periodicity pitch was first described in 1841 by Seebeck [37]. His observations of a temporally based pitch were inconsistent with the popular resonance theory, and the furor that ensued has been described by Schouten [38], who reintroduced the phenomenon in 1940.

The manner in which periodicity results in a perception of pitch was shown rather clearly in an experiment by Thurlow and Small [40]. They found that if a high-frequency tone is interrupted periodically, then the subject will perceive a pitch corresponding to the frequency whose period is equal to the interruption rate. Thus, if the high-frequency tone is interrupted every 10 msec (the period of a 100 Hz tone), then subjects will match the pitch of the interrupted high-frequency tone to that of a 100 Hz tone. Perhaps the best-known example of periodicity pitch is the perception of the "missing fundamental" [37,38]. Consider a complex periodic tone containing energy only above 1200 Hz, spaced as shown in Fig. 12.5a. This power spectrum shows energy at 1200 Hz, 1400 Hz, 1600 Hz, etc., all of which are higher harmonics of 200 Hz. Thus, there is no energy available to stimulate the more apical area of the basilar membrane, which would respond to the 200 Hz fundamental frequency. Nevertheless, subjects presented with this complex tone will match its pitch to that of a 200 Hz tone. In other words, the pitch of this complex periodic tone corresponds to its fundamental frequency (200 Hz) even though no energy is physically present at that frequency. It appears that the auditory system is responding to the period of the complex periodic tone (5 msec), which results in a pitch perception based upon that period (1/5 msec = 200 Hz). If the components were separated by 100 Hz (i.e., 2000, 2100, 2200, 2300 Hz), then the waveform would have a period of 10 msec, corresponding to 100 Hz. With a large enough number of harmonics, periodicity pitches can be perceived as high as roughly 1400 Hz [41,42].

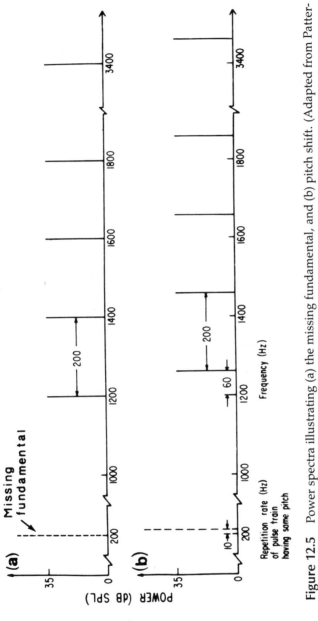

Figure 12.5 Power spectra illustrating (a) the missing fundamental, and (b) pitch shift. (Adapted from Patterson [39], with permission of *J. Acoust. Soc. Am.*)

We might now ask which harmonics are most important in determining the pitch of complex tones. The results of several classic experiments by Plomp [41] and Ritsma [43,44] indicated that roughly the first three to five harmonics provide this information. It is understandable, in view of the nature of the critical bandwidth, that the higher harmonics will contribute less than the lower ones. Recall that the critical band widens as frequency increases. Thus, the lower harmonics will fall more than a critical bandwidth apart, so that they will be perceived separately from one another. However, the higher harmonics will fall within a (wider) critical bandwidth of each other, so that they will not contribute separately to the pitch of the complex tone. More recently, frequency difference limen and pitch matching experiments by Moore and colleagues [45,46] confirmed that the lowest several harmonics are the dominant ones in a complex sound; and also demonstrated that an harmonic which has a substantially higher level than its neighbors can dominate the pitch of the complex sound.

An especially interesting observation is the pitch shift of the missing fundamental [38,39,47–51]. Suppose we have a complex periodic tone composed of exact harmonics of 200 Hz, as in Fig. 12.5a (1200 Hz, 1400 Hz, 1600 Hz, etc.). The resulting missing fundamental has a pitch of 200 Hz. Interestingly, if the frequencies making up the complex are increased to, say, 1260 Hz, 1460 Hz, 1660 Hz, etc. (Fig. 12.5b), then there will be a slight increase (shift) in the pitch of the missing fundamental, even though these frequencies are still all multiples of 200 Hz. In the first case, the harmonics are exact multiples of 200 Hz, so that there is exactly 5 msec between equivalent peaks (Fig. 12.6) in the fine structure of the

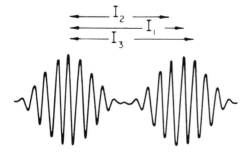

Figure 12.6 Comparison of the interval I_1 between equivalent peaks on repetitions of a waveform. Pitch ambiguity results when the pitch-extracting mechanism compares the peak of one repetition to peaks not equivalent to it on the next repetition of the waveform (I_2 and I_3). (From Schouten et al., [47], with permission of *J. Acoust. Soc. Amer.*)

repeated waveform. The upward shift of the harmonics by 60 Hz results in a slightly shorter interval between the equivalent peaks as the waveform is repeated, so that the pitch shifts upwards a bit. Ambiguities of pitch would result when the nearly but not exactly equivalent peaks are compared, as in the figure.

This fine structure or "peak picking" explanation was suggested by Schouten and colleagues [38,47], and by deBoer [48], among others. A problem, however, is that a mechanism that picks out aspects of the fine structure requires that phase changes must alter the pitch of the complex waveform. Unfortunately, there is considerable disagreement in the literature [39,49–55] as to whether the phase of a complex tone affects its pitch or timbre. It probably does not. (We may define timbre as those aspects of a complex sound's spectral content that enable us to differentiate, say, between middle C played on a violin, a piano, and a French horn. Plomp [56] defines timbre as the sensory attribute that enables one to judge differences between complex sounds having the same pitch, loudness, and duration.)

In light of this conclusion, Whightman [55] has suggested a mathematical model explaining these aspects of pitch on the basis of pattern recognition. Pattern recognition may be thought of as the extraction of those similar attributes of a stimulus which allow it to be recognized as a member of a class in spite of variations in details. For example, the letter "A" is recognized whether it is printed upper- or lowercase, in italics, or even in this author's illegible penmanship (see Fig. 12.2). In Whightman's model the waveform is first coarsely analyzed at a peripheral level, and the result is then subjected to a Fourier analysis. The resulting neural pattern is examined by a pitch extractor that looks for important features shared by stimuli having the same pitch. The details of the model are of course well beyond the current scope; the reader is referred to Plomp [56,57], Ritsma [58], and Whightman [50,55] for detailed reviews of such models.

Place theory would suggest that the missing fundamental is due to energy present at the fundamental frequency as a result of distortions. In other words, the difference tone f_2-f_1 missing fundamental since, for example, $1100 - 1000 = 100$ Hz. However, this supposition is quite unlikely because the missing fundamental differs from combination tones in several dramatic ways. For example, the missing fundamental is heard at levels as low as about 20 dB of SPL [40,59] whereas difference tones are not heard until the primary tones are presented at levels of 60 dB SPL or more [6,22]. Furthermore, if a probe tone is presented to a subject at a frequency close to a difference tone (which is actually represented at a place along the basilar membrane), then aural beats are heard. However, beats do not occur when the probe is added to the missing fundamental [38].

Even stronger evidence against the supposition that the missing fundamental is the result of energy at the apex of the cochlea due to distortions (or other means) comes from masking studies [59–61]. These experiments demonstrated that masking of the frequency range containing the missing fundamental does not obliterate its audibility. In other words, real low-frequency tones and difference tones can be masked, but the missing fundamental cannot be. Of course, this result supports a neural basis for periodicity pitch perception.

The concept that the missing fundamental results from an interaction among the harmonics within the cochlea is further weakened by studies which preclude this by using dichotic stimulation [62] or by presenting the harmonics sequentially rather than simultaneously [65]. Dichotic stimulation refers to the presentation of different stimuli to the two ears (see Chap. 13). Houtsma and Goldstein [62] presented one harmonic to each ear and asked their subjects to identify melodies based upon the perception of missing fundamentals. If the missing fundamental were really the result of interacting harmonics in the cochlea, then the subjects in this dichotic experiment would not hear it because only one tone was available to each cochlea. They found that the missing fundamental was perceived when the harmonics were presented separately to the two ears. This finding indicates that the phenomenon occurred within the central auditory nervous system, since this is the only region where the harmonics were simultaneously represented.

More recently, Hall and Peters [65] showed that subjects could hear the missing fundamental when presented with three harmonics one after the other rather than simultaneously. Their stimuli were sequences of three harmonics (e.g., 600, 800, and 1000 Hz) each lasting 40 msec and separated by 10 msec pauses. An interaction among the harmonics was precluded because they were present at different times. These stimuli were presented alone (in quiet) and also in the presence of a noise. Pitch discrimination and matching tests revealed that their subjects heard the pitches of the harmonics in quiet, but that they heard the missing fundamental in noise. They argued that the presence of the noise made it difficult for the auditory system to operate in an "analytic mode," i.e., to extract unambiguous spectral information. It thus switched to a "synthetic mode," in which the analysis time is increased. This enabled the combining of information (from different frequency locations) over time, so that the missing fundamental can be heard. In any case, the residue pitch was perceptible without the interaction of the component harmonics.

Just the surface layer of the topic of pitch perception, and only a fleeting allusion to pitch perception models, have been covered here. There are several works that the interested reader should consult for an in-depth understanding of pitch and the models of its perception [e.g., 9–12,63,64,66–69]. The overall topic is covered extensively in a recent review by Moore and Glasberg [68].

REFERENCES

1. S. S. Stevens, J. Volkmann, and E. B. Newman, A scale for the measurement of the psychological magnitude pitch, *J. Acoust. Soc. Amer. 8*, 185–190 (1937).
2. S. S. Stevens and J. Volkmann. The relation of pitch to frequency: A revised scale, *Amer. J. Psych. 53*, 329–353 (1940).
3. J. Beck and W. A. Shaw, Magnitude estimations of pitch. *J. Acoust. Soc. Amer. 34*, 92–98 (1962).
4. J. Beck and W. A. Shaw, Single estimates of pitch magnitude. *J. Acoust. Soc. Amer. 35*, 1722–1724 (1963).
5. B. Scharf, Critical bands, in *Foundations of Modern Auditory Theory* (J. V. Tobias, ed.), Vol. I, Academic Press, New York, 1970, pp. 157–202.
6. G. Bekesy, *Experiments in Hearing*, McGraw-Hill, New York, 1960.
7. T. S. Littler, *The Physics of the Ear*, Pergamon, London 1965.
8. W. D. Ward, Musical perception, in *Foundations of Modern Auditory Theory* (J. V. Tobias, ed.), Vol. I, Academic Press, New York, 1970, pp. 405–447.
9. E. Terhardt, Pitch, consonance, and harmony. *J. Acoust. Soc. Amer. 55*, 1061–1069 (1974).
10. E. Terhardt, Calculating virtual pitch, *Hearing Research 1*, 155–182 (1979).
11. E. Terhardt, G. Stoll, and M. Seewann, Pitch of complex signals according to virtual-pitch theory: Tests, examples, and predictions, *J. Acoust. Soc. Am. 71*, 671–678 (1982a).
12. E. Terhardt, G. Stoll, and M. Seewann, Algorithm for extraction of pitch and pitch salience from complex tonal signals, *J. Acoust. Soc. Am. 71*, 679–688 (1982b).
13. R. Plomp and W. J. M. Levelt, Tonal consonance and critical bandwidth. *J. Acoust. Soc. Amer. 38*, 548–560 (1965).
14. R. Plomp and H. J. M. Steeneken, Interference between two simple tones, *J. Acoust. Soc. Amer. 43*, 883–884 (1968).
15. A. Kameoka and M. Kuriyagawa, Consonance theory. Part I: Consonance of dyads. *J. Acoust. Soc. Amer. 45*, 1451–1459 (1969).
16. S. S. Stevens, The relation of pitch to intensity. *J. Acoust. Soc. Amer. 6*, 150–154 (1935).
17. W. B. Snow, Changes of pitch with loudness at low frequencies. *J. Acoust. Soc. Amer. 8*, 14–19 (1936).
18. C. T. Morgan, W. R. Garner, and R. Galambos, Pitch and intensity. *J. Acoust. Soc. Amer. 23*, 658–663 (1951).

19. W. D. Ward, The subjective octave and the pitch of pure tones, Ph.D. Dissertation, Harvard University, Cambridge, Mass., 1953.

20. A. Cohen, Further investigations of the effects of intensity upon the pitch of pure tones, *J. Acoust. Soc. Amer. 33*, 1363–1376 (1961).

21. E. G. Boring, *Sensation and Perception in the History of Experimental Psychology*, Appleton-Century, New York, 1942.

22. R. Plomp, Detectability threshold for combination tones. *J. Acoust. Soc. Amer. 37*, 1110–1123 (1965).

23. J. L. Goldstein, G. Buchsbaum, and M. Furst, Compatability between psychophysical and physiological measurements of aural combination tones, *J. Acoust. Soc. Amer. 63*, 474–485 (1978).

24. M. Lawrence and P. J. Yantis, Onset and growth of aural harmonics in the overloaded ear, *J. Acoust. Soc. Amer. 28*, 852–858 (1956).

25. M. F. Meyer, Aural harmonics are fictitious. *J. Acoust. Soc. Amer. 29*, 749 (1957).

26. R. Chocolle and J. P. Legouix, On the inadequacy of the method of beats as a measure of aural harmonics. *J. Acoust. Soc. Amer. 29*, 749–750 (1957).

27. M. Lawrence and P. J. Yantis, In support of an "inadequate" method for detecting "fictitious" aural harmonics, *J. Acoust. Soc. Amer. 29*, 750–751 (1957).

28. E. Zwicker, Der Ungewöhnliche Amplitudengang der Nichtilinearen Vertzerrungen des Ohres, *Acoustica 5*, 67–74 (1955).

29. J. L. Goldstein, Auditory nonlinearity, *J. Acoust. Soc. Amer. 41*, 676–689 (1967).

30. J. L. Hall, Nonmonotonic behavior of distortion product $2f_1$–f_2; Psychophysical observations, *J. Acoust. Soc. Amer. 58*, 1046–1050 (1975).

31. E. Zwicker, Dependence of level and phase of the ($2f1$–$f2$)-cancellation tone on frequency range, frequency difference, and level of primaries, and subject, *J. Acoust. Soc. Am. 70*, 1277–1288 (1981).

32. G. F. Smoorenburg, Audibility region of combination tones. *J. Acoust. Soc. Amer. 52*, 603–614 (1972).

33. J. L. Hall, Auditory distortion products f_2–f_1 and $2f_1$–f_2. *J. Acoust. Soc. Amer. 51*, 1863–1871 (1972).

34. J. L. Hall, Monaural phase effect: Cancellation and reinforcement of distortion products f_2–f_1 and $2f_1$–f_2, J. Acoust. Soc. Amer. 51, 1872–1881 (1972).

35. L. R. Humes, Cancellation level and phase of the ($f2$–$f1$) distortion product, *J. Acoust. Soc. Am. 78*, 1245–1251 (1985a).

36. L. R. Humes, An excitation-pattern algorithm for the estimation of ($2f1$–$f2$) and ($f2$–$f1$) cancellation level and phase, *J. Acoust. Soc. Am. 78*, 1252–1260 (1985b).

37. A. Seebeck, Beohachtungen über einige Bedingungen der Entstehung von Tönen, *Ann. Phys. Chem. 53*, 417–436 (1841).

38. J. F. Schouten, The residue, a new concept in subjective sound analysis, *Proc. Kon. Ned. Akad. 43*, 356–365 (1940).

39. R. D. Patterson, The effects of relative phase and the number of components on residue pitch, *J. Acoust. Soc. Amer. 53*, 1565–1572 (1973).

40. W. R. Thurlow and A. M. Small, Pitch perception of certain periodic auditory stimuli, *J. Acoust. Soc. Amer. 27*, 132–137 (1955).
41. R. Plomp, Pitch of complex tones. *J. Acoust. Soc. Amer. 41*, 1526–1533 (1967).
42. B. C. J. Moore, Some experiments relating to the perception of complex tones, *Quart. J. Exp. Psych. 25*, 451–475 (1973).
43. R. J. Ritsma, Frequencies dominant in the perception of the pitch of complex tones, *J. Acoust. Soc. Amer. 42*, 191–198 (1967).
44. F. A. Bilsen and R. J. Ritsma, Repetition pitch mediated by temporal fine structure at dominant spectral regions, *Acoustica 19*, 114–116 (1967).
45. B. C. J. Moore, B. R. Glasberg, and M. J. Shailer, Frequency and intensity limens for harmonics within complex tones, *J. Acoust. Soc. Am. 75*, 550–561, (1984).
46. B. C. J. Moore, B. R. Glasberg, and R. W. Peters, Relative dominance of individual partials in determining the pitch of complex tones, *J. Acoust. Soc. Am. 77*, 1853–1860 (1985).
47. J. F. Schouten, R. Ritsma, and B. Cardozo, Pitch of the residue, *J. Acoust. Soc. Amer. 34*, 1418–1424 (1962).
48. E. deBoer, On the residue in hearing, Ph.D. Dissertation, University of Amsterdam, Amsterdam, 1956.
49. G. Smoorenburg, Pitch perception of two-frequency stimuli, *J. Acoust. Soc. Amer. 48*, 924–942 (1971).
50. F. L. Whightman, Pitch and stimulus fine structure, *J. Acoust. Soc. Amer. 54*, 397–406 (1973).
51. T. J. F. Buunen, J. M. Festen, F. A. Bilsen, and G. van den Brink, Phase effects in a three-component signal, *J. Acoust. Soc. Amer. 55*, 297–303 (1974).
52. R. C. Mathes and R. Miller, Phase effects in monaural perception. *J. Acoust. Soc. Amer. 19*, 780–797 (1947).
53. J. C. R. Licklider, Influence of phase coherence upon the pitch of complex periodic sounds. *J. Acoustic Soc. Amer. 27*, 996 (1957).
54. R. Ritsma and F. Engel, Pitch of frequency-modulated signals. *J. Acoust. Soc. Amer. 36*, 1637–1644 (1964).
55. F. L. Whightman, The pattern-transformation model of pitch. *J. Acoust. Soc. Amer. 54*, 407–416 (1973).
56. R. Plomp, Timbre as a multidimensional attribute of complex tones, in *Frequency Analysis and Periodicity Detection in Hearing* (R. Plomp and G. F. Smoorenburg, eds.), Sijtthoff, Leiden 1970, pp. 397–414.
57. R. Plomp, Auditory psychophysics, *Ann. Rev. Psych. 26*, 207–232 (1975).
58. R. Ritsma, Periodicity detection, in *Frequency Analysis and Periodicity Detection in Hearing* (R. Plomp and G. F. Smoorenburg, eds.), Sijtthoff, Leiden 1970, pp. 250–266.
59. A. M. Small and R. A. Campbell, Masking of pulsed tones by bands of noise, *J. Acoust. Soc. Am. 33*, 1570–1576 (1961).
60. J. C. R. Licklider, Periodicity pitch and plate pitch. *J. Acoust. Soc. Amer. 26*, 945 (1954).
61. R. D. Patterson, Noise masking of a change in residue pitch. *J. Acoust. Soc. Amer. 45*, 1520–1524 (1969).

62. A. J. M. Houtsma and J. L. Goldstein, The central origin of the pitch of complex tones: Evidence from musical interval recognition. *J. Acoust. Soc. Amer. 51*, 520–529 (1972).

63. J. L. Goldstein, A. Gerson, P. Srulovicz, and M. Furst, Verification of an optimal probabilistic basis of aural processing in pitch of complex tones, *J. Acoust. Soc. Amer. 63*, 486–497 (1978).

64. A. Gerson and J. L. Goldstein, Evidence for a general template in central optimal processing for pitch of complex tones, *J. Acoust. Soc. Amer. 63*, 498–510 (1978).

65. J. W. Hall and R. W. Peters, Pitch for nonsimultaneous successive harmonics in quiet and noise, *J. Acoust. Soc. Am. 69*, 509–513 (1981).

66. P. Srulovicz and J. L. Goldstein, A central spectrum model: A synthesis of auditory-nerve timing and place cues in monaural communication of frequency spectrum, *J. Acoust. Soc. Am. 73*, 1266–1276 (1983).

67. B. C. J. Moore, *An Introduction to the Psychology of Hearing, Second Edition*, Academic Press, London, 1982.

68. B. C. J. Moore and B. R. Glasberg, The role of frequency selectivity in the perception of loudness, pitch and time, in *Frequency Selectivity in Hearing* (B. C. J. Moore, ed.), Academic Press, London, 1986, pp. 251–308.

69. W. A. Yost and C. S. Watson (eds.), *Auditory Processing of Complex Sounds*, Erlbaum, New Jersey, 1987.

13

Binaural Hearing

We will now examine several aspects of binaural hearing—i.e., of hearing with two ears rather than one. We shall see that binarual hearing offers a number of important advantages over monaural hearing which have obvious implications for daily living. The binaural processing of signals clearly involves the neural interaction of inputs from the two ears (see Chaps. 5 and 6). Furthermore, the importance of relatively low-frequency signal processing which we have already seen operating in pitch perception (Chap. 12) is a recurring theme in binaural hearing.

BINAURAL SUMMATION

Although Sivian and White [1] did not find significant differences between the minimal audible field (MAF) for the better ear and binaural MAF, subsequent studies demonstrated that the intensity needed to reach threshold is lower when listening with two ears than with one. The essential finding is that, if one first corrects for any difference in monaural threshold between the two ears, so that they are equal in terms of sensation level (SL), then the binaural threshold will be approximately 3 dB better (lower) than the monaural thresholds [2–5]. For example, to correct for the difference between a monaural threshold of 11 dB in the right ear and one of 16 dB in the left, the binaural stimulus would be presented 5 dB higher in the left ear. The resulting binaural threshold would be about 3 dB below these equated monaural thresholds. Hirsh [6] refers to this threshold advantage that occurs when listening with two ears as "binaural summation at threshold." (Recall that 3 dB is a doubling of power, 10 log 2/1 = 3 dB; so that "summation" implies a 2:1 advantage). Similar binaural advantages have been demonstrated when the stimulus is white noise [7] or speech [2,3].

Loudness is also enhanced by binaural hearing. Based upon loudness level measurements, Fletcher and Munson [8] concluded that a stimulus presented at a given SPL will sound twice as loud binaurally as monaurally. "Binaural summation of loudness" [6] was shown as a function of SL by Caussé and Chavasse [9], who performed loudness balances between binaurally and monaurally presented tones. At SLs close to threshold, they found that a binaural tone had to be about 3 dB lower in intensity than a monaural tone in order to produce the same sensation of loudness. This binaural advantage increased gradually with SL so that equal loudness was produced by a binaural tone 6 dB softer than the monaural stimulus at about 35 dB SL. This difference remained essentially constant at approximately 6 dB for higher sensation levels.

Perfect binaural summation means that a sound is twice as loud binaurally as it is monaurally. That loudness summation actually occurs at the two ears was questioned by Reynolds and Stevens [10]. They found that the ratio of binaural to monaural loudness increased as a power function of stimulus level (with an exponent of approximately 0.066). Thus, although both binaural and monaural loudness increased as power functions of SPL, the rate of binaural loudness growth was steeper (exponent of 0.6) than of monaural growth (exponent 0.54). Reynolds and Stevens attributed this binaural advantage, or at least part of it, to processes in the central nervous system.

It thus appears that the nature of binaural summation is somewhat uncertain, particularly the problem of whether there is actually binaural *summation* of loudness, per se. For example, some findings have suggested that a tone is twice as loud binaurally as it is monaurally [11], whereas others have reported less than perfect binaural summation [12]. Marks [13] reported on the binaural summation of loudness for 100, 400, and 1000 Hz tones using magnitude estimation (and also loudness matches for corroboration). His findings are summarized in Fig. 13.1. The circles and squares show the loudness estimates for the left and right ears, respectively. The dotted lines show what the binaural estimates should be if summation is perfect. Notice that the actual binaural loudness estimates (shown by the triangles) fall almost exactly along the predicted functions. This indicates essentially perfect binaural summation at each frequency. More recently, Marks [14] demonstrated complete binaural summation of loudness at 1000 Hz, as revealed by a two to one ratio of the loudness of a binaural tone to the monaural one.

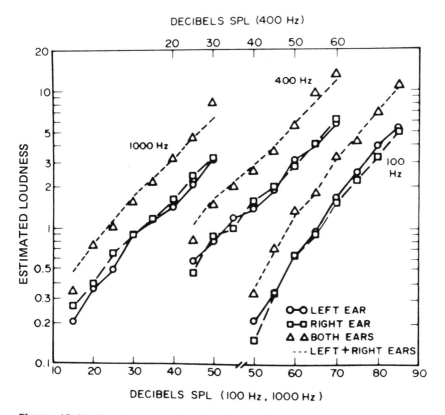

Figure 13.1 Loudness magnitude estimates for each ear and binaurally at 100, 400, and 1000 Hz. The dotted lines are predicted values for perfect summation. See text. (From Marks [13], with permission of *J. Acoust. Soc. Amer.*)

DIFFERENTIAL SENSITIVITY

Various studies suggest that differential sensitivity for both intensity [15–18] and frequency [18–20] is better binaurally than when listening with only one ear. A problem, however, has been that the small differences detected between monaural and binaural difference limens (DLs) may have been the result of loudness summation. Pickler and Harris [20] highlighted this problem. They found that the frequency DL was better binaurally than monaurally at low SLs. Recall from Chap. 9 that the effect of intensity upon differential sensitivity is greatest at low SLs, and that binaural hearing enhances sensitivity (or loudness) by roughly 3–6 dB. Thus, the smaller binaural DL may be due to summation rather than to some binaural mechanism for discrimination. To test this idea, Pickler

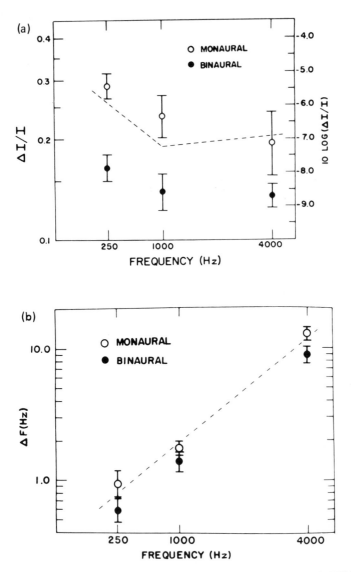

Figure 13.2 (a) Mean values of binaural and monaural $\Delta I/I$. Dotted line shows predicted monaural values from Jesteadt et al. [21]. (b) Mean binaural and monaural values of Δf. Dotted line shows predicted monaural DLs from Wier et al. [22]. (From Jesteadt et al. [18], with permission of *J. Acoust. Soc. Amer.*)

and Harris adjusted the binaural signal level to account for the loudness advantage, and also tested DLs at a high level where differential sensitivity should not be affected by intensity. In both cases the difference between monaural and binaural DLs disappeared. It was thus unclear whether the binaural DL is smaller than it is monaurally, or whether the difference just reflects a level difference.

This enigma was essentially resolved in a recent study by Jesteadt et al. [18]. They obtained intensity and frequency DLs at 70 dB SPL for 250, 1000, and 4000 Hz tones using a two-interval forced-choice method. Their results are shown in Fig. 13.2. Note that binaural differential sensitivity is uniformly better (the DL is smaller) than monaural, and that the difference is largely the same regardless of frequency. The ratio of the monaural to the binaural DL is on the order of 1.65 for intensity and 1.44 for frequency. The binaural-monaural differences obtained by Jesteadt et al. are not attributable to a loudness advantage for binaural hearing because a difference of about 30 dB would have been needed to produce the observed binaural DL advantages [18,19]; and binaural summation is equivalent to only about 3–6 dB.

BINAURAL FUSION AND BEATS

Even though the sounds of daily life reach the two ears somewhat differently in terms of time, intensity, and spectrum, we still perceive a single image. As Cherry [23] points out, we perceive one world with two ears. More precisely, the similar but nonidentical signals reaching the two ears are fused into a single, coherent image (gestalt). This process is called binaural fusion.

Binaural fusion experiments require earphone listening because this allows us to precisely control the stimuli presented to the two ears, as well as how these signals are related. Generally, the experimenter is looking for a combination of stimuli that results in a fused image lateralized to the center (midline) of the head. The essential finding is that, although completely dissimilar signals are not fused, the auditory system does achieve binaural fusion as long as the signals presented to the two ears are similar in some way [24–28]. The low frequencies, below roughly 1500 Hz, appear to be the most important. Thus, if each ear is presented with a 300 Hz tone at the same time, the subject will perceive a fused image in the center of his head.

A second example will demonstrate an important property of binaural fusion. If two different high-frequency tones are presented one to each ear, they will be heard as two separate signals. However, if a single low-frequency tone is superimposed upon both high frequencies so that they are caused to modulate at the frequency of the low tone, the listener will report a fused image [27]. This result shows that the auditory system uses the low frequency envelopes of the complex signals (their macrostructures) for fusion even though the details of the signals (their microstructures) are different. Fusion of speech can be shown to occur, for example, when only the high-frequency components of the speech waveform are directed to one ear and only the lows are presented to the other [28]. Even though neither ear alone receives enough of the speech signal for identification, the resulting fused image is readily identified.

The binaural fusion mechanism has been described in terms of a mathematical model by Cherry and Sayers [25,26]. The details of the model are beyond the current scope; however, its basis is that the central auditory nervous system carries out a running cross-correlation between the inputs to the two ears. In other words, the signals entering the ears are viewed as statistical events, and the fusion mechanism operates by looking for commonalities between the inputs coming from the two ears on an ongoing basis.

A very interesting phenomenon occurs when one tone is presented to the right ear and a second tone of slightly different frequency is presented to the left. The result is the perception of beats (see Chap. 12) in the fused image. Recall that beats occur when one combines two tones slightly different in frequency because phase differences between the tones result in alternating increases and decreases in amplitude. The intriguing aspect of binaural beats is that they occur even though the two signals are acoustically completely isolated from one another. Obviously, binaural beats must result from some interaction between the neural codings of the signals from the two ears, taking place within the central nervous system. (Cells have been identified in the superior olive that are responsive to the envelope of binaural beats [29]. They are probably at least partially involved in subserving the perception of binaural beats.)

Binaural beats differ from monaural beats in several ways [30–31]. Whereas monaural beats can be heard for interacting tones across the audible frequency range, binaural beats are associated with the lower frequencies, and the best responses are for tones between about 300 and 600 Hz. Binaural beats can still be heard even if the frequency difference between the ears is relatively wide, although the perception of the image changes with frequency separation (see below). Furthermore, binaural beats can also be perceived if there is a substantial intensity difference between the ears, and even if one of the tones is presented at a level below the behavioral threshold for that ear. (Recall from Chap. 5 that phase locking to stimulus cycle occurs at the very lowest levels at which an auditory neuron responds.)

Licklider et al. [30] reported that perceptual differences occur as the frequency separation widens between the ears. When identical frequencies are presented to two ears, the listener hears a fused image. When the frequencies are 2–10 Hz apart, the subject reports loudness fluctuations, which give way to a perception of "roughness" when the frequency difference reaches about 20 Hz. As the frequency separation becomes wider and wider, the fused image appears first to split into two smooth tones, and these tones then migrate in perceived location to the respective ears.

DIRECTIONAL HEARING

How do we determine the direction of a sound source? Intuitively, we know that some sort of comparison between the two ears must be involved.* The question is to determine what cues are used. Although we are most often concerned with binaural listening in a sound field (stereophony), we must often resort to the use of earphones to precisely control experimental conditions, as described above. Interestingly, however, stereophonic and headphone listening result in different perceptions of space. Sounds heard in a sound field seem to be *localized* in the environment. However, sounds presented thruogh a pair of earphones are perceived to come from within the head, and their source appears to be *lateralized* along a plane between the two ears. Thus, identical sounds impinging at the same time upon the two ears appear to come from directly in front of (or behind) the listener, unless he is listening through earphones, in which case the source seems to be in the center of the head. This difference between extracranial localization and intracranial lateralization is easily experienced by comparing the way the same stereo record sound through speakers and through headphones.

The basic framework of directional hearing cue was described in 1907 by Rayleigh [33]. It is often called the duplex theory because it involves interaural time differences between the ears at lower frequencies and interaural intensity differences at higher frequencies. Consider the arrangement in Fig. 13.3a, which shows the directional cues available in binaural listening. The signal from the speaker, which is off to the right, must follow a longer path to the far (left) ear than to the near (right) ear. As Fig. 13.3b shows, low frequencies have wavelengths that

---

*See Chap. 3 for a discussion of monaural and midline localization cues.

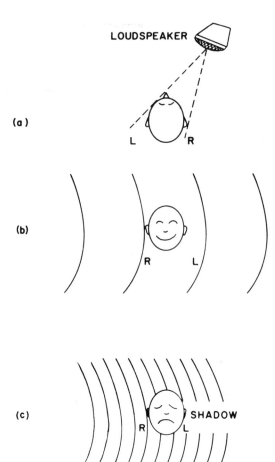

Figure 13.3 (a) Relationship between a loudspeaker and the two ears. (b) Low frequencies bend around the head due to their large wavelengths λ. (c) High frequencies have wavelengths smaller than head diameter so that an acoustic shadow results at the far ear.

are longer than the path around the head, so that they "bend around" the head to the far ear (diffraction). However, higher frequencies (Fig. 13.3c) have wavelengths smaller than the head, so that they are "blocked" in the path to the far (left) ear. This "head shadow" causes a reduction in the intensity of the signal at the far ear. We would thus expect lower frequencies to be localized on the basis of time or phase differences between the ears as the signal bends around the head;

whereas localization of high frequencies would depend upon intensity differences due to the head shadow. (Recall Fig. 3.3, which shows the effects of azimuth angle on the sound pressure at the eardrum.)

Time of arrival differences between the two ears, which we will call interaural time differences (ITDs), are useful localization cues as long as the wavelength of the tone is larger than the distance the signal must travel from the near (right) ear to the far (left) ear. The conventional approach to this issue is sometimes called the Woodworth model [34]. While it turns out that this model is contradicted by well-established findings (see below), it is covered here because it illustrates the traditional notion and is associated with Feddersen et al.'s classic study [35]. It models the head as a solid sphere around which the ear-to-ear distance approximates 22–23 cm (roughly 8.75 inches). This results in a time delay of roughly 660 μsec for the sound to get from the near ear to the far ear; which in turn corresponds to a frequency of 1500 Hz. The greatest time delay occurs when a sound source is directly to one side or the other (90° azimuth), for which the ITD would be 660 μsec. This situation is denoted by the peak of the curve in Fig. 13.4, in which the crosses are the calculated values. Below 1500 Hz, where the wavelength is greater than the distance around the head, the phase difference at the two ears results in an unequivocal localization cue. However, the phase discrepancy becomes ambiguous (except for the first wavelength) as the frequency increases to 1500 Hz, where its wavelength approximates the distance around the head, resulting in localization errors. Further increases in frequency will cause the tonal wavelength to become shorter than the size of the head. The resulting head shadow will then produce intensity differences between the ears, which we will call interaural intensity differences (IIDs). The IIDs thus provide localization cues for the higher frequencies.

Feddersen et al. [35] measured the interaural time and intensity differences for human heads as functions of angle around the head (azimuth) and frequency. The circles in Fig. 13.4 show their results for interaural time differences. Notice that there is no difference in the arrival time at the two ears when the signals (clicks) come from directly in front of the listener (0°) or directly behind (180°) since the ears are equidistant from the sound source in both cases. Interaural arrival time differences develop as the loudspeaker is moved around the head, bringing it closer to one ear than the other. The time difference between the ears increases to a maximum when the loudspeaker is directly in front of one ear (90° azimuth), where the distance (and therefore the time delay) between the ears is greatest. As the speaker continues to move around the head, the interaural time difference (ITD) becomes smaller, reaching

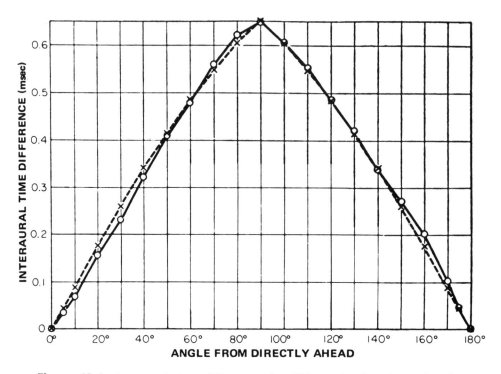

Figure 13.4 Interaural time differences for different loudspeaker azimuths. Circles are measurements of Feddersen et al. [35]. Crosses are calculated differences based on a solid sphere [34]. See text. (From Feddersen et al. [35], permission of *J. Acoust. Soc. Amer.*)

zero when the speaker is directly behind the head (180° azimuth), where once again the ears are equidistant from the sound source. Notice that the maximum ITD measured at 90° azimuth is about 660 μsec. Their values agree with the calculations based on the solid sphere model discussed above.

Subsequent observations have contradicted the predictions of Woodworth's sphere model to describe ITDs, and have shown it to be misleading. Kuhn [36] demonstrated that ITDs do not change with frequency below 500 Hz or above 3000 Hz, and that the ITDs below about 500 Hz are on the order of 800–820 μsec instead of the 660 μsec value called for by the Woodford model. His findings have been supported by experiments in cats by Roth et al. [37], and have been confirmed by the recent data of Bronkhorst and Plomp [38]. Moreover, the ITDs for the higher frequencies came close to the 660 μsec value predicted by the sphere

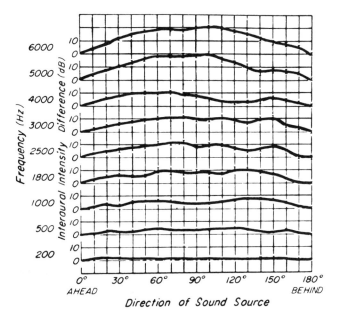

Figure 13.5 Interaural intensity differences as a function of frequency and azimuth (see text). (From Feddersen et al. [35], with permission of *J. Acoust. Soc. Amer.*)

model. Taken together with other findings [37,39,40], the implication is that the Woodworth model does not explain the nature of low frequency ITDs, but applies only to the higher frequencies and to the leading edges of clicks and click-like signals, for which the major directional cues are not the phase-derived ITDs. Moreover, a growing body of findings has demonstrated that directional hearing for high frequency complex sounds, which is known to be principally based upon IIDs (see below), is also affected by interaural time differences.*

Figure 13.5 shows the interaural intensity differences (IIDs) obtained by Feddersen et al. There were no intensity differences between the ears when the sound source was directly in front of (0°) or behind (180°) the head. However, IIDs occurred when the loudspeaker was closer to one ear than the other, with a maximum when it was directly in front of one

_____

*Discussions of these and related relevant issues, including distinctions among various types of ITDs related to acoustical properties well beyond the current scope may be found in several sources [36,37,41–45].

[handwritten margin note: IID's MAIN METHOD OF DIRECTION FINDING]

ear (90°). Note in particular that the IIDs were negligible at 200 Hz, and increased with frequency, reaching as much as 20 dB at 6000 Hz.

The importance of IIDs in high-frequency localization and of ITDs in low-frequency directionality was first demonstrated in 1907 by Lord Rayliegh [33]. However, the classic paper by Stevens and Newman [46] probably represents the first modern rigorous experimentation on directional hearing. Since echoes and reverberation (see below) introduce major complications into the localization of a sound source, Stevens and Newman sat their subjects in a chair elevated about 12 feet above the roof of the Harvard Biological Laboratories building. This made the test environment as anechoic (echo-free) as possible, by essentially removing all reflecting surfaces except for the roof below. The sound source was a loudspeaker mounted on a boom arm extended 12 feet from the listener (6 feet for low frequencies). Rotating the boom allowed the speaker to be placed at any azimuth angle. The loudspeaker was moved to the subject's right in 15° steps from 0° to 180°, and the task was to listen for the signal and report its apparent direction. We have already seen that interaural time and intensity differences are nil at 0° and 180° azimuth. This fact resulted in constant front-back reversals. Stevens and Newman therefore considered front-back reversals as correct responses; and the location of the sound source was judged relative to 0° or 180°, whichever was closer. In other words, since front and back were virtually indistinguishable, 30° right (30° off center from 0°) and 150° (30° off center from 180°) were considered to be equivalent responses. We will return to the issue of front-back confusions after discussing interaural differences.

Stevens and Newman's findings are shown as a function of frequency in Fig. 13.6. Localizations were accurate below 1000 Hz and above 4000 Hz, with the greatest errors between about 2000 and 4000 Hz. In terms of azimuth, the smallest errors were on the order of 4.6°, and occurred when the sound sources were off to one side. Furthermore, Stevens and Newman observed that noiselike sounds were better localized than tones. They attributed this result to quality (spectral) differences as well as to IIDs for the high-frequency energy in these noises.

Sandel et al. [47] asked subjects to localize sounds in an anechoic room. Their heads were held immobile to produce localization cues from head movements. Loudspeakers were placed at 0° azimuth and at 40° right and left. The stimuli were presented from one or two speakers. Two novel aspects of this study are notable. First, the use of two speakers permitted the generation of "phantom" sound sources between the speakers or off to one side, depending upon the phases of the signals. Second, an "acoustic pointer" was used to show the perceived location of the sound source. That is, the subject controlled the location of a

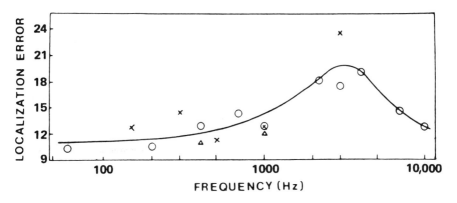

Figure 13.6 Localization error as a function of frequency. (Adapted from Stevens and Newman [46], with permission of *Amer. J. Psych.*)

speaker that rotated on a boom around his head. A noise from this speaker alternated with the presentations of the test tones. The subject indicated the perceived location of the sound source by placing the noise loudspeaker (pointer) at the same angle around his head.

There were systematic localization errors between about 1500 and 5000 Hz. When these errors were eliminated from the data, Sandel et al. found that ITDs accounted for that localization of tones below about 1500 Hz, but that the only available cues at high frequencies were IIDs. There were many random errors at 1500 Hz, showing the localization cues are ambiguous around this frequency. These results essentially confirm those of Stevens and Newman.

Before proceeding, let us briefly return to the issue of front-rear confusions, which was demonstrated by Stevens and Newman. These confusions make sense because, after all, interaural intensity or time differences are the same whether the source is before us or in the rear. Yet, we are able to tell whether sounds come from in front of us or from behind. How, then, do we know whether a sound source is in front or in back of us? The answer appears to lie in the spectral differences produced at high frequencies by the pinnae [48–50]. These effects were shown quite ludicly in recent experiments by Musicant and Butler [50]. They found that subjects could best differentiate between the front and back quadrants when the stimuli included high frequencies (above 4000 Hz), and that their performance dropped considerably when the various depressions of the pinnae were occluded. They also found that the pinna of the ear closer to the source makes the stronger contribution toward front-back localization accuracy. Front-rear localization was also possible when a low-pass noise with a 4000 Hz cutoff was used. Musicant and Butler suggested that diffraction around the torso is the most likely source of the underlying spectral differences in the latter case.

Another way to examine localization is to find the smallest difference in location between two sound sources that results in a different perceived location. Since the two sound sources are viewed relative to the head, this is the same as asking what is the smallest angle (or difference in azimuth) that a listener can discriminate. Mills [51–53] studied this phenomenon in depth, and called it the minimal audible angle (MAA). Specifically, he tested the MAA as a function of frequency when the sound sources were located in front of the subject (0°), and when they were 30°, 60°, and 75° off to the side. He found that the MAA was smallest (best) for the frequencies below about 1500 Hz and above approximately 2000 Hz, and was largest (poorest) between these frequencies. This result reflects the ambiguity of localization cues in the vicinity of 1500 Hz, thus confirming the previously mentioned findings. Mills also found that MAAs were most acute (1–2°) when the sound sources were directly in front of the head, and that they increased dramatically to very high values when the sources were at the side of the head. This result occurs because small changes in location in front of the head result in large interaural differences (especially ITDs). However, when the sources are off to one side of the head (facing one ear), the interaural differences remain largely the same in spite of reasonably large changes in angle between the loudspeakers. We might thus conceive of a "cone of confusion" (Fig. 13.7) to one side of the head, within which the interaural differences do not vary when the sound sources change location [53]. This image demonstrates the importance of head movements in localization, since these movements keep changing the position of the

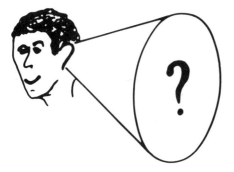

Figure 13.7   Cone of confusion (see text). (Modified after Mills [53].)

cone of confusion—the zone of ambiguity—thereby minimizing its detrimental effect.

The MAA described by Mills involved the discrimination of two stimuli presented sequentially. Perrott [54] expanded upon the concept of the MAA using stimuli that were presented at the same time, describing the concurrent minimum audible angle (CMAA). As for the MAA, the CMAA is also most acute for sound presented directly in front of the subject and least sensitive when the stimuli are presented off to one side. However, the CMAA is also affected by spectral differences between the two sounds whose locations are to be discriminated. Subjects were unable to distinguish a difference in the angular locations of the stimuli when their frequencies differed by only 15 Hz. When the signals differed in frequency by 43 Hz, the size of the CMAA increased from 4.5 degrees when the two signals were presented from 0° azimuth to an angle of about 45° when they were presented from 67° off to the left. On the other hand, signals 101 Hz apart had CMAAs which were about 10° no matter whether the two sources were from straight ahead (zero azimuth) up to 55° off center. The CMAA then increased dramatically to about 30° when these signals were presented from 67° to the left. (An intermediate relationship between CMAA and azimuth was obtained for signals differing in frequency by 72 Hz.) As Perrott has pointed out, the CMAA involves the issue of sound source identification ("what") as well as that of localization ("where"). One should refer to Perrott [54], as well as to Perrott and Musicant [55] and Perrott and Tucker [56] for further discussions of the MAA and the perception of motion.

Since earphones allow us to precisely control and manipulate the signals presented to the ears, lateralization experiments using them clarify and expand upon what we know about directional cues. Before discussing these studies, it is wise to point out a distinction between time and phase differences. Recall that low frequencies need a longer time period t than high frequencies for completion of one full cycle (period is the reciprocal of frequency, $t = 1/f$). We are concerned with the effects of delaying the onset of a stimulus at one ear relative to the other. If we impose the same delay upon three different frequencies, the delay will correspond to different phases of their cycles (Fig. 13.8). In other words, the higher the frequency, the greater the phase difference due to a given time delay. Thus, if we impose a time delay upon a broad-band noise or click, there will be more of a phase difference for the higher-frequency components of the signal than for the low.

Several studies [57–59] have examined the effects of interaural time (phase) and intensity cues upon lateralization. While exact procedures vary, the general approach is to present two stimuli to the subject that

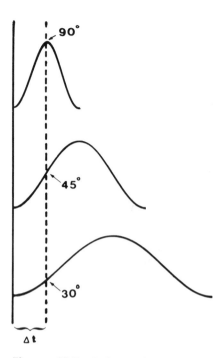

Figure 13.8 Relation between time delay Δt and phase shift for different frequencies.

differ with respect to interaural time (phase) or intensity, and to determine whether this interaural disparity results in a perceptible change in lateralization. The findings essentially agree with the localization data. That is, ITDs are most important up to about 1300 Hz, and IIDs take over as the primary lateralization cue for higher frequencies.

Yost [60] performed a particularly interesting lateralization experiment analogous to Mills' MAA studies. He presented subjects with two stimuli. The first included a particular interaural time (actually phase) difference Θ. This difference, of course, resulted in a lateralization toward one side of the head analogous to the azimuth position of the stimuli in Mills' work. The second stimulus was the same except that the phase difference between the ears was larger by a slight amount $\Delta\Theta$. Thus, it was $\Theta + \Delta\Theta$. The subjects had to detect the value of $\Delta\Theta$ by discriminating between the two stimuli (Θ versus $\Theta + \Delta\Theta$). We might think of the phase difference Θ as analogous to azimuth, and of $\Delta\Theta$ as the MAA. For any value of Θ, the smaller the value of $\Delta\Theta$ needed for a change in apparent lateralization, the better the discrimination of interaural phase. Yost's findings are summarized in Fig. 13.9. Note that $\Delta\Theta$ is smallest (best) when Θ is 0° or 360°. These values of Θ are midline lateralizations because 0° and 360° correspond to zero phase disparity between the ears. Thus, the most acute interaural phase discriminations are made at the midline. On the other hand, interaural phase discrimination was poorest ($\Delta\Theta$ was largest) when Θ was 180°, i.e., when the signals were lateralized directly to one side. These findings are consistent with the MAA data.

Fig. 13.9 also shows that $\Delta\Theta$ is essentially the same for all frequencies up to 900 Hz. Interaural phase discrimination was significantly poorer at 2000 Hz, where it was constant at about 30°. Interaural phase had no effect at all for 4000 Hz (not shown on the graph). Thus, interaural phase was shown to be an important cue at low frequencies but unimportant for high, in a manner consistent with the sound field data.

Recall that Stevens and Newman [46] found better localization accuracy for noiselike sounds than for tones. Since noises contain considerable transient information, this suggests that transient sounds provide excellent directional cues. If so, then we would expect improved lateralization as more transient cues are made available to the listener. In

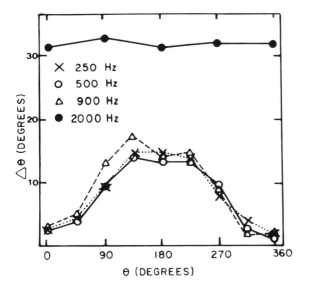

Figure 13.9 Changes in interaural phase ($\Delta\Theta$) required in order to detect a difference in lateralization from a standard (reference) phase difference (Θ). (Adapted from Yost [60], with permission of *J. Acoust. Soc. Am.*)

other words, very short-term events (e.g., clicks), which provide a transient cue only at their onset and offset, should require larger ITDs for lateralization than longer events (e.g., noises), which provide ongoing transient disparities between the ears. Klumpp and Eady [57] found that the ITD required to achieve 75% correct lateralizations was 28 μsec for a single click. The ITDs were reduced to 11 μsec for a 2 sec burst containing 30 clicks in rapid succession, and to 9–10 μsec for a 1.4 sec noise. Tobias and Zerlin [61] found smaller ITDs as the duration of a noise burst was increased from 10 msec to 700 msec. The ITD was only 6 μsec for noise bursts that lasted 700 msec or more. (Tobias [62] pointed out that this is puzzling, because synaptic delays average about 100 μsec.) Furthermore, Tobias and Schubert [63] found that very small ongoing ITDs could offset much larger onset ITDs. Thus, lateralization acuity improves substantially when ongoing transient ITDs are provided by a noise or a click train.

Klumpp and Eady [57] found that ITDs of about 10 μsec resulted in correct lateralizations of noises that contained low freqencies. However, high-frequency noise bands required substantially larger ITDs (44 μsec for 2400–3400 Hz; 62 μsec for 3056–3344 Hz). Yost et al. [64] found that the lateralization of clicks was unaffected by removing their high frequencies by filtering or masking. Removing the low-frequency components, however, substantially interfered with the correct lateralization of the clicks.

Lateralization experiments have revealed that discrimination for IIDs is constant as a function of frequency within a range of about 2 dB, but with a curious increase in the size of the IID at 1000 Hz [45,65,66]. These findings are illustrated in Fig. 13.10 from a recent study by Yost and Dye [45]. The excellent interaural level discrimination at high frequencies is expected from the previous discussion, and would be capitalized upon in the real world as a consequence of the level differences produced by the head shadow. However, the acute interaural level discrimination for low frequencies may be somewhat confusing. In order to explain this, Grantham [66] suggested that the low frequency intensity cues might be converted into time information by a threshold-latency mechanism [cf., 72, 120]. The "bump" in the function at 1000 Hz would the reflect the transition from one process to the other. In other words, interaural level discrimination becomes slightly poorer around 1000 Hz because the frequency is too high for maximum utilization of the threshold-latency based timing information, and too low to make optimal use of the intensity differences.

Three sets of findings are shown in Fig. 13.10, depending upon whether the standard stimulus against which the discrimination was

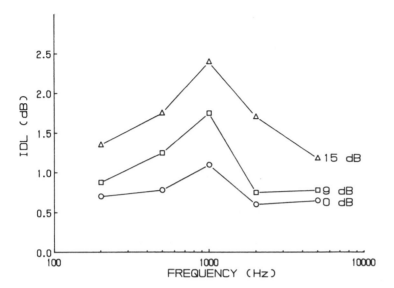

Figure 13.10   Thresholds for interaural differences in level (IDL) in dB as a function of frequency from 200–5000 Hz. (Note that the scale of the ordinate is from 0–2.5 dB.) These findings were obtained when the standard stimulus itself was lateralized at midline (circles, marked 0 dB), halfway between midline and the left ear (squares, marked 15 dB), and at the left ear (triangles, marked 15 dB). The 0, 9, and 15 dB values are the interaural intensity differences needed to place the standard image at these locations (see text). (From Yost and Dye [45], with permission of *J. Acoust. Soc. Am.*)

made was itself heard (lateralized) at the midline, halfway between midline and the left ear, or at the left ear. These three lateralizations of the standards signal were achieved by using IIDs of 0, 9 and 15 dB, respectively [67]. A comparison of these three curves makes it clear that IID discrimination is most acute at midline (circles, labeled 0 dB), is least sensitive when the standard is lateralized off to one side (triangles, labeled 15 dB), and is at some intermediate value when the discrimination is made between the midline and at the left ear (squares, labeled 9 dB).

Transient energy is also associated with the onset and offset of tone bursts. Yost [68] found that this transient energy enabled his subjects to lateralize a high-frequency (4050 Hz) tone burst on the basis of an ITD (71 μsec). Low-pass filtering did not detract from this performance; but the 4050 Hz tone burst could not be lateralized when the low-frequency segments of the associated transient were filtered out. The experiments show the importance of low-frequency information in the lateralization of wide-band and transient signals. It is interesting to note at this point that ITDs can subserve lateralizations of high-frequency tones if they are modulated by a lower frequency. Henning [69] demonstrated that a 3900 Hz tone can be lateralized on the basis of ITDs if it is modulated at 300 Hz. In this case, it appears that the lateralization is based upon the 300 Hz envelope rather than the 3900 Hz carrier tone.

TIME-INTENSITY TRADES

Having seen that both interaural time and intensity differences serve as lateralization cues, we might ask whether there is a trading relationship between them. In other words, can an ITD favoring one ear be offset by an IID favoring the other? This area has been extensively studied because of its theoretical implications.

Individual studies have varied considerably in technique. However, the basic experiment is to vary the interaural intensity of a signal in order to offset a given ITD, or vice versa. The subject's task is generally to adjust the IID (or ITD) until a midline image is perceived. A standard comparison signal presented without interaural differences may be used as a midline marker to assist the subject in achieving the lateralization.

Time-intensity trading studies are marked by inconsistent results between subjects. This fact, plus the nature of the findings, draws us to conclude that lateralization is actually a complex process rather than a simple interaction of time and intensity cues. Harris [70] performed time-intensity trades for high- and low-pass filtered clicks. Instead of a consistent trading ratio, he observed a ratio of 25 μsec/dB for clicks containing energy below 1500 Hz, and of 90 μsec/dB for clicks containing above 1500 Hz. In another study, Moushegian and Jeffress [71] found that the trading ratio for a 500 Hz tone was about 20–25 μsec/dB for two subjects but only on the order of 2.5 μsec/dB for another subject.

A series of experiments by Jeffress, Hafter, and colleagues [72–75] has contributed substantially to our understanding of the lateralization mechanism. For a variety of stimuli, these workers found that subjects often reported two lateralized images instead of just one. Furthermore, the two images are associated with different trading ratios. One image is particularly dependent upon ITDs (especially for frequencies below 1500 Hz), but is essentially unaffected by IIDs. This is the "time image." The other is an "intensity image" that is responsive to both IIDs and ITDs at all audible frequencies. Typical trading ratios (click stimuli) are on the order of 2–35 μsec/dB for the time image and 85–150 μsec/dB for the intensity image [73]. It may be that the large intersubject differences reported by Harris [70] and by Moushegian and Jeffress [71] were due to responses to the time image by some subjects and to the intensity image by others.

A rather straightforward mechanism was proposed by Jeffress and McFadden [74] for the two lateralization images. In this model, the time image depends upon a comparison of the signals at the two ears on a cycle-by-cycle basis—i.e., it depends on an interaural comparison of the fine structures of the signals. The intensity image, on the other hand, depends upon a comparison of the envelopes (gross structures) at the two ears. In this case, the amplitudes of the peaks of the waveform envelopes serve as the interaural intensity cues, and the ITDs between envelope peaks are the timing cues. We have already seen that neurons in the auditory nerve respond to both stimulus intensity and cycle (Chap. 5), and that brainstem neurons are responsive to ITDs and/or IIDs (Chap. 6). This situation provides a neurophysiological basis for the two mechanisms.

PRECEDENCE EFFECT, LOCALIZATION, AND REVERBERATION

Consider two apparently unrelated situations. The first involves listening to a monaural record album or a news broadcast through both speakers of a home stereo system. Thus, identical signals are coming from both speakers. Sitting equidistant from the speakers causes us to perceive a phantom sound source between them. However, sitting closer to one speaker (so that the signal reaches our ears sooner from that direction than the other) gives us the impression that all of the sound is coming from the closer speaker. This occurs even though the other speaker is still on.

The second situation involves listening to someone talking in a hard-walled room. The sounds reaching our ears will be composed of the direct sound from the talker's lips plus reflections of these sounds from the walls. Because they take an indirect route (via the walls), the reflected sounds reach our ears later and from different directions than the direct sound. Nevertheless, we localize the sound source based on the direction of the direct sound, not the reflections. In addition, although the reflections will "color" the quality of what we hear, we perceive only the earlier-arriving direct sound. (This applies to reflections arriving within a certain time after the direct sound. Longer-lasting reflections are perceived as reverberation, and discrete reflections arriving a certain time after the direct sound are heard as echoes. We shall discuss this further below.)

These situations illustrate the precedence effect, also known as the Haas phenomenon and the principle of the first wavefront. As a broad generality, the precedence effect states that within a certain time frame, the earlier-arriving signal (wavefront) will dominate over a later-arriving signal (e.g., echo) in determining what we hear. This effect was first described in detail by Wallach et al. [76] and Haas [77,78] in 1949, although it had been known for some time earlier [79].

The classic experiment by Wallach et al [76] illustrates the precedence effect. Figure 13.11 shows two clicks (A and B) delivered to the left ear and two others (C and D) presented to the right ear. The entire set of clicks was presented within 2 msec, so that they were perceived as a single fused image. Notice that there are two opposing ITDs at the onset and offset of the composite signal. The onset disparity t_1 favors the left ear, whereas the offset time difference t_2 favors the right. The question is which of these opposing ITDs is more important in lateralizing the fused image. The onset disparity t_1 was set to a certain interval so that the click would be lateralized left, and then the offset disparity t_2 was adjusted to give a centered image. If t_1 and t_2 were equally important directional cues, then a centered image would occur when the two delays were equal ($t_1 = t_2$). However, Wallach et al. found that a much larger offset delay t_2 was needed to overcome a small onset delay t_1. For example, t_2 had to be about 400 μsec to counteract an opposing t_1 of about 50 μsec. This result demonstrates the importance of the first arriving signal in determining the location of the sound source. The precedence effect was maintained even if the level of the second click pair was as much as 15 dB greater than the first.

The findings just described were obtained as long as the interval t_3 between the click pairs was from 2 to 40 msec, depending on the stimuli. Longer durations of t_3 caused the subject to hear two separate signals, one at each ear.

Haas [77,78] presented speech stimuli from two loudspeakers. If the signal from one speaker was delayed up to 35 msec, then the stimulus was perceived to come only from the leading loudspeaker. Longer delays caused the listener to detect the presence of the second (delayed) sound, although the signal was still localized toward the leading side.

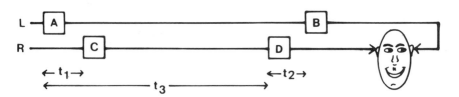

Figure 13.11   The precedence effect (see text).

Delays longer than about 50 msec caused the listener to hear a distinct echo from the second loudspeaker. Thus, these findings correspond to the effect of the intervals t_3 in the study of Wallach et al.

The precedence effect serves us not only in sound source localization, but also by suppressing the effects of reflections arriving soon after the direct sound. This occurs because the reflections are integrated with the direct sound into a single fused image, at least for delays up to about 30 msec. These reflections would otherwise interfere with our perception of the direct sound, and particularly with speech intelligibility. This was demonstrated by Lochner and Burger [80], who found that speech discrimination was unaffected by reflections arriving up to 30 msec after the direct sound. However, later-arriving reflections were not integrated with the direct sounds, and resulted in reduced intelligibility. Similarly, Nabelek and Robinette [81] found that speech recognition was reduced by single echoes arriving 20 msec or more after the direct stimulus. Reflections that arrive beyond the time when the precedence effect is operative result in distortions of the speech signal because they tend to mask the direct signal [81–84]. Gelfand and Silman [84] found that the speech sound confusions associated with small-room reverberation were similar to those associated with masking or filtering of the speech signal. This result confirms that the reflections distort the speech signal via a masking mechanism.

MASKING LEVEL DIFFERENCES *(READ FOR EXAM)*

The term "masking level difference" (MLD) may be a bit confusing at first glance. Obviously it refers to some sort of difference in masking. Let us see how. Consider a typical masking experiment (Chap. 10) in which a signal S is barely masked by a noise N. This can be done in one ear (monotically), as in Fig. 13.12a, or by presenting an *identical* signal and noise to both ears (diotically), as in Fig. 13.12b. Identical stimuli are obtained by simply directing the output of the same signal and noise sources to both earphones (in phase). For brevity and clarity, we will adopt a shorthand to show the relationships among the stimuli and ears. The letter "m" will denote a monotic stimulus and "o" will refer to a diotic stimulus. Thus, SmNm indicates that the signal and noise are presented to one ear, and SoNo means that the same signal and the same noise are simultaneously presented to both ears. Either of these conditions can be used as our starting point.

Suppose that we add an identical noise to the unstimulated ear of Fig. 13.12a, so that the signal is still monotic but the noise is now diotic (SmNo), as in Fig. 13.12c. Oddly enough, the previously masked signal

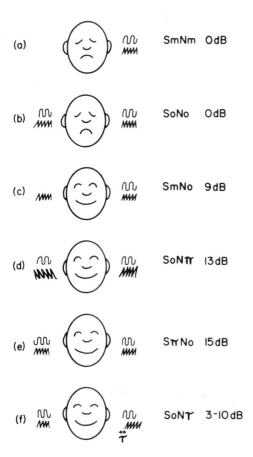

(a)   SmNm   0 dB

(b)   SoNo   0 dB

(c)   SmNo   9 dB

(d)   SoNπ   13 dB

(e)   SπNo   15 dB

(f)   SoNτ   3-10 dB

Figure 13.12   Masking level differences (MLDs) for various conditions.

now becomes audible again! Starting this time from the masked situation
in Fig. 13.12b (SoNo), we can make the signal audible again by reversing
the phase of (inverting) the noise between the ears (Fig. 13.12d) or by
reversing the phase of the signal between the ears (Fig. 13.12e). The
phase reversal is indicated by the Greek letter π, since the stimuli are
now 180° (or one radian, π) out of phase between the ears. (The phase
reversal is accomplished by simply reversing the + and − poles at one of
the earphones.) These new conditions are thus called SoNπ and SπNo,
respectively. Note that the binaural advantage occurs only when the
stimuli are in some way *different* at the two ears (dichotic). These fascinat-
ing observations were first reported in 1948 by Hirsh [85] for tonal signals and by Licklider [86] for speech.

MASKING LEVEL DIFFERENCE

We may now define the MLD as the difference (advantage) in masked threshold between dichotically presented stimuli and signals that are presented monotically (or diotically). It is not surprising to find that the MLD is also referred to as binaural unmasking, as binaural release from masking, or as the binaural masking level difference (BMLD). We shall express the magnitide of the MLD as the difference in dB between a particular dichotic arrangement and either the SmNm or SoNo conditions. Other MLD conditions are discussed below.

The size of the MLD varies from as large as about 15 dB for the SπNo condition [87] to as little as 0 dB, depending upon a variety of parameters. Typical MLD magnitudes associated with various dichotic arrangements [88] are shown in Fig. 13.12. It is a universal finding that the MLD becomes larger as the spectrum level of the masking noise is increased, especially when the noise is presented to both ears (No) at the same level [85, 89–92].

The largest MLDs are obtained when either the signal (SπNo) or the noise (SoNπ) is opposite in phase at the two ears. The large MLDs obtained from these antiphasic conditions have been known since it was first described [85] in 1948, and have been repeatedly confirmed [93,94]. Recall from Chap. 5 that the firing patterns of auditory nerve fibers are phase-locked to the stimulus, particularly at low frequencies. Thus, the large MLDs associated with antiphasic conditions may be related to this phase-locking in the neural coding of the stimuli [87]. Furthermore, since the degree of phase-locking is greatest at low frequencies, and decreases as frequency becomes higher, we would expect the size of the MLD to be related to stimulus frequency as well.

Figure 13.13 shows the relationship between MLD size and stimulus frequency for a variety of studies, as summarized by Durlach [95]. As expected, the MLD is largest for low frequencies—about 15 dB for 250 Hz—and decreases for higher frequencies until a constant of about 3 dB is maintained about 1500–2000 Hz. (Look at the individual data points in Fig. 13.13 rather than at the smooth line, which is a statistical approximation of the actual results.) It is a bit intriguing to observe that the MLD (at least for SπNo) does not fall to zero above 1500 Hz, since we have seen that phase information is essentially useless for high frequencies. However, these findings have been confirmed repeatedly [85,96–100]. One is drawn to recall in this context that statistically significant phase-locking is maintained as high as 5000 Hz (Chap. 5).

There is very good agreement about the size of the MLD for the frequencies above 250 Hz. At lower frequencies there is a great deal of variation in the MLD sizes reported by different studies [85,91,96,98,101]. This is shown in Fig. 13.13 by the substantial spread among the data

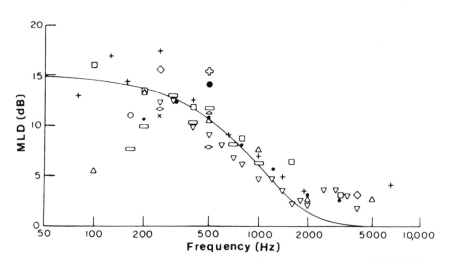

Figure 13.13 Magnitude of the MLD ($S_\pi N_0 - S_0 N_0$) as a function of frequency for many studies. [Adapted from Durlach [95], Binaural signal detection: equalization and cancellation theory, in *Foundations of Modern Auditory Theory, II* (J. V. Tobias, ed.), © 1972 by Academic Press.]

points for the lower frequencies. Much of this variation in the lower frequencies may be explained on the basis of differences in noise level. In particular, Dolan [91] showed that the MLDs at 150 and 300 Hz increase with the spectrum level of the masker, attaining a value of approximately 15 dB when the noise spectrum level is 50 dB or more. Thus, the MLD becomes rather stable once moderate levels of presentation are reached.

We have been assuming that the noises at the two ears (SoNo) are derived from the same noise source, insuring that the waveforms are exactly the same at both ears. Another way to indicate identical wave forms is to say that the noises are perfectly correlated. Had we used two separate noise generators, then the noises would no longer be perfectly correlated. We would then say that the noises are uncorrelated (Nu). Robinson and Jeffress [102] added noises from the same (correlated) and different uncorrelated generators to study how noise correlation affects the size of the MLD. They found that the MLD resulting from uncorrelated noises is on the order of 3–4 dB, and that the MLD becomes larger as the degree of correlation decreases. The MLD resulting from uncorrelated noise may contribute to our ability to overcome the effects of reverberation. This relation was demonstrated by Koenig et al. [105], who found that room reverberation decorrelates the noise reaching the two ears, resulting in an MLD of about 3 dB.

Since only a certain critical bandwidth contributes to the masking of a tone (Chap. 10), it is not surprising that the MLD also depends upon the critical band [104,105] around a tone. In fact, the MLD actually increases as the noise band narrows [106,107]. As it turns out, a very narrow band of noise looks much like a sinusoid that is being slowly modulated in frequency and amplitude. If we present such a narrow-band noise to both ears and delay the wavefront at one ear relative to the other, then the degree to which the noises are correlated will change periodically as a function of the interaural time delay.

With this in mind, consider the arrangement in Fig. 13.12f. The noises presented to the two ears are from the same generator, but the noise is delayed at one ear relative to the other (Nτ). The interaural time delay decorrelates the noises in a manner dependent upon the time delay. This situation (SoNτ) results in MLDs which are maximal when the time delay corresponds to half-periods of the signal, and minimal when the time delays correspond to the period of the signal [101,108]. Figure 13.14 shows example at several frequencies. The effect is clearest at 500 Hz. The period of 500 Hz is 2 msec, and the half-period is thus 1 msec. As the figure shows, the MLDs are largest at multiples of the half-period (in the vicinity of 1 msec and 3 msec for 500 Hz) and are smallest at multiples of the full period (about 2 msec and 4 msec for 500 Hz). Also notice that successive peaks tend to become smaller and smaller.

Licklider [86] reported MLDs for speech about the same time that the phenomenon was described for tones [85]. Interestingly enough, the unmasking of speech is associated with the MLDs for pure tones within the spectral range critical for speech perception [110–112]. This was shown quite clearly in a study by Levitt and Rabiner [111] which used monosyllabic words as the signal S and white noise as the masker N. The subjects were asked to indicate whether the test words were detectible in the presence of the noise while different parts of the speech spectrum were reversed in phase between the ears. They found MLDs (SπNo) on the order of 13 dB when the frequencies below 500 Hz were reversed in phase, indicating that the MLD for speech detection is primarily determined by the lower frequencies in the speech spectrum.

The MLD for speech detection obviously occurs at a minimal level of intelligibility. That is, a signal whose intelligibility is zero (see Chap. 14) may still be barely detectable. Increasing the presentation level of the words would result in higher intelligibility, i.e., a larger proportion of the words would be correctly repeated. The level at which half of the words are correctly repeated may be called the 50% intelligibility level; the 100% intelligibility level is the test level at which all of the words are repeated correctly. We may now note an interesting aspect of MLDs for

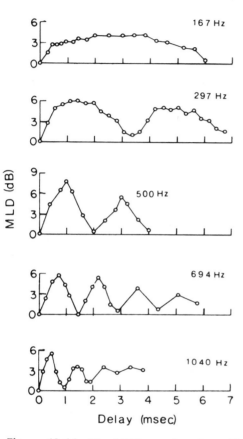

Figure 13.14 The MLD as a function of interaural time delay. (Adapted from Rabiner et al. [101], with permission of *J. Acoust. Soc. Am.*)

speech: The speech MLD is quite large at near-detection levels. However, MLDs for speech are smallest at higher presentation levels where overall intelligibility is good [88,109–112].

Levitt and Rabiner [111,112] suggested the term "binaural intelligibility level difference" (BILD or ILD) to indicate the amount of unmasking for speech intelligibility. The ILD is the difference between the levels at which a particular percentage of the test words are correctly repeated for a dichotic condition and for SoNo. Levitt and Rabiner [111] found that the ILD was on the order of only 3–6 dB for an intelligibility level of 50%. Thus, the release from masking increases from about 3 dB to 13 dB as the intelligibility level does down toward bare detection. At the lowest intelligibility level, where one can detect but not repeat the words, the ILD

MLD = MASKING LEVEL DIFFERENCE

and MLD for speech are synonymous. In this light, we may consider the MLD as the limiting case of the ILD [113].

Although the speech MLD depends on frequencies below 500 Hz, Levitt and Rabiner [111] found that the entire speech spectrum makes a significant contribution to the ILD. In a later paper [113], they presented a numerical method for predicting the ILD. The procedure assumes that the SπNo condition reduces the noise level in a manner that depends upon frequency and S/N ratio. That is, the lower frequencies are given greater relative importance at low S/N ratios where overall intelligibility is poor. This technique makes predictions which are in close agreement with the empirical data [86,109,111].

Some work has also been done on MLDs for differential sensitivity and loudness [114,115]. We shall not go into detail in these areas, except to point out that MLDs for loudness and discrimination of intensity occur mainly at near-detection levels, and become insignificant well above threshold. This situation, of course, is analogous to what we have seen for ILDs as opposed to MLDs for speech signals. However, Marks [14] recently reported that binaural loudness summation for a 1000 Hz tone under MLD-like masking conditions was substantially greater than a doubling of loudness over the monaural condition.

MLD Models

Several models [95,96,98,116–119] try to explain the mechanism of MLDs. These models do not account for all known facets of MLDs, but they do provide good explanations of the phenomenon and actually allow one to make predictions about the results of experiments as yet undone. We will take a brief look as the two most established models, the Webster-Jeffress lateralization theory [96,116] and Durlach's equalization-cancellation model [95,98].

The Webster-Jeffress theory attributes MLDs to interaural phase and intensity differences. Recall that only a certain critical band contributes to the masking of a tone, and that this limited-bandwidth concept also applies to MLDs. Basically, the lateralization model compares the test tone to the narrow band of frequencies in the noise that contribute to its masking. Changing phase between the ears (SπNo) results in a time-of-arrival difference at a central mechanism, which provides the detection cue. The vector diagrams in Fig. 13.15 show how this system might operate for SπNo versus SmNm. Figure 13.15a shows the interaction between the noise N and signal S amplitudes as vectors 7.5° apart. The resulting S + N amplitude is too small for detection. Fig. 13.15b shows the situation when the signal is reversed in phase at the two ears

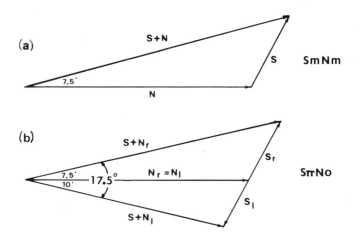

Figure 13.15 Vector diagrams for (a) SmNm and (b) S$_\pi$No (see text). [Adapted from Jeffress [116], Binaural signal detection: vector theory, in *Foundations of Modern Auditory Theory, II* (J. V. Tobias, ed.), © 1972 by Academic Press.]

(SπNo). Now, the right and left noise amplitudes are equal (N$_r$ = N$_l$), but the signal vectors for the two ears (S$_r$ and S$_l$) point in opposite directions due to the reversed phase. Thus, the signal in the right ear leads the noise in phase by 7.5° while in the left ear it lags in phase by 10°; so that the phase difference between the resulting S = N at the two ears is 17.5°. In other words, S + N at the right ear is now 17.5° ahead of that in the left. If the signal is a 500 Hz tone, this lag corresponds to a time-of-arrival advantage for the right S + N of 97 μsec. In addition, the lengths of the S + N vectors indicates an amplitude advantage which is also available as a detection cue, since the right S + N is now substantially longer (more intense) than the left. That is, the SπNo condition causes the combined S + N from the right ear to reach a central detection mechanism sooner and with greater amplitude. This causes a lateralization of the result (to

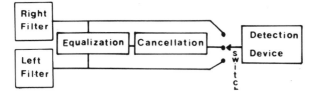

Figure 13.16 A simplified block diagram of Durlach's equalization–cancellation (EC) model.

the right in this example) which the model uses as the basis for detection of the signal.

Durlach's equalization-cancellation (EC) model is shown schematically in Fig. 13.16. The stimuli pass through critical band filters at the two ears, and then follow both monaural and binaural routes to a detection device, which decides whether the signal is present. The detection device switches between the three possible channels (two monaural and one binaural), and will use the channel with the best S/N ratio as the basis for a response. The monaural channels go straight to the detection mechanism. The binaural channel, however, includes two special stages.

In the first stage, the inputs from the two ears are adjusted to be equal in amplitude (the equalization step). Then the inputs from the two ears are subtracted one from the other in the cancellation step.* Of course, if the signal and noise were identical in both ears (SoNo), then the entire binaural signal would be cancelled. In this case the detection device would choose between the monaural inputs so that no MLD resulted. However, for the SπNo condition, the subtraction cancels the in-phase noise and actually enhances the out-of-phase signal. Thus, if the EC model works perfectly, the S/N ratio will be improved infinitely. In reality, the mechanism operates less than perfectly, so that cancellation is not complete. This imperfection is due to atypical stimuli which necessitate unusual types of equalization, or to random jitter in the process, which causes the cancellation mechanism to receive inputs that are imperfectly equalized.

REFERENCES

1. L. J. Sivian and S. D. White, On minimal audible fields, *J. Acoust. Soc. Amer.* 4, 288–321 (1933).
2. J. Keys. Binaural versus monaural hearing. *J. Acoust. Soc. Amer. 19*, 629–631 (1947).
3. W. A. Shaw, E. B. Newman, and I. J. Hirsh, The difference between monaural and binaural thresholds. *J. Exp. Psycho. 37*, 229–242 (1947).
4. R. Caussé and P. Chavasse, Récherches sur les seuil de l'audition binauriculaire comparé au seuil monauriculaire en fonction de la fréquence, *Comp. R. Soc. Biol. 135*, 1272–1275 (1941).
5. R. Caussé and P. Chavasse, Différence entre le seuil de l'audition binauriculaire et le seuil monauriculaire de la fréquence, *Comp. R. Soc. Biol. 136*, 301 (1942).

---

*Recall the rules for algebraic subtraction $(+1) - (+1) = 0$, as for the in-phase noise; $(+1) - (-1) = +2$, as for the out-of-phase signal.

6. I. J. Hirsh, Binaural summation: A century of investigation, *Psych. Bull. 45*, 193–206 (1948).

7. I. Pollack, Monaural and binaural threshold sensitivity for tones and white noise, *J. Acoust. Soc. Amer. 20*, 52–58 (1948).

8. H. Fletcher and W. Munson. Loudness: Its definition, measurement and calculation, *J. Acoust. Soc. Amer. 5*, 82–108 (1933).

9. R. Caussé and P. Chavasse, Différence entre l'ecoute binauriculaire et monauriculaire por la perception des intensités supraliminaires. *Comp. R. Soc. Biol. 139*, 405 (1942).

10. G. S. Reynolds and S. S. Stevens, Binaural summation of loudness. *J. Acoust. Soc. Amer. 32*, 1337–1344 (1960).

11. R. P. Hellman and J. Zwislocki, Monaural loudness function at 1000 cps, and interaural summation, *J. Acoust. Soc. Amer. 35*, 856–865 (1963).

12. B. Scharf and D. Fishken, Binaural summation of loudness: Reconsidered. *J. Exp. Psych. 86*, 374–379 (1970).

13. L. E. Marks, Binaural summation of loudness of pure tones, *J. Acoust. Soc. Amer. 64*, 107–113 (1978).

14. L. E. Marks, Binaural versus monaural loudness: Supersummation of tone partially masked by noise, *J. Acoust. Soc. Am. 81*, (1987).

15. B. G. Churcher, A. J. King, and H. Davies, The minimal perceptible change of intensity of a pure tone, *Phil. Mag. 18*, 927–939 (1934).

16. J. D. Harris, Loudness discrimination, *J. Speech Hearing Dis.*, Monograph Suppl 11 (1963).

17. R. C. Rowland and J. V. Tobias, Interaural intensity difference limens, *J. Speech Hearing Res. 10*, 745–756 (1967).

18. W. Jesteadt, C. C. Wier, and D. M. Green, Comparison of monaural and binaural discrimination of intensity and frequency, *J. Acoust. Soc. Amer. 61*, 1599–1603 (1977).

19. E. G. Shower and R. Biddulph, Differential pitch sensitivity of the ear, *J. Acoust. Soc. Amer. 3*, 275–287 (1931).

20. A. G. Pickler and J. D. Harris, Channels of reception in pitch discrimination, *J. Acoust. Soc. Amer. 27*, 124–131 (1955).

21. W. Jesteadt, C. C. Wier, and D. M. Green. Intensity discrimination as a function of frequency and sensation level, *J. Acoust. Soc. Amer. 61*, 169–177 (1977).

22. C. C. Wier, W. Jesteadt, and D. M. Green. Frequency discrimination as a function of frequency and sensation level, *J. Acoust. Soc. Amer. 61*, 178–184 (1977).

23. C. Cherry, Two ears—but one world, in *Sensory Communication* (W. A. Rosenblith, ed.), MIT Press, Cambridge, Mass., 1961, pp. 99–117.

24. E. C. Cherry, Some experiments upon the recognition of speech with one and two ears, *J. Acoust. Soc. Amer. 25*, 975–979 (1953).

25. E. C. Cherry and B. McA. Sayers, "Human cross-'correlator'"—A technique for measuring certain parameters of speech perception. *J. Acoust. Soc. Amer. 28*, 889–895 (1956).

26. B. McA. Sayers and E. C. Cherry, Mechanism of binaural fusion in the heating of speech. *J. Acoust. Soc. Amer. 29*, 973–987 (1957).

27. D. M. Leakey, B. McA. Sayers, and E. C. Cherry, Binaural fusion of low- and high frequency sounds. *J. Acoust. Soc. Amer. 30*, 222–223 (1958).

28. D. E. Broadbent, A note on binaural fusion, *Quart. J. Exp. Psych. 7*, 46–47 (1955).

29. J. S. Wernick and A. Starr, Electrophysiological correlates of binaural beats in superior-olivary complex of cat, *J. Acoust. Soc. Amer. 40*, 1276 (1966).

30. J. C. R. Licklider, J. C. Webster, and J. M. Hedlun. On the frequency limits of binaural beats. *J. Acoust. Soc. Amer. 22*, 468–473 (1950).

31. J. V. Tobias, Application of a "relative" procedure to the binaural-beat problem, *J. Acoust. Soc. Amer. 35*, 1442–1447 (1963).

32. J. J. Groen, Super- and subliminate binaural beats, *Acta Otol. 57*, 224–230 (1964).

33. Lord Rayleigh, Our perception of sound duration, *Phil. Mag. 13*, 214–232 (1907).

34. R. S. Woodworth, *Experimental Psychology*, Holt, Rhinehart, and Winston, New York, 1938.

35. W. E. Feddersen, T. T. Sandel, D. C. Teas, and L. A. Jeffress, Localization of high-frequency tones, *J. Acoust. Soc. Am. 29*, 988–991 (1957).

36. G. F. Kuhn, Model for the interaural time differences in azimuthal plane, *J. Acoust. Soc. Am. 62*, 157–167 (1977).

37. R. L. Roth, R. K. Kochhar, and J. E. Hind, Interaural time differences: Implications regarding the neurophysiology of sound localization, *J. Acoust. Soc. Am. 68*, 1643–1651 (1980).

38. A. W. Bronkhorst and R. Plomp, The effect of head-induced interaural time and level differences on speech intelligibility in noise, *J. Acoust. Soc. Am. 83*, 1508–1516 (1988).

39. B. Nordlund, Physical factors in angular localization, *J. Acoust. Soc. Am. 54*, 75–93 (1962).

40. L. A. Abbagnaro, B. B. Bauer, and E. L. Torick, Measurements of diffraction and interaural delay of a progressive sound wave caused by the human head—II, *J. Acoust. Soc. Am. 58*, 693–700 (1975).

41. L. Brillouin, *Wave Propagation and Group Velocity*, Academic, New York, 1960.

42. J. Blauert, *Special Hearing: The Psychophysics of Human Sound Localization*, MIT Press, Cambridge, 1983.

43. L. R. Bernstein and C. Trahiotis, Detection of interaural delay in high-frequency noise, *J. Acoust. Soc. Am. 71*, 147–152 (1982).

44. L. R. Bernstein and C. Trahiotis, Lateralization of sinusoidally amplitude-modulated tones: Effects of spectral locus and temporal variation, *J. Acoust. Soc. Am. 78*, 514–523 (1985).

45. W. A. Yost and R. H. Dye, Jr., Discrimination of interaural differences of level as a function of frequency, *J. Acoust. Soc. Am. 83*, 1846–1851 (1988).

46. S. S. Stevens and E. B. Newman, *The localization of actual sources of sound*, *Amer. J. Psycho. 48*, 297–306 (1936).

47. T. T. Sandel, D. C. Teas, W. E. Feddersen, and L. A. Jeffress, Localization of sound from single and paired sources, *J. Acoust. Soc. Amer. 27*, 842–852 (1955).

48. J. Blauert, Sound localization in the median plane, *Acoustica 22*, 205–213 (1969/70).

49. S. Weinrich, The problem of front-back localization in binaural hearing, *Scand. Audiol. Suppl. 15*, 135–145 (1982).

50. A. Musicant and R. Butler, The influence of pinnae-based spectral cues on sound localization, *J. Acoust. Soc. Am. 75*, 1195–1200 (1984).

51. A. W. Mills, On the minimal audible angle. *J. Acoust. Soc. Amer. 30*, 237–246 (1958).

52. A. W. Mills, Auditory perception of spatial relations, *Proc. Int. Cong. Tech. Blind*, Vol. 2, Am. Found, Blind, New York, 1963.

53. A. W. Mills, Auditory localization, In *Foundations of Modern Auditory Theory* (J. V. Tobias, ed.), Vol. 2, Academic Press, New York, 1972, pp. 301–348.

54. D. R. Perrott, Concurrent minimum audible angle: A re-examination of the concept of auditory spacial acuity, *J. Acoust. Soc. Am. 75*, 1201–1206 (1984).

55. D. R. Perrott and A. Musicant, Minimum audible movement angle: Binaural localization of moving sources, *J. Acoust. Soc. Am. 62*, 1463–1466 (1977).

56. D. R. Perrott and J. Tucker, Minimum audible movement angle as a function of signal frequency and the velocity of the source, *J. Acoust. Soc. Am. 83*, 1522–1527 (1988).

57. R. G. Klumpp and H. R. Eady, Some measurements of interaural time difference thresholds, *J. Acoust. Soc. Amer. 28*, 859–860 (1956).

58. J. Zwislocki and R. S. Feldman, Just noticeable differences in dichotic phase. *J. Acoust. Soc. Amer. 28*, 860–864 (1956).

59. A. W. Mills, Lateralization of high-frequency tones. *J. Acoust. Soc. Amer. 32*, 132–134 (1960).

60. W. A. Yost, Discriminations of interaural phase differences, *J. Acoust. Soc. Amer. 55*, 1299–1303 (1974).

61. J. V. Tobias and S. Zerlin, Lateralization threshold as a function of stimulus duration, *J. Acoust. Soc. Amer. 31*, 1591–1594 (1959).

62. J. V. Tobias, Curious binaural phenomena, in *Foundations of Modern Auditory Theory* (J. V. Tobias, ed.), Vol. 2, Academic Press, New York, 1972, pp. 463–486.

63. J. V. Tobias and E. D. Schubert, Effective onset duration of auditory stimuli, *J. Acoust. Soc. Amer. 31*, 1595–1605 (1959).

64. W. A. Yost, F. L. Whightman, and D. M. Green, Lateralization of filtered clicks, *J. Acoust. Soc. Amer., 50*, 1526–1531 (1971).

65. A. W. Mills, Lateralization of high-frequency tones, *J. Acoust. Soc. Am. 32*, 132–134 (1960).

66. D. W. Grantham, Interaural intensity discrimination: Insensitivity at 1000 Hz, *J. Acoust. Soc. Am. 75*, 1190–1194 (1984).

67. W. A. Yost, Lateral position of sinusoids presented with interaural intensive and temporal differences, *J. Acoust. Soc. Am. 70*, 397–409 (1981).

68. W. A. Yost, Lateralization of pulsed sinusoids based on interaural onset, ongoing, and offset temporal differences. *J. Acoust. Soc. Amer. 61*, 190–194 (1977).

69. G. B. Henning, Detectability of interaural delay in high-frequency complex waveforms. *J. Acoust. Soc. Amer. 55*, 84–90 (1974).

70. G. G. Harris, Binaural interactions of impulsive stimuli and pure tones. *J. Acoust. Soc. Amer. 32*, 685–692 (1960).

71. G. Moushegian and L. A. Jeffress, Role of interaural time and intensity differences in the lateralization of low-frequency tones. *J. Acoust. Soc. Amer. 31*, 1441–1445 (1959).

72. R. H. Whitworth and L. A. Jeffress, Time vs. intensity on the localization of tones. *J. Acoust. Soc. Amer. 33*, 925–929 (1961).

73. E. R. Hafter and L. A. Jeffress, Two-image lateralization of tones and clicks, *J. Acoust. Soc. Amer. 44*, 563–569 (1968).

74. L. A. Jeffress and D. McFadden, Differences of interaural phase and level in detection and lateralization, *J. Acoust. Soc. Amer. 49*, 1169–1179 (1971).

75. E. R. Hafter and S. C. Carrier, Binaural interaction in low-frequency stimuli: The inability to trade time and intensity completely, *J. Acoust. Soc. Amer. 51*, 1852–1862 (1972).

76. H. Wallach, E. B. Newman, and M. R. Rosenzweig, The precedence effect in sound localization, *Amer. J. Psych. 62*, 315–336 (1949).

77. H. Haas, The influence of a single echo on the audibility of speech, *Library Com. 363*, Dept. Sci. Indust. Rest., Garston, Watford, England, 1949.

78. H. Haas, Über den Einfluss eines Einfachechos aud die Hörsamkeit von Sprache, *Acoustica 1*, 49–58 (1951). [English translation: *J. Audiol. Eng. Soc. 20*, 146–159 (1972).]

79. M. B. Gardner, Historical background of the Haas and/or precedence effect, *J. Acoust. Soc. Amer. 43*, 1243–1248 (1968).

80. J. P. A. Lochner and J. F. Burger, The influence of reflections on auditorium acoustics, *J. Sound Vib. 1*, 426–454 (1964).

81. A. K. Nabelek and L. Robinette, Influence of the precedence effect on word identification by normal hearing and hearing-impaired subjects, *J. Acoust. Soc. Amer. 63*, 187–194 (1978).

82. R. H. Bolt and A. D. MacDonald, Theory of speech masking by reverberation, *J. Acoust. Soc. Amer. 21*, 577–580 (1949).

83. H. Kurtović, The influence of reflected sound upon speech intelligibility, *Acoustica, 33*, 32–39 (1975).

84. S. A. Gelfand and S. Silman, Effects of small room reverberation upon the recognition of some consonant features, *J. Acoust. Soc. Amer. 66*, 22–29 (1979).

85. I. J. Hirsh, The influence of interaural phase on interaural summation and inhibition, *J. Acoust. Soc. Amer. 20*, 536–544 (1948).

86. J. C. R. Licklider, The influence of interaural phase relations upon the masking of speech by white noise, *J. Acoust. Soc. Amer. 20*, 150–159 (1948).

87. D. M. Green and G. R. Henning, Audition, *Ann. Rev. Psych. 20*, 105–128 (1969).

88. D. M. Green and W. A. Yost, Binaural analysis, in *Handbook of Sensory Physiology* (W. D. Keidel and W. D. Neff, eds.), Vol. V/2: *Auditory System*, Springer-Verlag, 1975, pp. 461–480.
89. H. C. Blodgett, L. A. Jeffress, and R. H. Whitworth, Effect of noise at one ear on the masking threshold for tones at the other, *J. Acoust. Soc. Amer. 34*, 979–981 (1962).
90. T. R. Dolan and D. E. Robinson, An explanation of masking-level differences that result from interaural intensive disparities of noise, *J. Acoust. Soc. Amer. 42*, 977–981 (1967).
91. T. R. Dolan, Effects of masker spectrum level on masking-level differences at low signal frequencies, *J. Acoust. Soc. Amer. 44*, 1507–1512 (1968).
92. D. McFadden, Masking-level differences determined with and without interaural disparities in masking intensity, *J. Acoust. Soc. Amer. 44*, 212–223 (1968).
93. L. A. Jeffress, H. C. Blodgett, and B. H. Deatheredge, The masking of tones by white noise as a function of interaural phases of both components, *J. Acoust. Soc. Amer. 24*, 523–527 (1952).
94. H. S. Colburn and N. I. Durlach, Time-intensity relations in binaural unmasking, *J. Acoust. Soc. Amer. 38*, 93–103 (1965).
95. N. I. Durlach, Binaural signal detection: Equalization and cancellation theory, in *Foundations of Modern Auditory Theory* (J. V. Tobias, ed.), vol. 2, Academic Press, New York, 1972, pp. 369–462.
96. F. A. Webster, The influence of interaural phase on masked thresholds. I. The role of interaural time-duration, *J. Acoust. Soc. Amer. 23*, 452–462 (1951).
97. I. J. Hirsh and M. Burgeat, Binaural effects in remote masking, *J. Acoust. Soc. Amer. 30*, 827–832 (1958).
98. N. I. Durlach, Equalization and cancellation theory of binaural masking-level differences. *J. Acoust. Soc. Amer. 35*, 1206–1218 (1963).
99. K. D. Schenkel, Über die Abhängigkeit der Mithörschwellen von der interauralen Phasenlage des Testchalls, *Acoustica 14*, 337–346 (1964).
100. D. M. Green, Interaural phase effects in the masking of signals of different durations, *J. Acoust. Soc. Amer. 39*, 720–724 (1966).
101. L. R. Rabiner, C. L. Lawrence, and N. I. Durlach, Further results on binaural unmasking and the EC model, *J. Acoust. Soc. Amer. 40*, 62–70 (1966).
102. D. E. Robinson and L. A. Jeffress, Effect of varying the interaural noise correlation on the detectability of tonal signals, *J. Acoust. Soc. Amer. 35*, 1947–1952 (1963).
103. A. H. Koenig, J. B. Allen, D. A. Berkley, and T. H. Curtis, Determination of masking-level differences in a reverberant environment, *J. Acoust. Soc. Amer. 61*, 1374–1376 (1977).
104. M. M. Sondhi and N. Guttman, Width of the spectrum effective in the binaural release of masking, *J. Acoust. Soc. Amer. 40*, 600–606 (1966).
105. B. E. Mulligan, M. J. Mulligan and J. F. Stonecypher, Critical band in binaural detection, *J. Acoust. Soc. Amer. 41*, 7–12 (1967).

106. P. J. Metz, G. von Bismark, and N. I. Durlach, I. Further results on binaural unmasking and the EC model. II. Noise bandwidth and interaural phase. *J. Acoust. Soc. Amer.* 43, 1085–1091 (1967).

107. F. L. Whightman, Detection of binaural tones as a function of masker bandwidth, *J. Acoust. Soc. Amer.* 50, 623–636 (1971).

108. T. L. Langford and L. A. Jeffress, Effect of noise cross-correlation on binaural signal detection, *J. Acoust. Soc. Amer.* 36, 1455–1458 (1964).

109. E. D. Schubert and M. C. Schultz, Some aspects of binaural signal selection, *J. Acoust. Soc. Amer.* 34, 844–849 (1962).

110. R. Carhart, T. Tillman, and K. Johnson, Release of masking for speech through interaural time delay, *J. Acoust. Soc. Amer.* 42, 124–138 (1967).

111. H. Levitt and I. R. Rabiner, Binaural release from masking for speech and grain in intelligibility, *J. Acoust. Soc. Amer.* 42, 601–608 (1967).

112. R. Carhart, T. Tillman, and P. Dallos, Unmasking for pure tones and spondees: Interaural phase and time disparities, *J. Speech Hearing Res. 11*, 722–734 (1968).

113. H. Levitt and L. R. Rabiner, Predicting binaural gain in intelligibility and release from masking for speech, *J. Acoust. Soc. Amer.* 42, 820–829 (1967).

114. G. B. Henning, Effect of interaural phase on frequency and amplitude discrimination, *J. Acoust. Soc. Amer.* 54, 1160–1178 (1973).

115. T. H. Townsend and D. P. Goldstein, Suprathreshold binaural unmasking, *J. Acoust. Soc. Amer.* 51, 621–624 (1972).

116. L. A. Jeffress, Binaural signal detection: Vectory theory, in *Foundations of Modern Auditory Theory* (J. V. Tobias, ed.), Vol. 2, Academic Press, New York, 1972, pp. 349–368.

117. E. R. Hafter, W. T. Bourbon, A. S. Blocker, and A. Tucker, Direct comparison between lateralization and detection under antiphasic masking, *J. Acoust. Soc. Amer.* 46, 1452–1457 (1969).

118. E. R. Hafter and S. C. Carrier, Masking-level differences obtained with a pulsed tonal masker, *J. Acoust. Soc. Amer.* 47, 1041–1048 (1970).

119. E. Osman, A correlation model of binaural masking level differences, *J. Acoust. Soc. Amer.* 50, 1494–1511 (1971).

120. R. M. Stern and H. S. Colburn, Theory of binaural interaction based on auditory-nerve data. IV. A model for subjective lateral position, *J. Acoust. Soc. Am.* 64, 127–140 (1978).

14

Speech Perception

Pure tones, clicks, and the like enable us to study specific aspects of audition in a precise and controllable manner. On the other hand, we communicate with each other by speech, which is composed of particularly complex and variable waveforms. A knowledge of how we perceive simpler sounds is the foundation upon which an understanding of speech perception must be built. As one might suppose, speech perception and intimately related areas constitute a voluminous subject encompassing far more than hearing science, per se. For this reason, more than a cursory coverage of the topic would be neither prudent nor profitable within the current context. The interested reader is referred to several references [1–6].

Speech perception and speech production are inherently interrelated. We must be able to speak what we can perceive, and we must have the ability to perceive the sounds that our speech mechanisms produce. Traditionally, the sounds of speech have been described in terms of the vocal and articulatory manipulations that produce them. We too shall begin with production. For the most part, our discussion will focus upon phonemes.

By a "phoneme" we mean a group of sounds that are classified as being the same by native speakers of a given language. Let us see what the "sameness" refers to. Consider the phoneme /p/* as it appears at the

---

*By convention, phonemes are enclosed between slashes and phonetic elements between brackets.

beginning and end of the word "pipe." There are actually several differences between the two productions of /p/ in this word. For example, the initial /p/ is accompanied by a release of a puff of air (aspiration) whereas the final /p/ is not. In other words, the actual sounds are different (they are distinct phonetic elements). In spite of this, native speakers of English will classify both as belonging to the family designated as the /p/ phoneme. Such phonetically dissimilar members of the same phonemic class are called allophones of that phoneme. Consider a second example. The words "beet" and "bit" (/bit/ and /bɪt/, respectively) sound different to speakers of English but the same to speakers of French. This happens because the phonetic elements [i] and [ɪ] are different phonemes in English, but are allophones of the same phoneme in French. Since the Frenchman classifies [i] and [ɪ] as members of the same phonemic family, he hears them as being the same, just as English speakers hear the aspirated and unaspirated productions of /p/ to be the same.

This last example also demonstrates the second important characteristic of phonemes. Changing a phoneme changes the meaning of a word. Thus, /i/ and /ɪ/ are different phonemes in English, because replacing one for the other changes the meaning of at least some words. However, [i] and [ɪ] are not different phonemes in French (i.e., they are allophones), because replacing one for the other does not change the meaning of words. Implicit in the distinction of phonetic and phonemic elements is that even elementary speech sound classes are to some extent learned. All babies the world over produce the same wide range of sounds phonetically; it is through a process of learning that these phonetic elements become classified and grouped into families of phonemes that are used in the language of the community.

SPEECH SOUNDS: PRODUCTION AND PERCEPTION

Our discussion of speech sounds will be facilitated by reference to the simplified schematic diagram of the vocal tract in Fig. 14.1. The "power source" is the air in the lungs, which is directed up and out under the control of the respiratory musculature. Voiced sounds are produced when the vocal cords (folds) are vibrated (see Flanagan [7] and Stevens and House [8] for detailed discussions.) The result of this vibration is a periodic complex waveform made up of a fundamental frequency on the order of 100 Hz in males and 200 Hz in females, with as many as 40 harmonics of the fundamental represented in the waveform [7] (see Fig. 14.2a). This complex periodic waveform is then modified by the resonance characteristics of the vocal tract. In other words, the vocal tract constitutes a group of filters which are added together, and whose effect

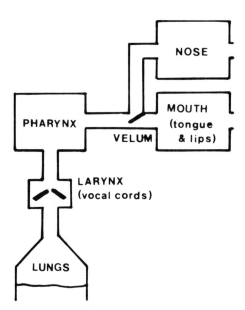

Figure 14.1   Schematic representation of the vocal tract.

is to shape the spectrum of the waveform from the larynx. The resonance characteristics of the vocal tract (Fig. 14.2b) are thus reflected in
the speech spectrum (Fig. 14.2c).

   Voiceless (unvoiced) sounds are produced by opening the airway
between the vocal folds so that they do not vibrate. Voiceless sounds are
aperiodic and noiselike, being produced by turbulences due to partial or
complete obstruction of the vocal tract.

Vowels

Speech sounds are generally classified broadly as vowels and consonants.
Vowels are voiced sounds* whose spectral characteristics are determined
by the size and shape of the vocal tract. Changing the shape of the vocal
tract changes its filtering characteristics, which in turn changes the frequencies at which the speech signal is enhanced or de-emphasized (Fig.
14.2). Examples of how the vocal tract is shaped for various English vow-

---

*Certain exceptions are notable. Whispered speech is all voiceless; and vowels
may also be voiceless in some contexts of voiceless consonants in connected
discourse. Also, the nasal cavity is generally excluded by action of the velum,
unless the vowel is in the environment of a nasal sound.

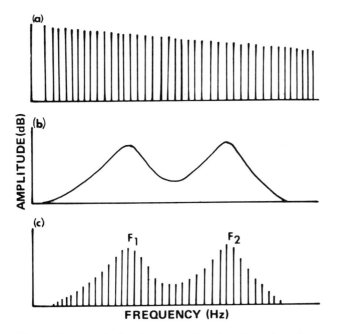

Figure 14.2   Idealized spectra showing that when the complex vocal waveform (a) is passed through the vocal tract filters (b) the resulting waveform (c) represents the acoustic characteristics of the vocal tract. Vocal tract resonances result in the formants (F_1, F_2).

els are shown in Fig. 14.3. As the figure shows, the vowel we hear is largely determined by the effects of tongue and lip position and movement. (Diphthongs such as /aɪ/ in "buy" and /oʊ/ in "toe" are heard when one vowel glides into another.) The resulting frequency regions where energy is concentrated are called formants, and are generally labeled starting from the lowest as F_1, F_2 etc. The lower formants (especially F_1 and F_2, as well as F_3) are primarily responsible for vowel recognition [10–12].

   In general, the formant frequencies depend upon where and to what extent the vocal tract is constricted [11,13,14]. The locations and degrees of these constrictions control the sizes and locations of the volumes in the vocal tract (Fig. 14.3). For example, elevation of the back of the tongue results in a larger volume between this point of constriction and the lips than does elevation of the tongue tip. We may thus describe a vowel from front to back in terms of the amount of tongue elevation. Lip rounding is another important factor. In English, front vowels (/i, ɪ, e, ɛ,

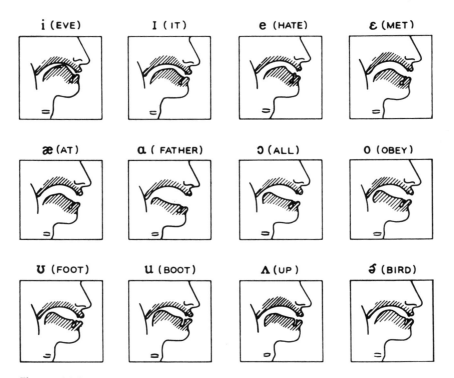

Figure 14.3 Articulation of various English vowels (see text). [From Flanagan [14], adapted from Potter et al. [9], *Visible Speech*, © 1947 by Bell Telephone Laboratories. Reprinted by permission.]

æ/) are produced with retraction of the lips, while the lips are rounded when the back vowels (/u, ʊ, o, ɔ, a/) are formed. Rounding the front vowel /i/ as in "tea" while keeping the high-front tongue placement results in the Frency /y/ as in "*tu*."

The degree of tenseness associated with the muscle contractions is also a factor in vowel production and perception, as in the differentiation of the tense (i) ("peat") from the lax /ɪ/ ("pit"). Tense vowels are generally more intense and longer in duration than their lax counterparts.

The middle vowels (/ʌ, ə, ɜ, ɝ, ɚ/) are produced when tongue elevation is in the vicinity of the hard palate. These include the neutral vowel /ə/ associated mainly with unstressed syllables (eg., "*a*bout" and "s*u*pport").

Without going into great detail, the frequency of the first format F_1 is largely dependent upon the size of the volume behind the tongue elevation, i.e., upon the larger of the vocal tract volumes. This volume must of course increase as the elevated part of the tongue moves forward.

Thus, front tongue elevation produces a larger volume behind the point of constriction, which in turn is associated with lower F_1 frequencies; whereas back tongue elevations decrease the size of this volume, thereby raising the frequency of F_1. The frequency of F_2 depends largely upon the size of the volume in front of the point of tongue elevation, becoming higher when the cavity is made smaller (when tongue is elevated closer to the front of the mouth). Lip rounding lowers the first two formants by reducing the size of the mouth opening.

Figure 14.4 shows sustained productions of several vowels in the form of sound spectrograms [9,15]. Frequency is shown up the ordinate, time along the abscissa, and intensity as relative blackness. Thus, blacker areas represent frequencies with higher energy concentrations and lighter areas indicate frequency regions with less energy. The formants are indicated by frequency bands much darker than the rest of the spectrogram. These horizontal bands represent frequency regions containing concentrations of energy and thus reflect the resonance characteristics of the vocal tract. The vertical striations correspond to the period of the speaker's fundamental frequency.

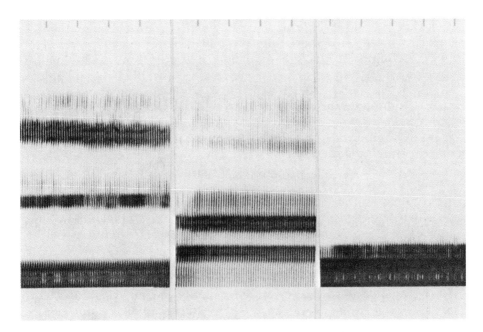

Figure 14.4 Spectrograms showing sustained production of the vowels /i/, /æ/ and /u/ (left to right). Timing marks along the top are 100 msec apart.

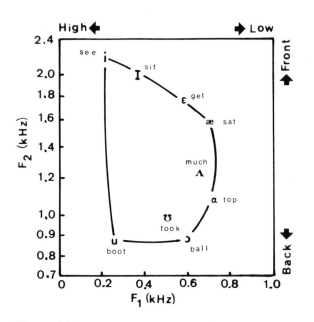

Figure 14.5 Approximate values of F_1 and F_2 are several vowels as they relate to tongue height and position. (Modified from Peterson and Barney [11].)

The relationship between tongue position and the frequencies of F_1 and F_2 are shown for several vowels in Fig. 14.5. However, it should be noted that these formant frequencies are approximations. Formant center frequencies and bandwidths tend to become higher going from men to women to children, which reflects the effect of decreasing vocal tract length. Furthermore, they vary among studies and between subjects.

Given these wide variations it is doubtful that vowels are identified on the basis of their formant frequencies, per se. The relationships among the formants, as well as the environment of the vowel and its duration, provide important cues [16–18]. It has been suggested that, for each individual speaker, the listener adjusts the "target" values of the formants according to the utterances of that speaker [19,20].

Consonants

The consonants are produced by either a partial or complete obstruction somewhere along the vocal tract. The ensuing turbulence causes the sound to be quasi-periodic or aperiodic and noiselike. The consonants are differentiated on the basis of manner of articulation, place of articulation, and voicing; i.e., on how and where the obstruction of the vocal tract occurs and on whether there is vocal cord vibration. Table 14.1

Table 14.1 Consonants of English

	Bilabial	Labiodental	Linguadental	Alveolar	Palatal	Velar	Glottal
Stops							
vl[a]	p			t		k	
vd[a]	b			d		g	
Fricatives							
vl	ʌ (*which*)	f	Θ (*thing*)	s	ʃ (*shoot*)		h
vd		v	ð (*this*)	z	ʒ (*beige*)		
Affricates							
vl					tʃ (*catch*)		
vd					dʒ (*dodge*)		
Nasals[b]				n	ŋ (*sing*)		
Semivowels[b]	w			l,r	j (*yes*)		

[a]vl, voiceless; vd, voiced.
[b]nasals and semivowels are voiced.

shows the English consonants, arranged horizontally according to place of articulation and vertically by manner and voicing. Examples are given where the phonetic and orthographic symbols differ.

The stops, fricatives, and affricates may be either voiced or voiceless, whereas the nasals and semivowels are virtually always voiced. The

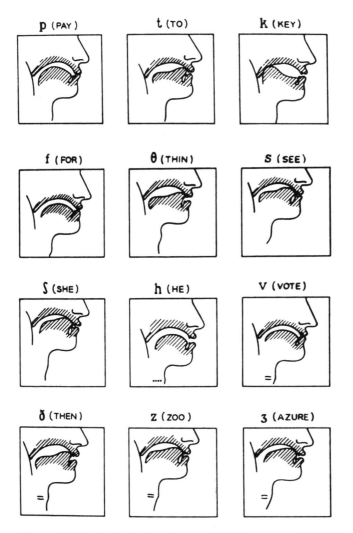

Figure 14.6 Articulation of some English stops and fricatives. (From Flanagan [14], adapted from Potter et al. [9], *Visible Speech*, © 1947 by Bell Telephone Laboratories. Reprinted by permission.)

nasal cavities are excluded from the production of all consonants except the nasals by elevation of the velum. Cross-sectional diagrams for the production of the stops, fricatives, and affricates are given in Fig. 14.6, and for the nasals and semivowels in Fig. 14.7. We shall briefly discuss the consonants in order of the manner of their articulation.

The stops (plosives) are produced by a transition (see below) from the preceding vowel, a silent period on the order of roughly 30 msec during which air pressure is impounded behind a complete obstruction somewhere along the vocal tract, a release (burst) of the built-up pressure, and finally a transition into the following vowel [21–24]. Of course, whether there is a transition from the preceding vowel and/or into the following vowel depends upon the environment of the stop consonant. Voiceless stops in the initial position are generally aspirated, or released with a puff of air. Initial voiced stops and all final stops tend not to be aspirated, although this does not apply always or to all speakers. The voiceless stops (/p,t,k/) and their voiced cognates (/b,d,g/) are articulated in the same way except for the presence or absence of voicing and/or aspiration (see Fig. 14.6). As a rule, the voiceless stops tend to have longer and stronger pressure buildups than do their voiced counterparts [25,26].

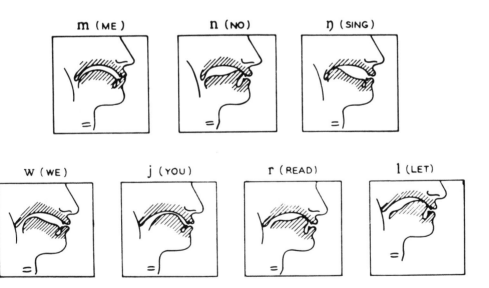

Figure 14.7 Articulation of some English nasals and semivowels (From Flanagan [14], adapted from Potter et al. [9], *Visible Speech,* © 1947 by Bell Telephone Laboratories. Reprinted by permission.)

The six stops are produced at three locations. The bilabials (/p,b/) are produced by an obstruction at the lips; the alveolars (/t,d/) by the tongue tip against the upper gum ridge; and the velars (/k,g/) by the tongue dorsum against the soft palate. Whether the sound is heard as voiced or voiceless is of course ultimately due to whether there is vocal cord vibration. However, cues differ according to the location of the stop in an utterance. The essential voicing cue for initial stops is voice onset time (VOT), which is simply the time delay between the onset of the stop burst and commencement of vocal cord vibration [27,28]. In general, voicing onset precedes or accompanies stop burst onset for voiced stops but lags behind the stop burst for voiceless stops. For final stops and those which occur medially within an utterance, the essential voicing cue appears to be the duration of the preceding vowel [29]. Longer vowel durations are associated with the perception that the following stop is voiced. Voiceless stops are also associated with longer closure durations [30], faster formant transitions [31], greater burst intensities [24], and somewhat higher fundamental frequencies [32], than voiced stops.

Place of articulation (bilabial versus alveolar versus velar) for the stop is largely cued by the second formant (F_2) transition of the associated vowel [33,34], along with some contribution from the F_3 transitions [35]. By a formant transition we simply mean a change with time of the formant frequency in going from the steady-state frequency of the vowel into the consonant (or vice versa). Formant transitions may be seen for several initial voiced stops in Fig. 14.8. The F_2 transitions point in the direction of approximately 700 Hz for bilabial stops, 1800 Hz for the alveolars, and 3000 Hz for the velars [33]. These directions relate to the location of vocal tract obstruction. That is, a larger volume is enclosed behind an obstruction at the lips (/p,b/) than at the alveolus (/t,d/) or velum (/k,g/), so that the resonant frequency associated with that volume is lower for more frontal obstructions. Moving the point of obstruction backward reduces the cavity volume and thus increases the resonant frequency. Further place information is provided by the frequency spectrum of the stop burst. Stop bursts tend to have concentrations of energy at relatively low frequencies (500–1500 Hz) for the bilabials, at high frequencies (about 4000 Hz and higher) for the alveolars, and at intermediate frequencies (between around 1500 and 4000 Hz) for the velars [24].

There tends to be a considerable amount of variability in the formant cues because the configurations of the formant transitions change according to the associated vowels. For example, the second formant transition from the /d/ into the following vowel is different for /di/ and /du/. Recent

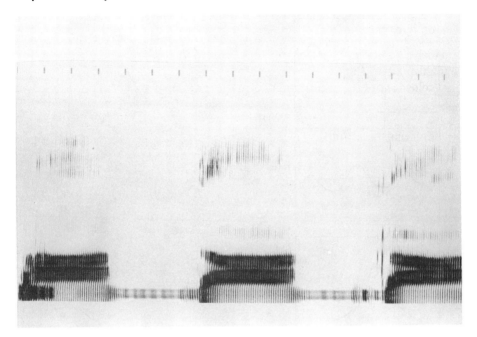

Figure 14.8 Spectrograms of /ba/, /da/ and /ga/ (left to right). Note second formant transitions.

acoustical and perceptual studies [36–41] have proposed invariant place of articulation features. For example, Stevens, Blumstein, and colleagues [36–39] have suggested that there are invariant patterns in the gross configurations of the spectra integrated over a period of roughly 20 msec in the vicinity of the consonant release. Figure 14.9 shows the general configurations of these onset spectra, which are diffuse and falling for labials, diffuse and rising for alveolars, and compact for velars. In addition to the perceptual findings, further support for this concept comes from experiments using computer models [42] and auditory nerve discharge patterns [43]; although there are inconsistent results as well [44].

The fricatives are produced by a partial obstruction of the vocal tract so that the air coming through becomes turbulent. The nature of the fricatives has been well described [45–54], and examples are shown by the spectograms in Fig. 14.10. Fricatives are distinguished from other manners of articulation by the continuing nature of their turbulent energy (generally lasting 100 msec or more); and vowels preceding fricatives tend to have greater power and duration, and somewhat longer fundamental frequencies, than vowels preceding stops. As is true for the stops,

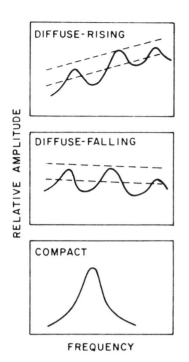

Figure 14.9 Invariant onset spectrum configurations associated with stop consonant place of articulation: alveolars, diffuse and rising; labials, diffuse and falling; velars, compact. (From Blumstein and Stevens [37], with permission of *J. Acoust. Soc. Am.*)

fricatives may be either voiced or voiceless, and voicing is similarly cued by VOT and by the nature of the preceding vowel. In addition, voiceless fricatives tend to have longer durations than their voiced counterparts.

Spectral differences largely account for place distinctions between the alveolar (/s,z/) and (palatal (/ʃ, ʒ/) fricatives. The palatals have energy concentrations extending to lower frequencies (about 1500–7000 Hz) than do the alveolars (roughly 4000–7000 Hz), most likely because of the larger volume in front of the point of vocal tract obstruction for /ʃ,ʒ/ than for /s,z/. On the other hand, /θ,ð/ and /f,v/ are differentiated mainly on the basis of formant transitions. Due to resonation of the entire vocal tract above the glottis, /h/ possesses more low frequencies than the more anterior fricatives. The amplitudes of /s/ and /ʃ/ are considerably greater than those of /f/ and /θ/. However, recent perceptual experiments by Behrens and Blumstein [54] have demonstrated that these amplitudes are less important than spectral properties in differentiating between

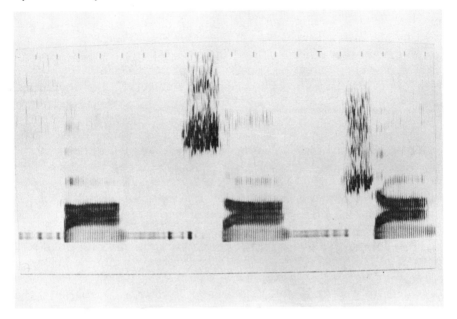

Figure 14.10   Spectrograms of /fa/, /s/, and /ʃa/ (left to right).

these two groups of fricatives. The affricates are produced by the rapid release of their stop components into their fricative components.

The nasals are produced by opening the port to the nasal cavities at the velum (Fig. 14.7). They are semivowels in that they are voiced and have some of the formant characteristics of vowels. However, they differ from other sounds by the coupling of the nasal and oral cavities. The characteristics of nasals have been described by Fujimura [55] and others [21,56–58]. The coupling of the nasal cavities to the volume of oral cavity behind the point of obstruction (the velum for /ŋ/, alveolus for /n/, and lips for /m/ constitutes a side-branch resonator. This results in anti-resonances at frequencies which become lower as the volume of the side branch (oral cavity) becomes larger. Thus, we find that antiresonances appear in the frequency regions of roughly 1000 Hz for /m/ (where the side branch is largest), 1700 Hz for /n/, and 3000 Hz for /ŋ/ (where the side branch is shortest). Furthermore, overall intensity is reduced, and for the first formant is lower than for the vowels, constituting a character-istic low-frequency nasal murmur. Place of articulation is cued by differ-ences in formant structure among the nasal consonants and by formant transitions for adjacent vowels. Recent findings by Kurowski and Blum-stein [58] suggested that there may be invariant patterns of spectral cues involving the nasal murmur and release, at least for the labial and alveolar places of articulation.

The semivowels are /w,j/ and /r,l/. The latter two are also called liquids. The semivowels have been described by O'Connor et al. [59], Lisker [60], and Fant [61]. The bilabial semivowel /w/ is produced initially in the same way as the vowel /u/, with a transition into the following vowel over the course of about 100 msec. For /j/, the transition into the following vowel is from /i/, and takes about the same amount of time as for /w/. The first formants of both /w/ and /j/ are on the order of 240 Hz, with the second formant transitions beginning below about 600 Hz for /w/ and above 2300 Hz for /j/. Furthermore, there appears to be relatively low-frequency frication-like noise associated with /w/ and higher-frequency noise with /j/, due to the degree of vocal tract constriction in their production.

The liquid semivowels (/r,l/) have short-duration steady-state portions of up to about 50 msec, followed by transitions into the following vowel over the course of roughly 75 msec. The /r/ is produced with some degree of lip rounding, and /l/ is produced with the tongue tip at the upper gum ridge so that air is deflected laterally. The first formants of the liquids are on the order of 500 Hz for /r/ and 350 Hz for /l/, which are relatively high; and the first and second formant transitions are roughly similar for both liquids. The major difference appears to be associated with the presence of lip rounding for /r/ but not /l/. Since lip rounding causes the third formant to be lower in frequency, /r/ is associated with a rather dramatic third formant transition upward in frequency which is not seen for /l/, at least not for transitions into unrounded vowels. The opposite would occur for /r/ and /l/ before a rounded vowel.

Categorical Perception

Liberman et al. [62] prepared synthetic consonant-vowel (CV) monosyllables composed of two formants each. They asked their subjects to discriminate between these pairs of synthetic CVs as the second formant transition was varied, and obtained a finding which has had a profound effect upon the study of speech perception. Subjects' ability to discriminate between the two CVs in a pair was excellent when the consonants were identifiable as different phonemes, whereas discrimination was poor when the consonants were identified as belonging to the same phonemic category. This observation of categorical perception has been confirmed by a variety of studies [27,63–76]. Figure 14.11 shows typical (idealized) results for a categorical perception experiment.

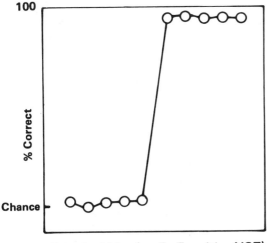

Figure 14.11   Idealized functions for a categorical perception experiment (see text).

The circles in Fig. 14.11 represent the percentage of correct discriminations between the CVs as a function of the difference between them along some continuum (such as the direction of F_2 transition or voice onset time). For small values along this continuum the subjects are essentially unable to discriminate between the two CVs beyond a chance rate. At a certain point, however, there is a dramatic jump in correct discrimination to near 100% performance. If we now ask the subject to identify each of the stimuli according to phonemic category, we find that the CVs identified as belonging to the same category are those which were poorly discriminated from one another, whereas those belonging to different categories are the ones that were easily discriminated.

This categorical perception of speech sounds was not found to occur when Liberman et al. [63] inverted the synthetic stimuli to form non-speech materials. Instead, discrimination among the nonspeech sounds occurred along a continuum without the peaks and troughs seen in the categorical perception of speech stimuli. Using VOT as the parameter to be discriminated, Abramson and Lisker [27,64,65] demonstrated that categorical perception occurs across languages, generally with voicing time offsets on the order of approximately 20 msec. In addition, similar categorical discriminations for VOT was shown to occur in both infants and adults [66]. These findings suggested that discriminability depends upon some kind of phonetic (rather than acoustic) categorization of the stimuli, and have been proposed as evidence that there is an innate special mode for the perception of speech [67]. As we shall see, however, more recent findings rather powerfully support an acoustically based discriminability related to whether the stimuli are perceived as simultaneous versus successive, and upon their perceived order [68].

Several findings cast doubt upon a phonetic basis for categorical perception. First, categorical perception has been demonstrated to occur for a variety of nonspeech materials [68–70]. Second, three categorical boundaries along the VOT parameter have been found to be discriminated by Spanish and Kikuyu infants [71,72]. This result contradicts the phonetic basis because there is only one phonetic boundary for voicing in Spanish and none for the labial stops in Kikuyu. Most impressive, however, is the finding by Kuhl and Miller [73] that chinchillas can be trained to discriminate along the VOT parameter, and that the "phoneme" boundaries derived from the chinchilla data are excellent approximations of the human findings. The absence of a phonetic system is a reasonable assumption. Thus, one is drawn toward some sort of psychoacoustic rather than phonetic discrimination as a basis for categorical perception. It is interesting to note here that Nelson and Marler [77] recently demonstrated the existence of categorical perception for birdsong among sparrows.

Pisoni [68] found that onset-time disparities between two tones were categorically perceived at boundaries comparable to those for stop consonant VOT. Further, he demonstrated that judgments of whether the onsets of the two tones were simultaneous or successive lined up remarkably well with the categorical perception data for these stimuli. That is, two events were heard when the onsets of the two tones were 20 msec apart, whereas a single onset was heard when they were less than 20 msec apart. Since these discrepancies are the same as those needed to perceive the temporal order of two stimuli [74,75], Pisoni proposed that this psychoacoustic phenomenon may well be the basis of categorical perception. For a comprehensive discussion of categorical perception. For a comprehensive discussion of categorical perception, the reader should refer to the recent recent by Repp [76].

POWER OF SPEECH SOUNDS

Several points about the power of speech sounds are noteworthy prior to a discussion of speech intelligibility. From the foregoing, we would expect to find most of the power of speech in the vowels; and since the vowels have a preponderance of low-frequency energy, we would expect the long-term speech spectrum to reflect this as well. This expectation is borne out by the literature [1]. The weakest sound in English is the voiceless fricative /θ/ and the strongest is the vowel /ɔ/ [1,78]. If /θ/ is assigned a power of one, then the relative power of /ɔ/ becomes 680 [1]. The relative power of the consonants range up to 80 for /ʃ/; are between 36 (/n/) and 73 (/ŋ/) for the nasals; are on the order of 100 for the semi-vowels; and range upward from 220 (/i/) for the vowels [1]. As one would expect, the more powerful sounds are detected and are more intelligible at lower intensities than are the weaker ones.

The long-term average spectrum of speech is shown in Fig. 14.12. This figure shows the general range of findings from several studies [79–81] in terms of relative level in dB. As expected, most of the energy in speech is found in the lower frequencies, particularly below about 1000 Hz. Intensity falls off as frequency increases above this range. It should be noted that the crosshatched region in the figure is the relative speech spectrum averaged over time for male and female speakers in several studies. The average overall sound pressure level of male speech tends to be on the order of 3 dB higher than for females. The spectrograms shown earlier in the chapter are examples of the short-term speech spectrum.

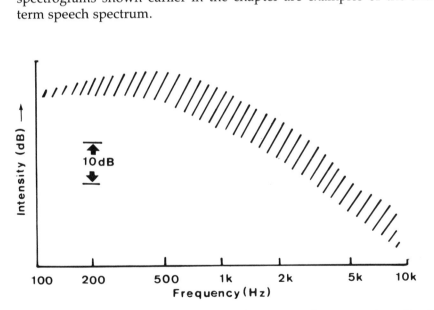

Figure 14.12 Long-term average speech spectrum from several studies (see text).

SPEECH INTELLIGIBILITY

In general, speech intelligibility refers to how well the listener receives and comprehends the speech signal. The basic approach to studying speech intelligibility is quite simple and direct. The subject is presented with a series of stimuli (syllables, words, phrases, etc.), and is asked to identify what he has heard. The results are typically reported as the percent correct, which is called the articulation or discrimination score [82–84]. The approach may be further broken down into open-set methods requiring the subject to repeat (or write) what was heard without prior knowledge of the corpus of test items [84–86]; and close-set methods which provide a choice of response alternatives from which the subject must choose [87,88]. These tests were originally devised in the development of telephone communication systems, and efforts were accelerated for obvious though unfortunate reasons during the second world war. The factors that contribute to speech intelligibility (or interfere with it) may be examined by obtaining articulation scores under various stimulus conditions and in the face of different kinds of distortions.

Intensity and Materials

It is a general finding for all speech materials that intelligibility improves as the level of the signal is increased from barely audible levels up to higher levels, at which discrimination reaches a maximum [1,81,83]. In other words, there is a psychometric function (Chap. 7) for speech intelligibility as well as for the other psychoacoustic phenomena we have discussed. As a rule, discrimination performance becomes asymptotic when maximum intelligibility is reached for a given type of speech material; however, discrimination may actually decrease in some cases if intensity is raised to excessive levels.

Intelligibility depends upon the nature of the speech materials used, and a general rule is that performance improves as the speech stimuli become more redundant in any of a variety of ways [84,89–92]. For example, Miller et al. [90] asked their subjects to discriminate (1) words in sentences, (2) digits from 0 to 9, and (3) nonsense (meaningless) syllables. A psychometric function was generated for each type of test material, showing percent correct performance as a function of signal-to-noise (S/N) ratio (Fig. 14.13). Note that the digits were audible at softer levels (lower S/N ratios) than were the words in sentences, which were in turn more accurately perceived than the nonsense syllables. We observe this result in several ways. First, at each S/N ratio in the figure

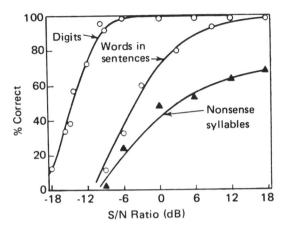

Figure 14.13 Psychometric functions showing the effects of test materials. (From Miller, Heise, and Lichten [90], with permission of *J. Exp. Psych.*)

percent correct performance is best for the digits, less good for the words in sentences, and poorest for the syllables. Conversely, the subjects were able to repeat 50% of the digits at a level 17 dB softer than that needed to reach 50% correct for the monosyllables. Second, a small increase in S/N ratio resulted in a substantial increase in digit discrimination but a much smaller improvement for the syllables, with improvement for word identification lying between these. Finally, notice that digit discrimination becomes asymptotic at 100% correct at low levels. On the other hand, words in sentences do not approach 100% intelligibility until the S/N ratio reaches 18 dB, and monosyllable discrimination fails to attain even 70% at the highest S/N ratio tested. Thus, we find that the most restricted (redundant) materials are more intelligible than the less redundant ones. In other words, we need only get a small part of the signal to tell one digit from another; whereas there is little other information for the subject to call upon if part of a nonsense syllable is unclear. (For example, if one hears "-en" and knows in advance that the test item is a digit, the test is inordinately easier than when the initial sound might be *any* of the 25 or so consonants of English.) Word redundancy falls between the exceptionally high redundancy of the digits and the rather minimal redundancy of the nonsense syllables. As expected, Miller and associates found that words were more intelligible in a sentence than than when presented alone, which also reflects redundancy afforded by the context of the test item.

In a related experiment, Miller et al. [90] obtained intelligibility measures for test vocabularies made up of 2, 4, 8, 16, 32 or 256 monosyllable words, as well as for an "unrestricted" vocabulary of approximately 1000 monosyllables. The results were similar to those just described. The fewer the alternatives (i.e., the more redundant or predictable the message), the better the discrimination performance. As the number of alternatives increases, greater intensity (a higher S/N ratio) was needed in order to obtain the same degree of intelligibility.

Frequency

How much information about the speech signal is contained in various frequency ranges? The answer to this question is not only important in describing the frequencies necessary to carry the speech signal (an important concept if communication channels are to be used with maximal efficiency), but also may enable us to predict intelligibility. Egan and Wiener [93] studied the effects upon syllable intelligibility of varying the bandwidth around 1500 Hz. They found that widening the bandwidth improved intelligibility, which reached 85% when a 3000 Hz bandwidth was available to the listener. Narrowing the passband resulted in progressively lower intelligibility; conversely, discrimination was improved by raising the level of the stimuli. That is, the narrower the band of frequencies, the higher the speech level must be in order to maintain the same degree of intelligibility.

French and Steinberg [81] determined the intelligibility of male and female speakers under varying conditions of low- and high-pass filtering. Discrimination was measured while filtering out the high frequencies above certain cutoff points (low-pass), and while filtering out the lows below various cutoffs (high-pass). Increasing amounts of either high- or low-pass filtering reduced intelligibility; and performance fell to nil when the available frequencies (the passband) were limited to those below about 200 Hz or above roughly 6000 Hz. As illustrated in Fig. 14.14, the high- and low-pass curves intersected at approximately 1900 Hz, where discrimination was about 68%. In other words, roughly equivalent contributions accounting for 68% intelligibility each were found for the frequencies above and below 1900 Hz. One must be careful, however, not to attach any magical significance to this frequency or percentage. For example, the crossover point dropped to about 1660 Hz for only male talkers. Furthermore, Miller and Nicely [94] showed that the crossover point depends upon what aspect of speech (feature) is examined. Their high- and low-pass curves intersected at 450 Hz for the

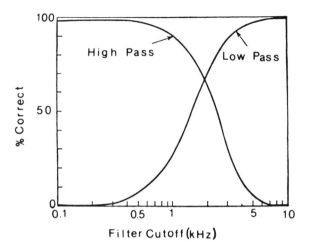

Figure 14.14   Syllable discrimination as a function of high- and low-pass filtering. (Adapted from French and Steinberg [81], with permission of *J. Acoust. Soc. Amer.*)

identification of nasality, 500 Hz for voicing, 750 Hz for frication, and 1900 Hz for place of articulation.

The results of filtering studies have provided a basis for methods of predicting speech intelligibility, an articulation index. The articulation index (AI) was introduced by French and Steinberg [81].* Since its origination, the AI has been improved upon and modified by others, particularly Beranek [95], Kryter [96–98], and Pavlovic et al. [99,100]. The actual calculations are not within the current scope, and the interested reader is referred to the original works by those authors for details, as well as to Janssen [101] for an example of a simplified approach. The basic concept of the AI involves the use of 20 contiguous frequency bands, each of which contributes the same proportion (5%) to the overall intelligibility of the message. These bands are then combined into a single number from 0 to 1.0, which is the articulation index. The AI has been shown to be a reasonably good predictor of actual speech recognition performance

---

*Another approach to estimating speech intelligibility is the Speech Transmission Index (STI), which is based upon the modulation transfer function. This technique was originated by Steeneken and Houtgast [102]. In addition to their work, the interested reader should also refer to recent papers by Humes et al. [103] and Anderson and Kalb [104] (see also Schmidt-Nielsen [105]).

for a variety of speech materials [96–98]. One should refer to a number of recent papers with respect to applying the AI to the speech intelligibility of the hearing impaired [e.g., 99,102,106,107].

Masking and Reverberation

The presentation of a noise has the effect of masking all or part of a speech signal. The general relationship between the effective level of the masker and the amount of masking for tones (Chap. 10) also holds true for the masking of speech by a broad-band noise [108]. That is, once the noise reaches an effective level, a given increment in noise level will result in an equivalent increase in speech threshold. Furthermore, this linear relationship between masker level and speech masking holds true for both the detection of the speech signal and intelligibility.

Recall from Chap. 10 that masking spreads upward a frequency, so that we would expect an intense low-frequency masker to be more effective in masking the speech signal than one whose energy is concentrated in the higher frequencies. This has been confirmed by Stevens et al. [109] and by Miller [110]. Miller also found that when noise bands were presented at lower intensities, the higher-frequency noise bands also reduced speech discrimination. This effect reflects the masking of consonant information concentrated in the higher frequencies.

Miller and Nicely [94] demonstrated that the effect of a wide-band noise upon speech intelligibility similar to that of low-pass filtering. This is expected, since a large proportion of the energy in the noise is concentrated in the higher frequencies. Both the noise and low-pass filtering resulted in rather systematic confusions among consonants, primarily affecting the correct identification of place of articulation. On the other hand, voicing and nasality, which rely heavily upon the lower frequencies, were minimally affected.

Reverberation is the persistence of acoustic energy in an enclosed space after the sound source has stopped; it is due to multiple reflections from the walls, ceiling, and floor of the enclosure (normally a room). It is a common experience that intelligibility decreases in a reverberant room, and this has been demonstrated experimentally as well [111–117]. The amount of discrimination impairment becomes greater as the reverberation time* increases, particularly in small rooms where the reflections are "tightly packed" in time. Excellent reviews of the phenomenon may be found in Nabelek [115] and Nabelek and Robinette [116].

---

*Reverberation time is the time it takes for the reflections to decrease 60 dB after the sound source has been turned off.

Common experience reveals that reverberation causes a reduction in speech intelligibility. In one sense, reverberation appears to act as a masking noise in reducing speech intelligibility [111,117]. This occurs because the reflected energy overlaps the direct (original) speech signal so that perceptual cues are masked. In addition, reverberation causes a smearing of the speech signal over time, thereby also causing confusions that are not typical of masking, per se. As an example of the masking effects, Gelfand and Silman [117] demonstrated that reverberation results in rather systematic consonant error patterns reminiscent of those associated with masking by noise and low-pass filtering. Their results also suggested that consonant error patterns are affected by the distribution characteristics of phonemes in the language [118], as well as by the alternatives imposed by the test being used. The manner in which reverberation affects the speech signal differently than masking is exemplified by the findings by Nabelek and colleagues [119,120]. They demonstrated that reverberation and noise produced different errors for vowels, often associated with the time course of the signal.

Amplitude Distortion

If the dynamic range of a system is exceeded, then there will be peak-clipping of the waveform. In other words, the peaks of the wave will be "cut off" as shown in Fig. 14.15. The resulting waveform approaches the appearance of a square wave, as the figure clearly demonstrates. The effects of clipping have been studied in detail by Licklider and colleagues [121–123], and the essential though surprising finding is that peak-clipping does not result in any appreciable decrease in speech intelligibility even though the waveform is quite distorted. On the other hand, if the peaks are maintained but the center portion of the wave is removed (center clipping), then speech intelligibility quickly drops to nil.

Interruptions and Temporal Distortion

Miller and Licklider [124] studied the effect of rapid interruptions upon word intelligibility. They electronically interrupted the speech waveform at rates from 0.1–10,000 times per second, and with speech-time fractions between 6.25% and 75%. The speech-time fraction is simply the proportion of the time that the speech signal is actually on. Thus, a 50% speech-time fraction means that the speech signal was on and off for equal amounts of time, while 12.5% indicates that the speech signal was actually presented 12.5% of the time.

For the lowest interruption rate, the signal was alternately on and off for several seconds at a time. Thus, the discrimination score was roughly

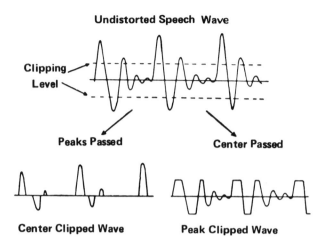

Figure 14.15 Effects of peak-clipping (right) and center clipping upon the speech waveform. "Clipping level" indicates the amplitude above (or below) which clipping occurs. (From *Language and Communication* by Miller [2], © 1951 by McGraw-Hill. Used with permission of McGraw-Hill Book Company.)

equal to the percent of the time that the signal was actually presented. The results for faster interruption rates are also shown in Fig. 14.16. When the speech-time fraction is 50%, performance was poorest when the signal was interrupted about one time per second. This is an expected finding because we would expect intelligibility to be minimal when the interruption is long enough to overlap roughly the whole test word. At much faster interruption rates, the subjects get many "glimpses" of the test word. That is, assuming a word duration of 0.6 sec and five interruptions per second, there would be about three glimpses of each word, and so forth for higher interruption rates. (The dip in the function between 200 and 2000 interruptions per second may be due to an interaction between the speech signal and the square wave that was used to modulate the speech signal to produce the interruptions.) Looking now at the remaining curves in Fig. 14.16, we find that the more the speech signal is actually on, the better is the discrimination; whereas when the speech-time fraction falls well below 50% intelligibility drops substantially at all interruption rates. Essentially similar findings have been reported in more recent work [125]. We see from such observation the remarkable facility with which the ear can "piece together" the speech signal, as well as the tremendous redundancy contained within the speech waveform.

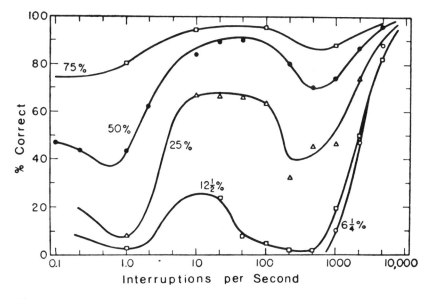

Figure 14.16 Discrimination as a function of interruption rate with speech-time fraction as the parameter. (Adapted from Miller and Licklider [124], with permission of *J. Acoust. Soc. Amer.*)

Other forms of temporal distortion also substantially decrease speech intelligibility—particularly speeding (or time-compression) of the speech signal [126–128]. Space and scope preclude any detailed discussion except to note that intelligibility decreases progressively with speeding (or time compression) of the speech signal. An excellent review may be found in Beasley and Maki [129].

DICHOTIC LISTENING

Dichotic listening involves the presentation of one signal to the right ear and another to the left ear. For an exceptional detailed review, see Berlin and McNeil [130]. This approach was introduced to the study of speech perception by Broadbent [131,132] as a vehicle for the study of memory, and was extended to the study of hemispheric lateralization for speech by Kimura [133,134]. Kimura asked her subjects to respond to different digits presented to the two ears. The result was a small but significant advantage in the perception of the digits at the right ear—the right ear advantage (REA). On the other hand, there was a left ear advantage when musical material was presented dichotically [135]. Since the primary and most efficient pathways are from the right ear to the left cerebral hemisphere, and from the left ear to the right hemisphere, these findings have been interpreted as indicating a right-eared (left hemispheric) dominance for speech and a left-eared (right hemispheric) dominance for melodic material. This appears to be the case for the overwhelming majority (about 95%) of right-handed individuals, and for roughly 70% of left-handed people as well.

A major breakthrough in the study of dichotic listening was the use of CV syllables as stimuli by Shankweiler and Studdert-Kennedy [136], and others [137–140]. The basic experiment is similar to Kimura's, except that the dichotic digits are replaced by a much more controllable pair of dichotic CV syllables. Most often, the syllables /pa, ka, ta, ba, da, ga/ are used.

The CV studies confirmed and expanded the earlier digit observations. Specifically, Shankweiler and Studdert-Kennedy found a significant REA for the CVs but not for vowels. They further found that the REA was larger when the consonants differed in both place of articulation and voicing (e.g., /pa/ versus /ga/) than when the contrast was out of place (e.g., /pa/ versus /ta/) or voicing (e.g., /ta/ versus /da/) alone. Similarly, Studdert-Kennedy and Shankweiler [137] found that errors were less common when the dichotic pair had one feature (place or voicing) in common than when both place and voicing were different. These findings support the concept of a final linguistic (phonetic) processor within the left hemisphere since (1) they suggest that the neural representations from the two ears are recombined at one location, and (2) the features appear to be independently processed. On the other hand, auditory (nonphonetic) features do not appear to be independently processed [141,142].

The contention that there is a specialized phonetic processor in the left hemisphere, as well as a preliminary auditory processor in both hemispheres, has been supported by electrophysiological studies by Wood and colleagues [143,144]. They presented their subjects with dichotic CVs differing in one of two ways. A phonetic difference between the CVs was provided in the standard way (/ba/ versus /ga/). An auditory (nonphonetic) difference was produced by presenting the same CV syllable to the two ears, with a difference in fundamental frequency. In other words, the tasks were phonetic (/ba/-/fa/) and auditory (high pitch-low pitch). In addition to the dichotic listening task, they also obtained auditory evoked potentials (see Chap. 7) from both hemispheres of their subjects. The responses to the auditory and phonetic materials were significantly different over the left hemisphere, but not over the right; thus supporting the presence of a phonetic process occurring in the left hemisphere that differs from the auditory processing of the materials.

The acoustic parameters of the REA were studied by Cullen et al. [140]. They demonstrated that the REA was maintained until (1) the stimuli were presented to the left ear at a level 20 dB higher than the right, (2) the S/N ratio in the right ear ear was 12 dB poorer than in the left, or (3) the CVs presented to the right ear were filtered above 3000 Hz while the left ear received an unfiltered signal. Thus, the REA is maintained until the signal to the right ear is at quite a disadvantage relative to the left. Interestingly, Cullen et al. demonstrated that when the right ear score decreased, the left ear score actually became proportionally better, so that the total percent correct (right plus left) was essentially constant. This suggests that there is a finite amount of information that can be handled at one time by the phonetic processor in the left hemisphere. The REA reflects the longer and noisier neural route (see Chap. 1) from the left ear to the left hemisphere processor for speech.

An interesting phenomenon occurs when the dichotic stimuli are presented with a time delay (lag) between the ears. If the CV delivered to one ear is delayed relative to the presentation of the CV to the other ear, then there is an advantage for the ear receiving the lagging stimulus, particularly for delays on the order of 30–60 msec [138,139]. This phenomenon is the "lag effect," and has been cited as evidence favoring the existence of a specialized phonetic processor. However, a lag effect has also been shown to occur for certain nonspeech (though speechlike) sounds, and there is evidence that the lag effect may rely upon the more general phenomenon of backward masking [145–148]. There is thus evidence implicating the perception of auditory as well as phonetic features in dichotic listening; an issue which remains to be fully resolved. In any case, the lag effect does appear to represent the interference with the perception of a stimulus by a following stimulus, and as such appears to be related to the time needed to complete the processing of the CV syllable [139].

REFERENCES

1. H. Fletcher, *Speech and Hearing in Communication*, Van Nostrand, New York, 1953.
2. G. A. Miller, *Language and Communication*, McGraw-Hill, New York, 1951.
3. I. Lehiste, *Readings in Acoustic Phonetics*, MIT Press, Cambridge, Mass., 1967.
4. M. E. Hawley, *Speech Intelligibility and Speech Recognition*, Dowden, Hutchinson, and Ross, Stroudsberg, Penn., 1977.

5. D. B. Pisoni, Speech perception: Some new directions in research and theory, *J. Acoust Soc. Am. 78*, 381–388 (1985).

6. A. M. Liberman and I. G. Mattingly, A specialization for speech perception,*Science 243*, 489–494 (1989).

7. J. L. Flanagan, Some properties of the glottal sound source, *J. Speech Hearing Res. 1*, 99–116 (1958).

8. K. N. Stevens and A. S. House, An acoustical theory of vowel productions and some of its implications, *J. Speech Hearing Res. 4*, 302–320 (1961).

9. R. K. Potter, G. A. Kopp, and H. C. Green, *Visible Speech*, Van Nostrand, New York, 1947.

10. G. E. Peterson, The information-bearing elements of speech, *J. Acoust. Soc. Amer. 24*, 629–637 (1952).

11. G. E. Peterson and H. L. Barney, Control methods used in a study of the vowels, *J. Acoust. Soc. Amer. 24*, 175–184 (1952).

12. P. Delattre, A. M. Liberman, F. S. Cooper, and L. J. Gerstman, An experimental study of the acoustic determinants of vowel color; Obsrevations on one- and two-formant vowels synthesized from spectrographic patterns, *Word 8*, 195–210 (1952).

13. K. N. Stevens and A. S. House, Development of a quantitative description of vowel articulation, *J. Acoust. Soc. Amer. 27*, 484–493 (1955).

14. J. L. Flanagan, *Speech Analysis, Synthesis and Perception*, Springer-Verlag, New York, 1972.

15. W. Koenig, H. K. Dunn, and L. Y. Lacy, The sound spectrograph, *J. Acoust. Soc. Amer. 17*, 19–49 (1946).

16. W. R. Tiffany, Vowel recognition as a function of duration, frequency modulation and phonetic context, *J. Speech Hearing Dis. 18*, 289–301 (1953).

17. K. N. Stevens and A. S. House, Perturbation of vowel articulations by consonantal context: An acoustical study, *J. Speech Hearing Res. 6*, 111–128 (1963).

18. B. Lindblom and M. Studdert-Kennedy, On the role of formant transitions in vowel recognition, *J. Acoust. Soc. Amer. 42*, 830–843 (1967).

19. P. Ladefoged and D. E. Broadbent, Information conveyed by vowels, *J. Acoust. Soc. Amer. 29*, 98–104 (1957).

20. P. Lieberman, On the evaluation of language: A unified view, *Cognition 2*, 59–94 (1973).

21. F. S. Cooper, P. C. Delattre, A. M. Liberman, J. M. Borst, and L. J. Gerstman, Some experiments on the perception of synthetic speech sounds, *J. Acoust. Soc. Amer. 24*, 597–617 (1952).

22. E. Fischer-Jorgensen, Acoustic analysis of stop consonants, *Misc. Phonetica 2*, 42–59 (1954).

23. A. M. Liberman, P. C. Delattre, L. J. Gerstman, and F. S. Cooper, Tempo of frequency as a cue for distinguishing classes of speech sounds, *J. Exp. Psych. 52*, 127–137 (1956).

24. M. Halle, G. W. Hughes, and J. P. A. Radley, Acoustic properties of stop consonants, *J. Acoust. Soc. Amer. 29*, 107–116 (1957).

25. D. J. Sharf, Duration of post-stress intervocalic stops preceding vowels, *Lang. Speech 5*, 26–30 (1962).

26. J. H. Arkebauer, T. J. Hixon, and J. C. Hardy, Peak intraoral air pressure during speech, *J. Speech Hearing Res. 10*, 196–208 (1967).

27. L. Lisker and A. S. Abramson, Cross-language study of voicing in initial stops: Acoustical measurements, *Word 20*, 384–422 (1964).

28. L. Lisker and A. S. Abramson, Some effects of context on voice onset time in English stops, *Lang. Speech 10*, 1–28 (1967).

29. L. J. Raphael, Preceding vowel duration as a cue to the perception of the voicing characteristics of word-final consonants in American English, *J. Acoust. Soc. Amer. 51*, 1296–1303 (1972).

30. L. Lisker, Closure duration and the intervocalic voiced-voiceless distinction in English, *Language 33*, 42–49 (1957).

31. I. H. Slis, Articulatory measurements on voiced, voiceless and nasal consonants, *Phonetica 24*, 193–210 (1970).

32. M. P. Haggard, S. Ambler, and M. Callow, Pitch as a voicing cue, *J. Acoust. Soc. Amer. 47*, 613–617 (1970).

33. A. M. Liberman, P. C. Delattre, F. S. Cooper, and L. J. Gerstman, The role of consonant-vowel transitions in the perception of the stop and nasal consonants, *Psych. Monogr. 68*, 1–13 (1954).

34. P. C. Delattre, A. M. Liberman, and F. S. Cooper, Acoustic loci and transitional cues for consonants, *J. Acoust. Soc. Amer. 27*, 769–773 (1955).

35. K. S. Harris, H. S. Hoffman, A. M. Liberman, P. C. Delattre, and F. S. Cooper, Effect of third formant transitions on the perception of the voiced stop consonants, *J. Acoust. Soc. Amer. 30*, 122–126 (1958).

36. K. N. Stevens and S. E. Blumstein, Invariant cues for place of articulation in stop consonants, *J. Acoust Soc. Am. 64*, 1358–1368 (1978).

37. S. E. Blumstein and K. N. Stevens, Acoustic invariance in speech production: Evidence from measurements of the spectral characteristics of stop consonants, *J. Acoust. Soc. Am. 66*, 1001–1017 (1979).

38. S. E. Blumstein and K. N. Stevens, Perceptual invariance and onset spectra for stop consonants indifferent vowel environments, *J. Acoust Soc. Am. 67*, 648–662 (1980).

39. S. E. Blumstein, E. Isaacs, and J. Mertus, The role of gross spectral shape as a perceptual cue to place of articulation in initial stop consonants, *J. Acoust Soc. Am. 72*, 43–50 (1982).

40. D. Kewley-Port, Time-varying features as correlates of place of articulation in stop consonants, *J. Acoust Soc. Am. 73*, 322–335 (1983).

41. D. Kewley-Port and P. A. Luce, Time-varying features of stop consonants in auditory running spectra: A first report, *Percept. Psychophys. 35*, 353–360 (1984).

42. C. L. Searle, J. Z. Jacobson, and S. G. Rayment, Stop consonant discrimination based on human audition, *J. Acoust Soc. Am. 79*, 799–809 (1979).

43. M. I. Miller and M. B. Sachs, Representation of stop consonants in the discharge patterns of auditory-nerve fibers, *J. Acoust Soc. Am. 74*, 502–517 (1983).

44. A. C. Walley and T. D. Carrell, Onset spectra and formant transitions in the adult's and child's perception of place of articulation in stop consonants, *J. Acoust Soc. Am. 73,* 1011–1022 (1983).

45. A. S. House and G. Fairbanks. The influence of consonant environment upon the secondary characteristics of vowels, *J. Acoust. Soc. Amer. 25,* 105–113 (1953).

46. G. W. Hughes and M. Halle, Spectral properties of fricative consonants, *J. Acoust. Soc. Amer. 28,* 303–310 (1956).

47. L. J. Gerstman, Perceptual dimensions for the friction portions of certain speech sounds, Unpublished Ph.D. Dissertation, NY: New York University, New York, 1957.

48. K. S. Harris, Cues for the discrimination of American English Fricatives in spoken syllables, *Lang. Speech 1,* 1–7 (1958).

49. P. Strevens, Spectra of fricative noise in human speech, *Lang. Speech 3,* 32–49 (1960).

50. J. M. Heinz and K. N. Stevens, On the properties of voiceless fricative consonants, *J. Acoust. Soc. Amer. 33,* 589–596 (1961).

51. W. Jassem, The formants of fricative consonants, *Lang. Speech 8,* 1–16 (1965).

52. J. A. Guerlekian, Recognition of the Spanish fricatives /s/ and /f/, *J. Acoust Soc. Am. 79,* 1624–1627 (1981).

53. A. Jongman, Duration of fricative noise as a perceptual cue to place and manner of articulation in English fricatives, *J. Acoust Soc. Am. 77,* Suppl. 1, S26 (1985).

54. S. Behrens and S. E. Blumstein, On the role of the amplitude of the fricative noise in the perception of place of articulation in voiceless fricative consonants, *J. Acoust Soc. Am. 84,* 861–867 (1988).

55. O. Fujimura, Analysis of nasal consonants, *J. Acoust. Soc. Amer. 34,* 1865–1875 (1962).

56. A. Malécot, Acoustic cues for nasal consonants, *Language 32,* 274–284 (1956).

57. A. S. House, Analog studies of nasal consonants, *J. Acoust. Soc. Amer. 22,* 190–204 (1957).

58. K. Kurowski and S. E. Blumstein, Acoustic properties for place of articulation in nasal consonants, *J. Acoust Soc. Am. 81,* 1917–1927 (1987).

59. J. D. O'Connor, L. J. Gerstman, A. M. Liberman, P. C. Delattre, and F. S. Cooper, Acoustic cues for the perception of initial /w,j,r,l/ in English, *Word 13,* 24–43 (1957).

60. L. Lisker, Minimal cues for separating /w,r,l,y/ in intervalic position, *Word 13,* 256–267 (1957).

61. G. Fant, *Acoustic Theory of Speech Perception,* Mouton, The Hague, 1970.

62. A. M. Liberman, K. S. Harris, H. S. Hoffman, and B. C. Griffith, The discrimination of speech sounds within and across phoneme boundaries, *J. Exp. Psych. 54,* 358–368 (1957).

63. A. M. Liberman, K. S. Harris, J. A. Kinney, and H. L. Lane, The discrimination of relative onset of certain speech and non-speech patterns, *J. Exp. Psych. 61,* 379–388 (1961).

64. A. S. Abramson and L. Lisker, Discriminability along the voicing continuum: Cross-language tests, in *Proceedings of the Sixth International Congress on Phonetic Science*, Academia, Prague, 1970, pp. 569–573.

65. L. Lisker and A. S. Abramson, The voicing dimension: Some experiments in comparative phonetics, *Proceedings of the Sixth International Congress on Phonetic Science*, Academia, Prague, 1970, pp. 563–567.

66. P. D. Eimas, P. Siqueland, P. Jusczyk, and J. Vigorito, Speech perception in infants, *Science 171*, 303–306 (1971).

67. A. M. Liberman, F. S. Cooper, D. P. Shankweiler, and M. Studdert-Kennedy, Perception of the speech code, *Psych. Rev. 74*, 431–461 (1967).

68. D. B. Pisoni, Identification and discrimination of the relative onset time of two component tones: Implications for voicing perception in stops, *J. Acoust. Soc. Amer. 61*, 1352–1361 (1977).

69. J. E. Cutting and B. S. Rosner, Categories and boundaries in speech and music, *Percept. Psychophysiol. 16*, 564–570 (1974).

70. J. D. Mitler, C. C. Wier, R. Pastore, W. J. Kelly, and R. J. Dooling, Discrimination and labeling of noise-buzz sequences with varying noise-lead times: An example of categorical perception, *J. Acoust. Soc. Amer. 60*, 410–417 (1976).

71. R. E. Lasky, A. Syrdal-Lasky, and R. E. Klein, VOT discrimination by four to six and a half month old infants from Spanish environments, *J. Exp. Child Psych. 20*, 213–225 (1975).

72. L. A. Streeter, Language perception of 2-month old infants shows effects of both innate mechanisms and experience, *Nature 259*, 39–41 (1976).

73. P. K. Kuhl and J. D. Miller, Speech perception by the chinchilla: Voice-voiceless distinctions in alveolar plosive consonants, *Science 190*, 69–72 (1975).

74. I. J. Hirsh and C. E. Sherrick, Perceived order in different sense modalities, *J. Exp. Psych. 62*, 423–432 (1961).

75. K. N. Stevens and D. H. Klatt, The role of formant transitions in the voiced-voiceless distinctions for stops, *J. Acoust. Soc. Amer. 55*, 653–659 (1974).

76. B. R. Repp, Categorical perception: Issues, methods, findings, in *Speech and Language: Advances in Basic Research and Practice (Vol. 10)*, (N. Lass, ed.), Academic Press, New York, 1984, pp. 243–335.

77. D. A. Nelson, and P. Marler, Categorical perception of a natural stimulus continuum: Birdsong, *Science 244*, 976–978 (1989).

78. C. F. Sacia and C. J. Beck, The power of fundamental speech sounds, *Bell Sys. Tech. J. 5*, 393–403 (1926).

79. H. K. Dunn and S. D. White, Statistical measurements on conversational speech, *J. Acoust. Soc. Amer. 11*, 278–288 (1940).

80. H. W. Rudmose, et al., Effects of high altitude on the human voice, OSRD Rept. 3106, Harvard University, Cambridge, Mass., 1944.

81. N. R. French and G. C. Steinberg, Factors governing the intelligibility of speech, *J. Acoust. Soc. Amer. 19*, 90–114 (1947).

82. G. A. Campbell, Telephonic intelligibility, *Phil. Mag. 19*, 152–159 (1910).

83. H. Fletcher and J. C. Steinberg, Articulation testing methods, *Bell Sys. Tech. J. 8*, 848–852 (1929).

84. J. P. Egan, Articulation testing methods, *Laryngoscope 58*, 955–981 (1948).

85. I. J. Hirsh, H. Davis, S. R. Silverman, E. G. Reynolds, E. Eldert, and R. W. Benson, Development of materials for speech audiometry, *J. Speech Hearing Dis. 17*, 321–337 (1952).

86. G. E. Peterson and I. Lehiste, Revised CNC lists for auditory tests, *J. Speech Hearing Dis. 27*, 62–70 (1962).

87. G. Fairbanks, Test of phonemic differentiation: The rhyme test, *J. Acoust. Soc. Amer. 30*, 596–600 (1958).

88. A. House, C. Williams, H. Hecker, and A. Kryter, Articulation-testing methods: Consonantal differentiations with a close-response set, *J. Acoust. Soc. Amer. 37*, 158–166 (1965).

89. C. V. Hudgens, J. E. Hawkins, J. E. Karlin, and S. S. Stevens, The development of recorded auditory tests for measuring hearing loss for speech, *Laryngoscope 57*, 57–89 (1947).

90. G. A. Miller, G. A. Heise, and W. Lichten, The intelligibility of speech as a function of the context of the test materials, *J. Ex. Psych. 41*, 329–335 (1951).

91. M. R. Rosenzweig and L. Postman, Intelligibility as a function of frequency of usage, *J. Exp. Psych. 54*, 412–422 (1957).

92. L. Hochhouse and J. R. Antes, Speech identification and "knowing that you know," *Percept. Psychophysiol. 13*, 131–132 (1973).

93. J. P. Egan and F. M. Wiener, On the intelligibility of bands of speech in noise, *J. Acoust. Soc. Amer. 18*, 435–441 (1946).

94. G. A. Miller and P. E. Nicely, An analysis of perceptual confusions among some English consonants, *J. Acoust. Soc. Amer. 27*, 338–352 (1955).

95. L. L. Beranek, The design of communication systems, *IRE Proc. 35*, 880–890 (1947).

96. K. D. Kryter, Methods for the calculation and use of the articulation index, *J. Acoust. Soc. Amer. 34*, 1689–1697 (1962).

97. K. D. Kryter, Validation of the articulation index, *J. Acoust. Soc. Amer. 34*, 1698–1702 (1962).

98. K. D. Kryter, *The Effects of Noise on Man, Second Edition*, Academic Press, New York, 1985.

99. C. V. Pavlovic, G. A. Studebaker, and R. L. Sherbecoe, An articulation index based procedure for predicting the speech recognition performance of hearing-impaired individuals, *J. Acoust Soc. Am. 80*, 50–57 (1986).

100. C. V. Pavlovic, Derivation of primary parameters and procedures for use in speech intelligibility predictions, *J. Acoust Soc. Am. 82*, 413–422 (1987).

101. J. H. Janssen, A method for the calculation of the speech intelligibility under conditions of reverberation and noise, *Acoustica 7*, 305–310 (1957).

102. H. J. M. Steeneken and T. Houtgast, A physical method for measuring speech-transmission quality, *J. Acoust Soc. Am. 67*, 318–326 (1980).

103. L. E. Humes, D. D. Dirks, T. S. Bell, C. Ahlstrom, and G. E. Kincaid, Application of the Articulation Index and the Speech Transmission Index to the recognition of speech by normal hearing and hearing-impaired listeners, *J. Speech Hear. Res. 29*, 447–462 (1986).

104. B. W. Anderson and J. T. Kalb, English verification of the STI method for estimating speech intelligibility of a communications channel, *J. Acoust Soc. Am. 81*, 1982–1985 (1987).

105. A. Schmidt-Nielsen, Comments on the use of physical measures to assess speech intelligibility, *J. Acoust Soc. Am. 81*, 1985–1987 (1987).

106. C. A. Kamm, D. D. Dirks, and T. S. Bell, Speech recognition and the articulation index for normal and hearing impaired listeners, *J. Acoust Soc. Am. 77*, 281–288 (1985).

107. C. V. Pavlovic, Articulation index predictions of speech intelligibility in hearing aid selection, *Asha 30*, (6/7), 63–65 (1988).

108. J. E. Hawkins and S. S. Stevens, The masking of pure tones and of speech by white noise, *J. Acoust. Soc. Amer. 22*, 6–13 (1950).

109. S. S. Stevens, J. Miller, and I. Truscott, The masking of speech by sine waves, square waves, and regular and modulated pulses, *J. Acoust. Soc. Amer. 18*, 418–424 (1946).

110. G. A. Miller, The masking of speech, *Psych. Bull. 44*, 105–129 (1947).

111. R. H. Bolt and A. D. MacDonald, Theory of speech masking by reverberation, *J. Acoust. Soc. Amer. 21*, 577–580 (1949).

112. A. K. Nabelek and J. M. Pickett, Reception of consonants in a classroom as affected by monaural and binaural listening, noise, reverberation and hearing aids, *J. Acoust. Soc. Amer. 56*, 628–639 (1974).

113. H. Kurtović, The influence of reflected sound upon speech intelligibility, *Acoustica 33*, 32–39 (1975).

114. S. A. Gelfand and I. Hochberg, Binaural and monaural speech discrimination under reverberation, *Audiology 15*, 72–84 (1976).

115. A. K. Nabelek, Reverberation effects for normal and hearing-impaired listeners, in *Hearing and Davis: Essays Honoring Hallowell Davis* (S. K. Hirsh, D. H. Eldredge, I. J. Hirsh, and S. R. Silverman, eds.), Washington University Press, St. Louis, 1976, pp. 333–341.

116. A. K. Nabelek and L. N. Robinette, Reverberation as a parameter in clinical testing, *Audiology 17*, 239–259 (1978).

117. S. A. Gelfand and S. Silman, Effects of small room reverberation upon the recognition of some consonant features, *J. Acoust. Soc. Amer. 66*, 22–29 (1979).

118. P. B. Denes, On the statistics of spoken English, *J. Acoust. Soc. Amer. 35*, 892–904 (1963).

119. A. K. Nabelek and T. R. Letowski, Vowel confusions of hearing-impaired listeners under reverberant and nonreverberant conditions, *J. Speech Hear. Dis. 50*, 126–131 (1985).

120. A. K. Nabelek and P. A. Dagenais, Vowel errors in noise and in reverberation by hearing impaired listeners, *J. Acoust. Soc. Am. 80*, 741–748 (1986).

121. J. C. R. Licklider, Effects of amplitude distortion upon the intelligibility of speech, *J. Acoust. Soc. Amer. 18*, 429–434 (1946).

122. J. C. R. Licklider, D. Bindra, and I. Pollack, The intelligibility of rectangular speech waves, *Amer. J. Psych. 61*, 1–20 (1948).

123. J. C. R. Licklider and I. Pollack, Effects of differentiation, integration, and infinite peak clipping upon the intelligibility of speech, *J. Acoust. Soc. Amer. 20*, 42–51 (1948).

124. G. A. Miller and J. C. R. Licklider, The intelligibility of interrupted speech, *J. Acoust. Soc. Amer. 22*, 167–173 (1950).

125. G. L. Powers and C. Speaks, Intelligibility of temporally interrupted speech, *J. Acoust. Soc. Amer. 54*, 661–667 (1973).

126. C. Calearo and A. Lazzaroni, Speech intelligibility in relation to the speed of the message,*Laryngoscope 67*, 410–419 (1957).

127. G. Fairbanks and F. Kodman, Word intelligibility as a function of time compression, *J. Acoust. Soc. Amer. 29*, 636–641 (1957).

128. D. S. Beasley, S. Schwimmer, and W. F. Rintelmann, Intelligibility of time-compressed CNC monosyllables, *J. Speech Hearing Res. 15*, 340–350 (1972).

129. D. S. Beasley and J. E. Maki, Time- and frequency-altered speech, in *Handbook of Perception* (E. C. Carterette and M. P. Friedman, Eds.), Vol. 7: *Language and Speech*, Academic Press, New York, 1976, pp. 419–458.

130. C. I. Berlin and M. R. McNeil, Dichotic listening, in *Contemporary Issues in Experimental Phonetics* (N. J. Lass, Ed.), Academic Press, New York, 1976, pp. 327–387.

131. D. E. Broadbent, The role of auditory localization in attention and memory span, *J. Exp. Psych. 47*, 191–196 (1954).

132. D. E. Broadbent, Successive responses to simultaneous stimuli, *Quart. J. Exp. Psych. 8*, 145–152 (1956).

133. D. Kimura, Cerebral dominance and the perception of verbal stimuli, *Canadian J. Psych 15*, 166–171 (1961).

134. D. Kimura, Functional asymmetry of the brain in dichotic listening, *Cortex 3*, 163–178 (1967).

135. D. Kimura, Left-right differences in the perception of melodies, *Quart. J. Exp. Psych. 16*, 355–358 (1964).

136. D. Shankweiler and M. Studdert-Kennedy, Identification of consonants and vowels presented to the left and right ears, *Quart. J. Exp. Psych. 19*, 59–63 (1967).

137. M. Studdert-Kennedy and D. Shankweiler, Hemispheric specialization for speech perception, *J. Acoust. Soc. Amer. 48*, 579–594 (1970).

138. M. Studdert-Kennedy, D. Shankweiler, and S. Schulman, Opposed effects of a delayed channel on perception of dichotically and monotically presented CV syllables, *J. Acoust. Soc. Amer. 48*, 599–602 (1970).

139. C. I. Berlin, S. S. Lowe-Bell, J. K. Cullen, C. L. Thompson, and C. F. Loovis, Dichotic speech perception: An interpretation of right-ear advantage and temporal-offset effects, *J. Acoust. Soc. Amer. 53*, 699–709 (1973).

140. J. K. Cullen, C. L. Thompsen, L. F. Hughes, C. I. Berlin, and D. S. Samson, The effects of various acoustic parameters on performance in dichotic speech perception tasks, *Brain Lang. 1*, 307–322 (1974).

141. P. T. Smith, Feature-testing models and their application to perception and memory for speech, *Quart. J. Exp. Psych. 25*, 511–534 (1973).

142. J. R. Sawusch and D. Pisoni, On the identification of place and voicing features in synthetic stop consonants, *J. Phonetics 2*, 181–194 (1974).
143. C. C. Wood, Auditory and phonetic levels of processing in speech perception: Neurophysiological and information-processing analyses, *J. Exp. Psych. 104*, 1–33 (1975).
144. C. C. Wood, W. R. Goff, and R. S. Day, Auditory evoked potentials during speech perception, *Science 173*, 1248–1251 (1971).
145. C. J. Darwin, Dichotic backward masking of complex sounds, *Quart. J. Exp. Psych. 23*, 386–392 (1971).
146. D. Pisoni and S. D. McNabb, Dichotic interactions and phonetic feature processing, *Brain Lang. 1*, 351–362 (1974).
147. P. J. Mirabile and R. J. Porter, Dichotic and monotic interaction between speech and nonspeech sounds at different stimulus-onset-asynchronies, Paper at 89th meeting of the Acoustical Society of America, Austin, Texas, 1975.
148. R. J. Porter, Effect of delayed channel on the perception of dichotically presented speech and nonspeech sounds, *J. Acoust. Soc. Amer. 58*, 884–892 (1975).

Author Index

514 Author Index

Sundby, A., 123(90), 124(90), 125(90), *136*
Sutton, S., 375(69), *381*
Sweetman, R. H., 175(79), 177(79, 85), *208, 209*
Swets, J. A., 313(1, 2), 317(4), 316(5), 323(9), *323, 324,* 360(26), *378*
Syka, J., 256(39), *278*
Syrdal-Lasky, A., 470(71), 472(71), *487*

Takahashi, T., 62(19), *91*
Tanaka, Y., 164(58), *207*
Tanner, W. P., 360(26), *378*
Tanner, W. P., Jr., 316(5), *323*
Tasaki, I., 158(38, 39), 159(38), 161(38), 167(62), *206, 207,* 237(62, 66), *246*
Taylor, K., 184(99), *209*
Taylor, K. J., 180(96), 184(96), *209*
Taylor, M. M., 295(10, 11), 299(14), 303(11), *309*
Teas, D. C., 237(64), 239(68), *246,* 272(123), *283,* 427(35), 428(35), 429(35), 430(47), *451, 452*
Teffeteller, S., 363(39), *379*
Tempest, W., 327(5), *347*
Terhardt, E., 362(30), 364(30), *379,* 404(9, 10, 11, 12), 415(9, 10, 11, 12), *415*
Terkildsen, K., 117(46, 47), 118(52), *134*
ter Kuile, E., 153(19, 20), *205*
Thallinger, G., 66(27), *92*
Thalmann, I., 66(27), *92*
Thalmann, R., 66(27), *92*
Theodore, L. H., 316(7), *324*
Thompsen, R. F., 263(61), *279*

Thompson, C. L., 482(139, 140), 483(139, 140), *490*
Thompson, P. O., 360(23), *378*
Thurlow, W. R., 410(40), 413(40), *417*
Thwing, E. J., 396(62), *400*
Tietze, G., 125(94, 95), *137*
Tiffany, W. R., 462(16), *484*
Tillman, T., 445(110, 112), 446(110, 112), *455*
Tilney, L. G., 71(48, 50, 52, 54), 72(50), *93,* 195(149), *212*
Tilney, M. S., 71(52), *93*
Tobias, J. V., 421(17), 424(31), 436(61, 62, 63), *450, 451, 452*
Tonndorf, J., 105(23), 107(23), 109(23), 110(23, 27), 113(36, 37), 114(38), 115(38), 116(36), 117(36), *133, 134,* 144(8), 146(10), 149(11), 150(11), 151(18), 152(18), 170(18), 175(10, 80, 81, 83), 176(80, 81), 177(83), 184(98), 187(121), *205, 208, 209, 211*
Torick, E. L., 429(40), *451*
Townsend, T. H., 447(115), *455*
Trahiotis, C., 429(43, 44), *451*
Treisman, M., 302(23), *310*
Truscott, I., 478(109), *489*
Tsuchitani, C., 260(49), *278*
Tsuchitani, C. C., 247(2), *276*
Tubis, A., 197(156), 201(170), *213,* 329(25), *348*
Tucker, A., 447(117), *455*
Tucker, J., 433(56), *452*
Tukey, J. W., 305(46), *311*
Tunturi, A. R., 262(56), *279*
Turner, C. W., 336(63), 339(63), 340(63), 341(63), *349*
Turner, R. G., 71(53), 72(53), *93,* 195(147), *212*

Subject Index

Speech transmission index, 477
Speech waveform, 344, 424, 456, 479, 480
Speeded speech, 481
Spike potential (*see* Action potential)
Spiral ganglia, 59, 78, 81, 258
Spiral ganglia frequency map, 218
Spiral ligament, 57, 59–62, 64, 73
Spontaneous acoustic emissions (*see* Otoacoustic emissions)
Spontaneous discharge rate (*see* Spontaneous rate)
Spontaneous firing rate (*see* Spontaneous rate)
Spontaneous rate (SR), 216, 218, 222, 229, 232–234
Spread of masking, 354–356, 363, 478
Squamous portion (of Temporal bone), 42–45
Square waves, 28, 29
Staircase method (*see* Up-down methods)
Standard zero reference levels (*see also* Hearing level), 329–332
Standing waves, 33–36, 148
Stapedius muscle and tendon, 50, 52–55, 111, 117, 118, 121, 130
Stapedius reflex (*see* Acoustic reflex)
Stapes, 41, 50–53, 55, 58, 60, 103, 108, 109, 116, 147, 148, 151, 183, 217
Statoacoustic nerve (*see* Auditory nerve)
Stellate cells, 248, 249
Step size, 287, 288, 290, 294–297
Stereocilia (*see* Cilia)
Stereophony, 425

Stevens' law (*see also* Power law), 388, 389
Stiffness, 37, 38,
Stiffness gradient (*see also* Basilar membrane, Traveling wave, Tuning), 60, 146–149
Stimulus novelty, 249
Stimulus-response matrix, 318, 319
Stop burst spectrum, 466
Stops, 464–469, 472
Strain, 7
Stress, 7
Stria vascularis, 73–77, 163
String, vibrating, 33–36
Styloid process (of temporal bone), 45
Subarachnoid space, 58
Successiveness (*see also* Perceived temporal order, Temporal resolution), 344, 345, 472
Summating potential (SP) (*see also* Receptor potentials), 170–175, 187
Summation tones, 408
Superior olivary complex (SOC), 54, 55, 85–87, 89, 90, 203, 247, 249, 252–254, 260, 261, 268, 369, 372, 424
Suprasylvian gyrus (*see* Auditory cortex)
Suprasylvian sulcus (*see* Auditory cortex)
Sylvian fringe area SF (*see* Auditory cortex)
Synapse, 144, 145, 157, 233
System International (SI), 2

Tectorial membrane, 61, 62, 64–66, 71, 72, 153–155, 164, 187, 202